Ovarian Cancer

A subject collection from *Cold Spring Harbor Perspectives in Medicine*

OTHER SUBJECT COLLECTIONS FROM *COLD SPRING HARBOR PERSPECTIVES IN MEDICINE*

Parkinson's Disease, Second Edition

Developmental Oncology: Principles and Therapy of Cancers of Children and Young Adults

Type 1 Diabetes: Advances in Understanding and Treatment 100 Years after the Discovery of Insulin, Second Edition

Cancer Metabolism: Historical Landmarks, New Concepts, and Opportunities

Modeling Cancer in Mice

Angiogenesis: Biology and Pathology, Second Edition

Retinal Disorders: Approaches to Diagnosis and Treatment, Second Edition

Breast Cancer: From Fundamental Biology to Therapeutic Strategies

Aging: Geroscience as the New Public Health Frontier, Second Edition

Combining Human Genetics and Causal Inference to Understand Human Disease and Development

Lung Cancer: Disease Biology and Its Potential for Clinical Translation

Influenza: The Cutting Edge

Leukemia and Lymphoma: Molecular and Therapeutic Insights

Addiction, Second Edition

Hepatitis C Virus: The Story of a Scientific and Therapeutic Revolution

The PTEN Family

Metastasis: Mechanism to Therapy

Genetic Counseling: Clinical Practice and Ethical Considerations

SUBJECT COLLECTIONS FROM *COLD SPRING HARBOR PERSPECTIVES IN BIOLOGY*

Telomeres and Telomerase

Evolution and Development of Neural Circuits

Machine Learning for Protein Science and Engineering

Glia, Second Edition

Speciation

The Biology of Lipids: Trafficking, Regulation, and Function, Second Edition

Synthetic Biology and Greenhouse Gases

Wound Healing: From Bench to Bedside

The Endoplasmic Reticulum, Second Edition

Sex Differences in Brain and Behavior

Regeneration

The Nucleus, Second Edition

Auxin Signaling: From Synthesis to Systems Biology, Second Edition

Stem Cells: From Biological Principles to Regenerative Medicine

Heart Development and Disease

Cell Survival and Cell Death, Second Edition

Calcium Signaling, Second Edition

Engineering Plants for Agriculture

Protein Homeostasis, Second Edition

Ovarian Cancer

A subject collection from *Cold Spring Harbor Perspectives in Medicine*

EDITED BY

James D. Brenton
University of Cambridge

Benjamin G. Neel
NYU Langone Medical Center

COLD SPRING HARBOR LABORATORY PRESS
Cold Spring Harbor, New York • www.cshlpress.org

Ovarian Cancer

A subject collection from *Cold Spring Harbor Perspectives in Medicine*
Articles online at www.perspectivesinmedicine.org

Executive Editor	John Inglis
Project Supervisor	Barbara Acosta
Editorial Assistant	Danett Gil
Permissions Administrator	Carol Brown
Production Editor	Diane Schubach
Production Manager/Cover Designer	Denise Weiss
Publisher	David Crotty

Front cover artwork: Top left, high-grade serous carcinoma is composed of a solid mass of cells with slit-like spaces. Nuclei are large, hyperchromatic, and pleomorphic with high mitotic activity (>12 mitoses per 10 high-power fields) (HES ×100). *Top middle,* low-grade serous carcinoma is composed of micro- or macropapillae lined by uniform small cells with limited nuclear pleomorphisms and low mitotic activity (<12 mitoses per 10 high-power fields), associated with psammoma bodies (HES ×100). *Top right,* endometrioid carcinoma is arranged in a cribriform pattern lined by cuboidal cells with eosinophilic cytoplasm and moderate nuclear atypia (HES ×200). *Bottom left,* the expansile pattern of mucinous carcinoma shows proliferation of complex glands arranged back-to-back with limited intervening stroma, exhibiting moderate cytologic atypia (HES ×200). *Bottom middle,* destructive pattern of mucinous carcinoma shows proliferation of irregular glands, nests, and cells with malignant cytology, infiltrating ovarian stroma (HES ×200). *Bottom right,* clear cell carcinoma shows papillae lined by cuboidal, hobnail cells with clear or eosinophilic cytoplasm and atypical nuclei. The papillae are round and small with a dense hyaline basement membrane material forming the core of the papillary stalk (HES ×200). (Cover reprinted from Devouassoux-Shisheboran M and Genestie C. 2015. Pathobiology of ovarian carcinomas. *Chin J Cancer* **34:** 50–55, with permission from the authors © 2015.)

Library of Congress Cataloging-in-Publication Data

Names: Brenton, James D., 1964- editor. | Neel, Benjamin G., editor.
Title: Ovarian cancer : a subject collection from Cold Spring Harbor Perspectives in Medicine / edited by James D. Brenton, University of Cambridge and Benjamin G. Neel, NYU Langone Medical Center.
Description: Cold Spring Harbor, New York : Cold Spring Harbor Laboratory Press, [2026] | Includes bibliographical references and index. | Summary: "Ovarian cancer is a devastating disease that is frequently fatal. This volume examines the molecular basis of the disease within the reproductive system, environmental and genetic risk factors, current treatments and the potential for targeted therapies"- Provided by publisher.
Identifiers: LCCN 2023048456 (print) | LCCN 2023048457 (ebook) | ISBN 9781621822356 (hardcover) | ISBN 9781621825128 (epub)
Subjects: LCSH: Ovaries--Cancer. | Ovaries--Cancer--Diagnosis. | Ovaries--Cancer--Treatment.
Classification: LCC RC280.O8 O885 2024 (print) | LCC RC280.O8 (ebook) | DDC 616.99/465--dc23/eng/20231227
LC record available at https://lccn.loc.gov/2023048456
LC ebook record available at https://lccn.loc.gov/2023048457

For a complete catalog of all Cold Spring Harbor Laboratory Press publications, visit our website at www.cshlpress.org.

Contents

Preface

EPITHELIAL OVARIAN CANCER (EOC) remains one of the most lethal gynecologic malignancies worldwide, because of its typically late-stage diagnosis, high recurrence rates, and limited long-term survival. Despite significant advances in molecular profiling, increased understanding of disease biology, efforts to improve early detection, and the development of new targeted therapeutics, the complexity and heterogeneity of these tumors still pose formidable challenges for clinicians and researchers. This volume arose out of a Banbury Conference on "Defeating Ovarian Cancer" in the Fall of 2014 and brings together a diverse range of experts to provide an integrative and contemporary account of the biology, pathogenesis, prevention, detection, and treatment of ovarian cancer, with a particular emphasis on histotype-specific insights and translational opportunities.

The opening chapter by Austria and Dubeau reframes our understanding of ovarian cancer biology through an embryological lens, challenging the previous and longstanding paradigm that ovarian surface epithelium is the primary cell-of-origin for EOC. By reviewing the developmental pathways of the Müllerian ducts, ovaries, and related structures, the authors lay the foundation for reclassifying many tumors as arising from extrauterine Müllerian epithelium, fundamentally altering approaches to prevention, risk assessment, and classification. The authors provide a firm foundation for the once-fringe view that fallopian tube epithelium is the cell-of-origin for the most lethal EOC subtype, high-grade serous carcinoma (HGSC).

This chapter is followed by focused discussions of rarer epithelial subtypes—low-grade serous and mucinous carcinomas—by Craig and colleagues, and clear cell carcinoma by Huang and Lin. These contributions highlight the distinctive molecular profiles, etiologic associations (e.g., the link between clear cell carcinoma and endometriosis), and therapeutic vulnerabilities that distinguish these malignancies from HGSC. Their inclusion supports the need for tailored strategies rather than a "one-size-fits-all" approach to EOC.

Pundel and Neel then review the state of models for HGSC—from genetically engineered mice to patient-derived organoids—offering critical tools for studying tumor biology and evaluating novel interventions. Sellers and co-authors review the current status of prevention efforts, synthesizing evidence from epidemiology, chemoprevention trials, and risk-reducing surgical strategies, while Sasamoto and Elias tackle the persistent challenge of early detection, surveying advances in imaging, biomarkers, and screening protocols. Färkkilä and collaborators delve into the tumor microenvironment, describing how single-cell and spatial profiling technologies can be used to reveal immune and stromal determinants of disease progression and response.

The later chapters turn to a comprehensive discussion of recent therapeutic advances. Miao, Matulonis, and Porter provide a state-of-the-art review of systemic therapy, from cytotoxic chemotherapy and anti-angiogenic agents to PARP inhibitors, antibody–drug conjugates, and emerging targeted modalities. Kurnit and Odunsi examine the expanding role of immunotherapy, updating research on checkpoint blockade, cancer vaccines, adoptive cell transfer, and rational combinations aimed at overcoming the immunosuppressive tumor milieu.

Overall, several unifying themes emerge. First, EOC is not—and should no longer be viewed as—a single disease. Rather, it is a collection of distinct entities that differ in cell-of-origin, causative mutational processes and molecular alterations, clinical behavior, and therapeutic responsiveness. Second, the integration of developmental biology, molecular pathology, and advanced modeling is essential for understanding EOC pathogenesis and rationally revealing novel vulnerabilities. Third, progress in the clinic will increasingly depend on translating high-dimensional data—genomic, transcriptomic, proteomic, and spatial—into actionable diagnostics and therapeutics. Finally, prevention and early detection remain critical frontiers, offering the best hope for reducing mortality in this challenging malignancy.

This book is intended as both a reference for established investigators and a guide for trainees and clinicians seeking a deep and nuanced understanding of the state of the field. By spanning disciplines from embryology to immuno-oncology, and from population science to molecular therapeutics, we hope to reflect the collaborative, multidisciplinary, and integrative effort that is required to confront and ultimately conquer this dreaded disease. The editors are grateful to the contributing authors for their scholarly rigor and to the broader research community for their relentless pursuit of discoveries that will ultimately improve the lives of women affected by ovarian cancer.

James D. Brenton
Benjamin G. Neel

Embryological Insights into the Origin of Epithelial Cancers of the Female Reproductive Tract

Theresa Austria and Louis Dubeau

Department of Pathology and USC/Norris Comprehensive Cancer Center, Keck School of Medicine of University of Southern California, Los Angeles, California 90033, USA

Correspondence: ldubeau@usc.edu

The embryology of the female reproductive organs is reviewed focusing on aspects relevant to the histogenesis of reproductive neoplasms. The evidence reviewed suggests that (1) there is no embryological link between the ovarian surface epithelium and the coelomic epithelium; (2) the ovarian surface epithelium is not composed of pluripotent cells that readily differentiate into various components of the reproductive tract before or after birth; (3) there is no embryological link between the ovarian surface epithelium and the Müllerian ducts, from which internal female reproductive organs other than the ovaries, including the endocervix, endometrium, and fallopian tubes, are derived; and (4) there is an embryological link between the Müllerian ducts and the renal collecting system, perhaps accounting for clear cell differentiation in some gynecological malignancies. Implications for our understanding of the origin of the tumors historically classified as ovarian epithelial neoplasms are discussed.

The last two decades witnessed fundamental changes in our views on the origin and histogenesis of the tumors historically classified as ovarian neoplasms. These tumors were widely presumed to originate in the epithelial cell layer covering the ovary until as recently as the early 21st century. This theory, originally based on inaccurate embryological concepts, was favored because it readily accounted for a number of perplexing observations. Common histological subtypes of these cancers are defined by elements not regarded as normal components of the ovary, but of other female reproductive organs such as fallopian tubes, endometrium, and endocervix. This was readily explained by the idea that they originated from the ovarian surface epithelium because this epithelium, also referred to as germinal epithelium, was thought to be composed of pluripotent cells capable of differentiating into these other components. The most common subtype of the cancers historically classified as ovarian carcinomas is the high-grade serous subtype. Tumors belonging to this subtype are morphologically and biologically indistinguishable from high-grade serous carcinomas of the fallopian tubes described as far back as the late 19th century (Orthmann 1886). However, all serous carcinomas of the adnexal regions have been regarded, by convention, as of ovarian surface origin instead of fallopian tube

Cite this article as *Cold Spring Harb Perspect Med* doi: 10.1101/cshperspect.a040642

origin unless they spared the ovaries, which is rarely the case because of their close vicinity to the fallopian tubes (Finn and Javert 1949). This convention was adopted partly to account for the existence of high-grade serous carcinomas sparing both the ovaries and the fallopian tubes (August et al. 1985; Dalrymple et al. 1989; Fromm et al. 1990; Altaras et al. 1991) based on the notion that the coelomic epithelium, which covers all pelvic and abdominal surfaces, and the ovarian surface epithelium, are part of a continuum. This misapprehension led to the hypothesis that tumors like those of alleged ovarian surface origin can also develop outside the ovary, from the coelomic epithelium, and still to this day continue to be classified as primary peritoneal carcinomas. The same logic led to the notion that benign intraovarian epithelial cysts, which typically resemble the epithelial linings of either the fallopian tubes, endometrium, or endocervix (ovarian serous, endometrioid, or mucinous cystadenomas), arise from invaginations of the ovarian surface epithelium.

The idea that the ovarian surface epithelium is an important site of tumorigenesis was questioned in the late 20th century (Dubeau 1999). It nevertheless remained widely accepted until isolation of the *BRCA1* and *BRCA2* genes led to a surge in risk-reducing surgeries entailing removal of organs at elevated cancer risk in germline *BRCA1* and *BRCA2* mutation carriers. The distribution of early cancerous lesions in the surgically resected organs led to the realization that high-grade serous carcinomas, the cancer subtype associated with these carrier states, commonly originate not from the ovarian surface, but from the distal (fimbrial) end of the fallopian tubes (Colgan et al. 2001; Piek et al. 2001; Medeiros et al. 2006; Crum et al. 2007; Lee et al. 2007b). It is now clear that the role of the fallopian tube in the genesis of cancers historically classified as high-grade serous ovarian carcinomas has been utterly underestimated. Whether or not the ovarian surface epithelium plays any role in their development has become highly contentious. Nevertheless, the arguments that led pathologists of the early 20th century to formulate the theory that the ovarian surface epithelium is an important site of cancer development are as valid today as they were then. This review attempts to revisit these observations in light of current knowledge of the embryology of the female reproductive tract. The text is organized in separate sections, each focused on a specific issue of relevance to the origin of the epithelial neoplasms historically classified as of ovarian surface origin. A brief review of the embryology of the kidney is first needed due to its close association with development of the reproductive organs.

RELATIONSHIP BETWEEN THE EMBRYOLOGICAL DEVELOPMENT OF KIDNEYS AND REPRODUCTIVE ORGANS

The kidneys are derived from the intermediate mesoderm located in the dorsolateral aspect of the abdominal and pelvic cavities. Three renal organs, respectively named pronephros, mesonephros, and metanephros, develop sequentially. The most primitive kidney, the pronephros, is a rudimentary filtering organ that is never functional. It progressively degenerates in a craniocaudal direction until it is no longer present by the end of the fourth week of pregnancy, but it is nevertheless necessary for subsequent renal development. Indeed, the mesonephros, which is the first functional kidney, develops from the inferior pole of the pronephros while the mesonephric duct, also called Wolffian duct, is a direct extension of the pronephric duct (Fig. 1). The Wolffian duct, which carries fetal urine to the developing bladder, drives the development of the ureteric bud inferiorly to the mesonephros. The metanephros, which is the permanent kidney used after birth, develops from the ureteric bud and surrounding mesenchyme. This sequence of events is shown in Figure 1.

Although degeneration of the mesonephros begins in a craniocaudal direction as early as the fifth gestational week, this organ nevertheless plays important roles in the development of the reproductive organs in both genders. The gonadal ridges (also known as the genital ridges) form from the medial aspect of each mesonephros in the fifth week of gestation (Fig. 1) and eventually develop into the primitive gonads, from which the ovaries or testes subsequently

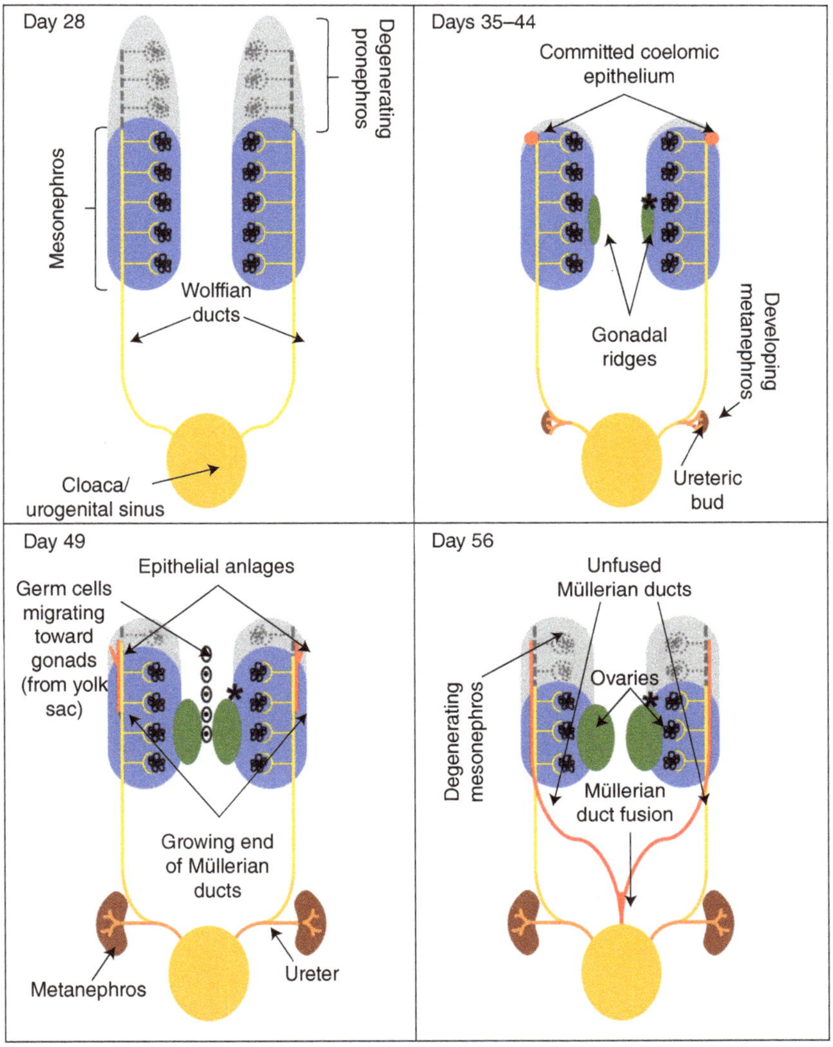

Figure 1. Relationship between the development of the renal and reproductive systems. (*Day 28*) The pronephros is largely degenerated and depicted by a gray shadow. The mesonephros is the only functioning renal organ. It contains filtration units that drain into the Wolffian ducts, which developed from the caudal ends of the pronephric ducts; the Wolffian ducts empty into the cloaca, which has already begun separating into two compartments, one connected to the gastrointestinal tract and another merging with the urogenital sinus to become the future urinary bladder and urethra. (*Days 35–44*) The ureteric bud begins developing on day 35. The metanephros develops from the ureteric bud and already functions as a kidney by the end of this 10-day period. The mesonephros is beginning to degenerate in a craniocaudal direction (depicted by a gray area); the gonadal ridges, precursors of the future ovaries, have already developed from the inferior and medial aspect of the mesonephros; areas of coelomic epithelium committed to differentiation into Müllerian ducts are seen over the superolateral aspect of the mesonephros. (*Day 49*) Germ cells have left the yolk sac (not shown here) and are migrating in the midline toward the developing gonads. Epithelial anlages have formed from the committed areas of the coelomic epithelium and started to develop into Müllerian ducts. (*Day 56*) Degeneration of the mesonephros is more extensive. The Müllerian ducts are fully developed and have begun fusing in the midline caudally. The asterisks depict the areas of transition between the gonadal ridges/primitive ovaries and the mesonephros that are enlarged in Figure 2.

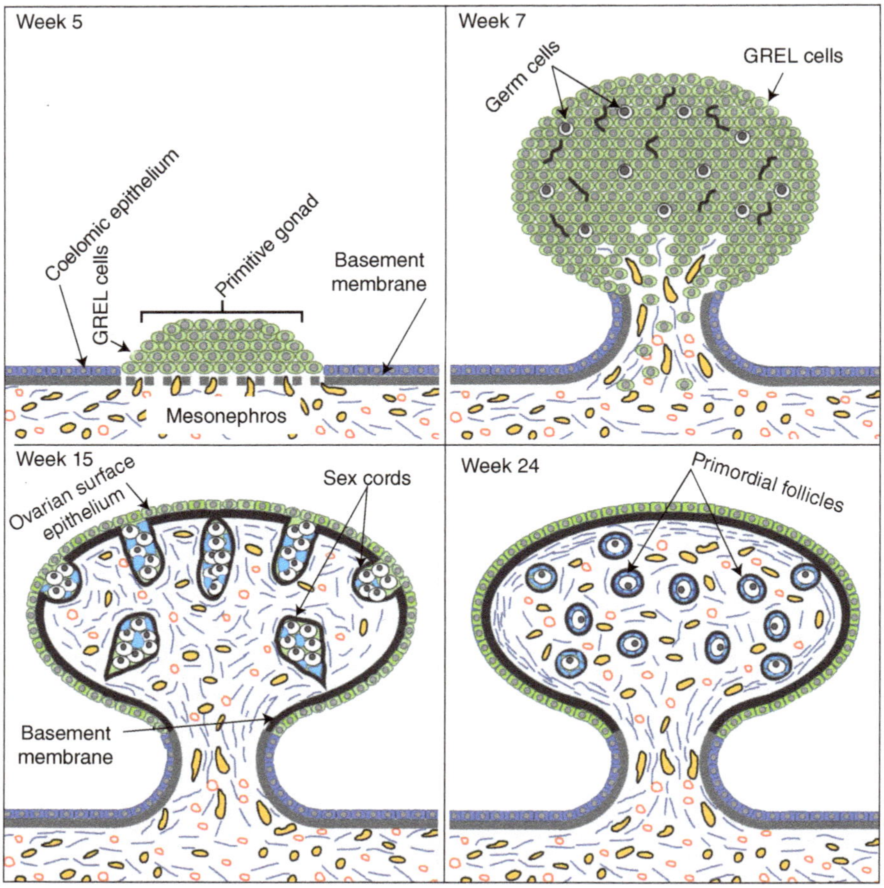

Figure 2. Contributions of the mesonephros and coelomic epithelium to ovarian development. (*Week 5*) Cells derived from the mesonephric mesenchyme have pierced through the coelomic basement membrane and began forming primitive gonads; note the absence of coelomic epithelium covering the primitive gonad as well as the absence of a basement membrane underneath the surface layer; the primitive gonad is formed entirely of gonadal ridge epithelial-like (GREL) cells. (*Week 7*) Germ cells entered the primitive gonad. (*Week 15*) The cells lining the ovarian surface, which are derived from mesonephric mesenchyme, are separated from the underlying cells by a basement membrane, completing the formation of a surface epithelial layer; GREL cells and ovarian germ cells accumulate below this surface epithelium leading to the formation of sex cords. (*Week 24*) The sex cords broke up into primordial follicles, each containing a single germ cell arrested at the G2 phase of the first mitotic division, which is surrounded by a single layer of granulosa cells, the origin of which is still being debated; the coelomic epithelium ends at the ovarian hilum and does not cover the ovarian surface.

develop (see next section). The craniolateral aspect of the mesonephros is the site of origin of another important structure that begins as an invagination of the coelomic epithelium covering the mesonephric surface. This invagination forms an epithelial anlage that subsequently develops into ductal structures called Müllerian (also called paramesonephric) ducts (Guioli et al. 2007; Orvis and Behringer 2007), which expand caudally in close association with the Wolffian ducts (Fig. 1). The caudal portion of the two Müllerian ducts eventually fuses in the midline and develops into the upper third of the vagina, cervix, and uterus while the cranial portion remains unfused and develops into the fallopian tubes (Fig. 1).

The Müllerian ducts initially develop in both sexes but later degenerate in males under the influence of the anti-Müllerian hormone (also called Müllerian-inhibiting substance) (Josso et al. 2001). The portion of the Wolffian ducts proximal to the ureteric bud transforms into the ducts of the male reproductive system including the rete testis, efferent ducts, epididymis, vas deferens, and into the ducts draining the seminal vesicles and prostate. The portion below the ureteric bud becomes the ureter in both sexes.

IS THE OVARIAN SURFACE EPITHELIUM AN EXTENSION OF THE COELOMIC EPITHELIUM?

High-grade serous carcinoma is the most common subtype of the cancers historically classified as ovarian carcinomas. Similar tumors can also arise either from the fallopian tube or in soft tissues sparing both the ovaries and the fallopian tubes. By convention, high-grade serous carcinomas have been historically classified as ovarian carcinomas if the ovaries were involved. The diagnosis of fallopian tube carcinoma was only used for cancers that involved these organs but spared the ovaries (Finn and Javert 1949). High-grade serous carcinomas sparing both the fallopian tubes and the ovaries continue, to this day, to be classified as primary peritoneal carcinomas (August et al. 1985; Dalrymple et al. 1989; Fromm et al. 1990; Altaras et al. 1991). This widely followed convention originated from the beliefs that (1) these tumors are biologically and clinically identical regardless of their site of origin, (2) the coelomic epithelium, an epithelial layer that covers most pelvic and abdominal surfaces including the peritoneum, is pluripotent and predisposed to changes in cellular differentiation via a process known as metaplasia, and (3) the ovarian surface epithelium is an extension of the coelomic epithelium, which is therefore also prone to undergo metaplasia. This logic accounted for the existence of cancers resembling fallopian tube carcinomas (or other gynecological carcinomas) that spared the reproductive organs. The question of whether the ovarian surface epithelium is indeed an extension of the coelomic epithelium is therefore relevant.

Figure 2 shows the relationship between the gonadal ridges, which are the precursors of the adult gonads in both sexes, and the mesonephros. While these ridges were originally thought to arise from a thickening of the coelomic epithelium covering the mesonephros, the current evidence shows that they instead are derived from the mesonephros immediately beneath the coelomic epithelium (Fig. 2; Hummitzsch et al. 2013, 2015; Rodgers and Hummitzsch 2014). An outgrowth of the mesonephric mesoderm pierces through the coelomic epithelium during this process (Fig. 2). There is no epithelium lining the surface of the early gonadal ridges. The entire gonadal ridge cell mass is composed of precursors of ovarian stroma as well as gonadal ridge epithelial-like (abbreviated GREL) cells (Hummitzsch et al. 2015). There is initially no basement membrane beneath the cells on the surface of the rudimentary gonads, further attesting to the absence of a true epithelial lining (Fig. 2). It is only later that a basal lamina is formed beneath the surface cells, giving rise to the ovarian surface epithelial layer (Hummitzsch et al. 2013; Rodgers and Hummitzsch 2014). The ovarian surface epithelium is therefore not derived from coelomic epithelium, invalidating the long-held hypothesis that these two epithelia are part of a continuum. A stem cell niche for the ovarian surface epithelium is located near the transition between this epithelium and the coelomic epithelium (Flesken-Nikitin et al. 2013), presumably at the boundary between this epithelium and the coelomic epithelium. Lineage-tracing studies showed that cells derived from this niche populate the ovarian surface epithelium but not the coelomic epithelium, further underscoring the differences between these two epithelia (Flesken-Nikitin et al. 2013).

IS THE OVARIAN SURFACE EPITHELIUM PLURIPOTENT?

The hypothesis that the ovarian surface epithelium is an important site of cancer development is partly based on the notion that it harbors pluripotent stem cells capable of differentiating into tissues similar to those lining other components of the reproductive tract such as the epithelial lining of fallopian tubes, endometrium, or endocervix. Pathologists of the last century hypothesized that such metaplastic changes were triggered by the rich hormonal milieu of the ovary and could take place in the epithelial cell layers lining either the ovarian surface or the coelomic epithelium, which were regarded as part of a single continuum (see previous section).

The idea that the ovarian surface epithelium is pluripotent originated from the initial belief that this epithelium is the source of all major components of the adult ovary including germ cells, follicular cells, and ovarian stromal cells. The ovarian surface epithelium has also been referred to as the germinal epithelium based on this notion. It is now established that ovarian stromal and follicular cells are instead of mesonephric origin as discussed in the previous section. It is also well-established that germ cells are not formed in the ovarian surface epithelium, as they first appear in the wall of the yolk sac and migrate to the gonadal ridges during the fifth week of pregnancy (Fig. 1; Chiquoine 1954; Gomperts et al. 1994; Saffman and Lasko 1999). Once in the ovary, their number expands via mitosis until they incorporate into sex cords. They later become incorporated into primordial follicles, characterized by a single oocyte arrested at the G2 phase of the cell cycle and surrounded by a single layer of primordial follicular cells (Fig. 2), which are precursors of granulosa cells in developing follicles in adults.

Our current understanding of the embryological origin of the cell types present in adult ovaries such as germ cells and others therefore does not support the hypothesis that they originate from the ovarian surface epithelial cell layer. Nevertheless, the pluripotency of the ovarian surface has been supported by recent observations. Stem cells with germ cell characteristics were detected outside ovarian follicles in normal rodent and human ovaries (Johnson et al. 2004; Zou et al. 2009; Zhang et al. 2011; White et al. 2012; Zhou et al. 2014), raising the possibility that the germ cell pool can be expanded in this organ after birth. The exact origin of such stem cells is still being debated. The initial suggestion that they are bone marrow–derived was challenged (Johnson et al. 2005; Eggan et al. 2006; Lee et al. 2007a). The possibility that they arise from the ovarian surface epithelium has been raised (Johnson et al. 2004; Zou et al. 2009). Cells expressing a reporter transgene construct driven by the *Oct4* promoter were isolated from the ovarian surface epithelium of adult mouse ovaries and subsequently shown to express germ cell markers as well as telomerase (Pacchiarotti et al. 2010). These cells, when transferred into oocyte-depleted ovaries in vivo, produced two generations of offspring (Zhang et al. 2011). Thus, the adult ovarian surface epithelium may indeed contain a population of stem cells that are capable of differentiating into germ cells under certain experimental conditions. To our knowledge, there is currently no evidence that such differentiation leads to expansion of the pool of germ cells or formation of ovarian follicules after birth. There is similarly no evidence that any component of the ovarian surface epithelium can differentiate into fallopian tube-like, endometrial-like, or endocervical-like epithelia, which has been a central component of the hypothesis that the surface epithelium is the source of serous, endometrioid, and mucinous ovarian tumors. While this hypothesis has also been buoyed by the argument that the ovarian surface epithelium could be embryologically related to these other components of the reproductive tract, evidence against the existence of such a relationship is presented in the next section.

IS THERE A LINK BETWEEN THE DEVELOPMENT OF THE OVARY AND THAT OF THE OTHER FEMALE REPRODUCTIVE ORGANS?

Major histological subtypes of the cancers historically referred to as ovarian carcinomas are similar to cancers arising in organs derived from the Müllerian ducts, which include all female internal reproductive organs other than the ovaries (Fig. 1). In addition, small cysts lined by epithelial cells similar to those lining the fallopian tube, endocervix, and endometrium are commonly found within the ovaries as well as in the paraovarian area where they can develop into benign tumors (ovarian serous or mucinous cystadenomas and endometriomas). The question of whether or not an embryological link exists between the development of the ovary and that of the other reproductive organs is therefore relevant to our understanding of the origin and histogenesis of these lesions. Such a link has been previously hypothesized based on the premise refuted elsewhere in this article that the Müllerian ducts as well as the ovarian surface epithelium were all originally derived from coelomic epithelium.

The first morphological sign of Müllerian duct development is a funnel-shaped invagination of the coelomic epithelial layer lining the dorsolateral edge of the mesonephros near the cranial end of each Wolffian duct (Fig. 1; Guioli et al. 2007; Orvis and Behringer 2007). A ductal structure develops and expands caudally from this epithelial anlage (Gruenwald 1941). While the most cranial segments of the two Müllerian ducts remain separated and eventually give rise to the fallopian tubes, the more caudal segments fuse in the midline and form the uterus, endocervix, and upper third of the vagina (Fig. 1). The extent of fusion varies among species. For example, the uterine body consists of two separate uterine horns in rodents because fusion of the Müllerian ducts in this species is confined to more caudal portions than in humans.

Regardless of the mammalian species, the caudal end of the fused Müllerian ducts connects to the sinovaginal bulbs within the urogenital sinus, resulting in the formation of the lower two-thirds of the vagina lined by stratified squamous epithelium (Bloomfield and Frazer 1927; Koff 1933). The upper third of the vagina is initially lined by columnar epithelium derived from the Müllerian ducts. The boundary between the stratified squamous and columnar epithelia later regresses toward the cervix, where it demarcates the exo- and endocervix.

The origin of the stratified squamous epithelium lining the upper third of the vaginal wall in adults has been controversial. The possibility that it is almost entirely derived from Müllerian ducts has been raised, at least in mice (Kurita 2010). The exact location of the boundary between columnar and stratified squamous epithelium continues to change after birth in response to local inflammation and is a common site of development of cervical squamous cell carcinoma. The drug diethylstilbestrol, used for pregnant women with a history of miscarriage or other complications of pregnancy from 1940 to 1971, prevents regression of the vaginal columnar epithelium in female fetuses. This drug led to a spike in the incidence of an otherwise rare vaginal cancer called clear cell vaginal carcinoma in adults who were exposed to it in utero (Herbst et al. 1971) and is therefore no longer prescribed to pregnant women.

Although the gonadal ridges from which the ovaries are derived and the Müllerian ducts both originate from the mesonephros at approximately the same embryonic age, they are formed independently of each other on opposite sides of the mesonephros. Furthermore, the Müllerian ducts develop from an infolding of coelomic epithelium (Fig. 1; Guioli et al. 2007; Orvis and Behringer 2007; Roly et al. 2018) while the gonadal ridges develop from mesonephric mesenchyme (Fig. 2; Hummitzsch et al. 2013; Rodgers and Hummitzsch 2014). Caudal extension of the Müllerian ducts from the original epithelial anlages is independent of ovarian development. Early embryologists noted that the Müllerian ducts in their early stages of development are so intimately associated with the Wolffian ducts that these two ducts can be found enclosed within the same basement membrane (Gruenwald 1941; Hashimoto 2003). An intact Wolffian duct is also necessary for normal Müllerian duct development while it plays no role in ovarian development (Gruenwald 1941; Ayers et al. 2015). The coelomic epithelium and its underlying mesenchyme are necessary for the caudal elongation of the Müllerian ducts but not for the development of the ovaries (Hummitzsch et al. 2013; Rodgers and Hummitzsch 2014). The development of Müllerian duct mesenchyme (Ayers et al. 2015) precedes and is driven by elongation of the caudal end of the Müllerian duct epithelium independently of the mesonephros (Fujino et al. 2009).

The embryological transcription factors driving the caudal expansion of the Müllerian ducts following the formation of the initial epithelial anlage are also different than those driving ovarian development. Extension of the Müllerian duct is dependent on the DMRT1 transcription factor (Ayers et al. 2015), which has no role in gonadal development. Expression of this transcription factor precedes that of the Müllerian duct in the coelomic epithelium and underlying stroma along the entire craniocaudal path of Müllerian duct development, as if a restricted portion of this epithelium were predetermined to contribute to their caudal extension (Ayers et al. 2015). Knockdown of DMRT1 in relevant segments of the coelomic epithelium prevents further extension of the Müllerian ducts (Ayers et al. 2015) but has no known effect on ovarian development. Differentiation of the various segments of the Müllerian ducts toward the fallopian tubal, uterine, and endocervical/vaginal elements is driven by the HOX family of transcription factors (Taylor et al. 1997; Lynch et al. 2004), which differ from the HOX genes involved in the development of the ovary (Cheng et al. 2005). There is therefore no evidence for any embryological link between the development of the ovaries and that of the other female reproductive organs.

EXTRAUTERINE MÜLLERIAN EPITHELIUM

The initial concept that extrauterine benign or malignant tumors resembling derivatives of the Müllerian ducts could develop from the coelomic epithelium simplified their histopathological classification and facilitated the development of experimental models by providing a common site of origin for this otherwise complex group of neoplasms. These tumors, regardless of whether or not the ovaries or fallopian tubes were involved, were regarded as a single broad pathological entity derived from the coelomic epithelium, albeit further divided into distinct histopathological subtypes. Pathologists of past centuries may have overlooked the significance of foci of histologically normal tissues showing Müllerian duct characteristics that are abundant in the paraovarian and paratubal regions and may also be seen well beyond these organs. The terms endosalpingiosis, endometriosis, and endocervicosis refer to structures lined by epithelia resembling, respectively, those lining the fallopian tubes, endometrium, and endocervix but located outside these organs. Their Müllerian origin is supported not only by their morphological appearance, but also by the demonstration of a Müllerian-specific gene-expression profile in endosalpingiosis (Esselen et al. 2014). These structures are abundant in the paratubal and paraovarian connective tissue (Sunde et al. 2020) and can also be found entrapped within lymph nodes or other pelvic organs including the ovary and bowel wall. The fact that they are most abundant around the fimbrial ends of the fallopian tubes supports the idea that they are derived from the most cranial portion of the Müllerian ducts. Whether endosalpingiosis, endometriosis, and endocervicosis are mere embryological remnants or have a functional role in adults is also unclear. However, not only has endosalpingiosis given rise to neoplastic growths (Bell and Scully 1990; Kadar and Krumerman 1995; Young and Clement 1996; Quddus et al. 1999; Carrick et al. 2003; McCoubrey et al. 2005), but oncogenic mutations have also been documented within these structures (Chui and Shih 2020). Several observations also support a role for endometriosis in the histogenesis of the tumors historically classified as endometrioid ovarian carcinomas (Heaps et al. 1990; Brinton et al. 1997; Ness and Cottreau 1999; Prefumo et al. 2002; Vignali et al. 2002; Ness 2003). The idea that endometriosis is a component of the extrauterine Müllerian system does not rule out the possibility that some endometriotic foci could also result from the implantation of retrograde menstrual flow, which has also been proposed as a potential mechanism for endometriosis.

The concept of extrauterine Müllerian epithelium was introduced as an entity that embodies all tissue types that show characteristics suggestive of embryological derivation from the Müllerian ducts located outside the confines of the uterus and its contiguous organs (Dubeau 2008). Components of this entity include endosalpingiosis, endometriosis, endocervicosis, and the extraluminal (fimbrial) portion of the fallopian tubes. The term "secondary Müllerian system" has also been used to designate some, but not all, of these components (Lauchlan 1994). The true origin of the group of neoplasms previously regarded as of coelomic epithelial origin would be more accurately conveyed if they were reclassified as extrauterine Müllerian tumors. Benign (cystadenomas) or malignant (carcinomas) serous tumors previously classified as of fallopian tube, primary peritoneal, or ovarian surface origin would be renamed serous extrauterine Müllerian cystadenomas or carcinomas (Tables 1 and

Table 1. Site of origin of benign gynecological epithelial tumors according to the coelomic and extrauterine Müllerian hypotheses

Tumor type	Location	As per the coelomic hypothesis	As per the extrauterine Müllerian hypothesis
Serous cystadenoma	Intraovarian	Serous metaplasia of ovarian surface epithelial inclusion cyst	Endosalpingiosis
	Extraovarian	Serous metaplasia of coelomic epithelium	
Endometrioid cystadenoma (endometrioma)	Intraovarian	Endometrioid metaplasia of ovarian surface epithelial inclusion cyst	Endocervicosis
	Extraovarian	Endometrioid metaplasia of coelomic epithelium	
Mucinous cystadenoma	Intraovarian	Mucinous metaplasia of ovarian surface epithelial inclusion cyst	Endocervicosis
	Extraovarian	Mucinous metaplasia of coelomic epithelium	

2). Tumors previously classified as endometriomas or ovarian endometrioid carcinomas would be reclassified as endometrioid extrauterine cystadenomas or carcinomas (Tables 1 and 2). Likewise, tumors previously classified as ovarian mucinous cystadenomas or carcinomas would be renamed as mucinous extrauterine Müllerian cystadenomas or carcinomas (Tables 1 and 2). Support for the notion that clear cell carcinomas should also be regarded as derivative of the extrauterine Müllerian epithelium is reviewed in the next section. Microscopic intraovarian serous or mucinous cysts, which are common and have been historically regarded as metaplastic surface inclusion cysts, should be regarded as mere examples of intraovarian endosalpingiosis, endometriosis, or endocervicosis. The exact histogenesis of these structures is not clear, but their presence in the ovary is unlikely to represent a specific association with ovarian development given that they can also be seen in a variety of other unrelated organs including lymph nodes and bowel wall.

Although the fallopian tubes are an integral component of the uterus, the epithelial lining of fallopian tube fimbriae is regarded as belonging to the serous compartment of extrauterine Müllerian epithelium distinguished from intrauterine serous epithelium. This is justified because the fimbriae give rise to cancers indistinguishable from those arising in endosalpingiosis. In addition, their management is dictated by clinicopathological parameters and staging criteria that do not apply to serous tumors developing from intrauterine Müllerian epithelium such as from the intraluminal portion of the tubes (a rare entity) or from serous metaplasia of the endometrium. The same argument supports distinguishing endometrioid and mucinous extrauterine Müllerian epithelial tumors from morphologically similar tumors arising from the endometrium and the endocervix.

EMBRYOLOGICAL INSIGHTS INTO THE ORIGIN OF OVARIAN CLEAR CELL CARCINOMAS

The notion that tumors historically classified as ovarian carcinomas are derived from extrauterine Müllerian epithelium accounts for the serous, endometrioid, and mucinous subtypes of these cancers. It does not readily account for the clear cell subtype, which has no normal counterpart in any of the reproductive organs. Clear cell differentiation is a common feature of cancers arising in the kidney, an organ with a close embryological relationship to the Müllerian ducts (Fig. 1). This raises the question of whether or not clear cell differentiation could reflect an embryological relationship between the Müllerian ducts and the renal tubules/collecting duct system. Indeed, the development of the Müllerian ducts is driven by

Table 2. Site of origin of malignant gynecological epithelial tumors according to the coelomic and extrauterine Müllerian hypotheses

Tumor type	Location	As per the coelomic hypothesis	As per the extrauterine Müllerian hypothesis
Serous	Involving the ovaries and/or the fallopian tubes	Ovarian surface epithelium	Either fimbrial end of fallopian tube or endosalpingiosis regardless of location
	Involving the fallopian tubes but sparing the ovaries	Fallopian tube epithelium	
	Sparing the ovaries and the fallopian tubes	Coelomic epithelium	
Endometrioid	Intraovarian Extraovarian	Ovarian surface epithelium Coelomic epithelium	Endometriosis regardless of location
Mucinous	Intraovarian Extraovarian	Ovarian surface epithelium Coelomic epithelium	Endocervicosis regardless of location
Clear cell	Intraovarian Extraovarian	Unknown Unknown	Endonephrosis regardless of location

transcription factors similar to those associated with renal development (Mueller 1994; Torres et al. 1995; Grote et al. 2006; Orvis and Behringer 2007) and is intimately related the Wolffian ducts (Gruenwald 1941), which in turn give rise to the ureteric buds from which the metanephros originates (Fig. 1). Clear cell carcinomas historically classified as of ovarian origin and renal clear cell carcinomas show some similarities not only in their gene-expression profiles (Zorn et al. 2005), but also in their response to chemotherapy (Anglesio et al. 2011), albeit they differ in their genetic profiles.

Direct evidence for an embryological link between the Müllerian ducts and the metanephros was reported (Liu et al. 2015). This study used the R26R reporter mouse line in which sequences encoding either one of two reporter genes (*LacZ* or *Gfp*) were inserted downstream of the constitutively active ROSA26 promoter (Friedrich and Soriano 1991). These reporter constructs also contain a stop codon flanked by two loxP sites, preventing reporter gene expression unless recombination occurs between these two sites due to transgenic expression of Cre recombinase (Friedrich and Soriano 1991). Once such recombination has taken place in any given cell, reporter gene expression becomes constitutive not only in that cell, but also in its daughter cells following mitosis even if Cre recombinase ceases to be expressed. Liu et al. (2015) achieved Müllerian-specific Cre recombinase expression using a transgenic construct in which a gene encoding this recombinase is downstream of the Müllerian-inhibiting substance type 2 receptor (*Mis2r*) promoter (Josso et al. 2001; Teixeira et al. 2001; Connolly et al. 2003). They documented reporter gene expression driven by this promoter in a segment of the renal tubules located near the boundary between the cortex and medulla in newborn female mice, but not in male littermates (Fig. 3). Confirmation that gender-specific Cre-mediated recombination had indeed taken place was achieved by enzymatic amplification of the reporter genes using primers on each side the loxP sites, followed by electrophoresis of the PCR products to evaluate their sizes (Fig. 3). Although the possibility of ectopic expression of the Cre transgene cannot be totally ruled out, this consistent gender-specific observation among littermates reduces its likelihood. These results strongly suggest the presence of a direct embryological link between a portion of the female adult renal collecting system and the Müllerian ducts. This conclusion is also supported by imaging studies of developing embryos (Kobayashi et al. 2004) and by the observation that congenital disorders associated with unilateral renal aplasia are often associated with the absence of

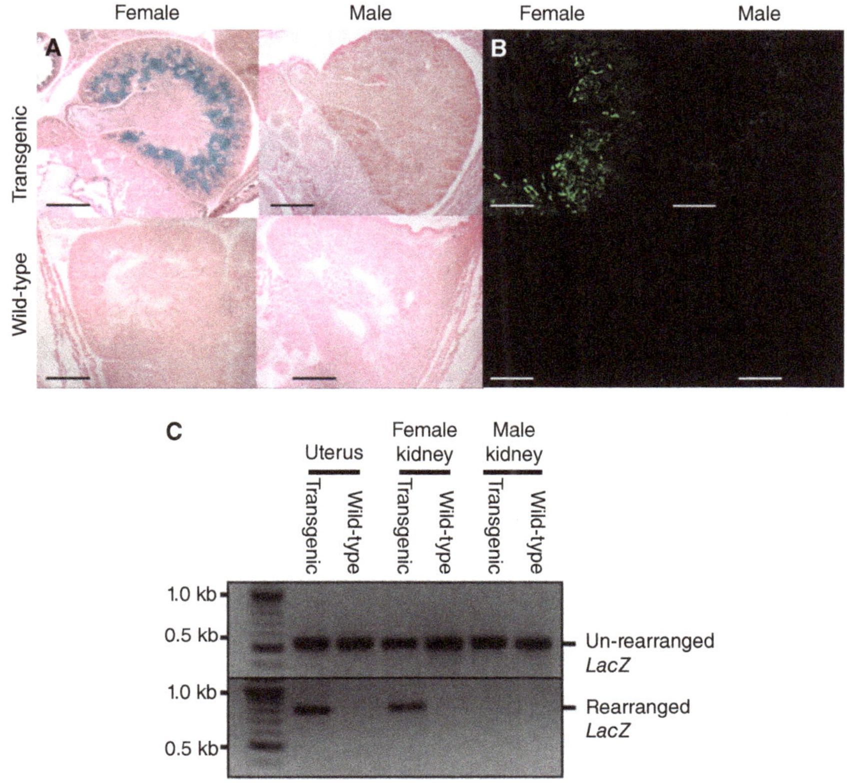

Figure 3. Sex-specific association between the Müllerian ducts and the collecting ducts of the metanephros. (*A*,*B*) Pelvic and lower abdominal tissues from male and female newborn *Mis2r-Cre;ROSA26*^{LacZ} (*A*) or *Mis2r-Cre; ROSA26*^{Gfp} (*B*). Reporter mice and controls lacking the *Mis2r-Cre* transgene were exenterated and embedded as whole mounts, sectioned with a microtome and either stained for *Lac*Z and counterstained with Nuclear Fast Red (*A*) or examined under a fluorescence microscope (*B*). Scale bar, 500 µm. (*C*) DNA was extracted from the kidneys of newborn *Mis2r-Cre;ROSA26*^{LacZ} transgenic mice and from littermates lacking the *Mis2r-Cre* transgene as well as from the uterus of *Mis2r-Cre; ROSA26*^{LacZ} mice (positive control). The DNA samples were subjected to PCR using primers flanking the *loxP* sites within the reporter construct and electrophoresed on 1% agarose gels in the presence of ethidium bromide. Presence or absence of *Mis2r-Cre*-mediated recombination in each DNA sample was evaluated by visualization of the PCR products under UV light. Such recombination was only seen in uteri and kidneys from transgenic females. (Reproduced from Liu et al. 2015 courtesy of a Creative Commons Attribution-NonCommercial-NoDerivatives 4.0 International license.)

the fallopian tube on the same side and presence of unicornus uterus on the other side (Gruenwald 1941). The presence of a developmental/environmental link between the Müllerian ducts and renal tubules may help explain gender differences in renal function in health and disease, which is a topic of great current interest in renal pathophysiology (Reckelhoff and Maric 2010).

These findings support the merit of regarding clear cell differentiation as an additional compartment of the extrauterine Müllerian epithelium alongside the serous, endometrioid, and mucinous compartments. The term endonephrosis used in Table 2 would appropriately designate nests of renal duct differentiation outside the kidneys. Clear cell ovarian carcinomas would be reclassified as clear cell extrauterine Müllerian carcinomas based on this concept. Further support for the notion that the origin of clear cell carcinomas of the reproductive tract is related to that of Müllerian tumors including serous, endometrioid, and mucinous carcinomas comes from the frequent admixture of these other tumor subtypes with clear cell carcinomas. Mixed tumors showing contiguous clear cell and endometrioid features are especially common.

CONCLUDING REMARKS

Early pathologists relied on embryological knowledge of their time to formulate a hypothesis about the histogenesis of a group of reproductive cancers that they regarded as originating from the ovarian surface epithelium. This theory, which remained widely accepted well into the early 21st century, is not compatible with current embryological knowledge reviewed in this article. The concept of extrauterine Müllerian epithelium provides a common embryological origin for all cancers historically classified as ovarian carcinomas as well as their benign counterparts. It also provides an experimental framework for further research on the biology of components of the extrauterine Müllerian epithelium, which may lead to novel strategies for cancer prevention.

REFERENCES

Altaras MM, Aviram R, Cohen I, Cordoba M, Weiss E, Beyth Y. 1991. Primary peritoneal papillary serous adenocarcinoma: clinical and management aspects. *Gynecol Oncol* **40:** 230–236. doi:10.1016/0090-8258(90)90283-Q

Anglesio MS, George J, Kulbe H, Friedlander M, Rischin D, Lemech C, Power J, Coward J, Cowin PA, House CM, et al. 2011. IL6-STAT3-HIF signaling and therapeutic response to the angiogenesis inhibitor sunitinib in ovarian clear cell cancer. *Clin Cancer Res* **17:** 2538–2548. doi:10.1158/1078-0432.CCR-10-3314

August CZ, Murad TM, Newton M. 1985. Multiple focal extraovarian serous carcinoma. *Int J Gynecol Pathol* **4:** 11–23. doi:10.1097/00004347-198501000-00002

Ayers KL, Cutting AD, Roeszler KN, Sinclair AH, Smith CA. 2015. DMRT1 is required for Müllerian duct formation in the chicken embryo. *Dev Biol* **400:** 224–236. doi:10.1016/j.ydbio.2015.02.001

Bell DA, Scully RE. 1990. Serous borderline tumors of the peritoneum. *Am J Surg Pathol* **14:** 230–239. doi:10.1097/00000478-199003000-00004

Bloomfield A, Frazer JE. 1927. The development of the lower end of the vagina. *J Anat* **62:** 9–32.

Brinton LA, Gridley G, Persson I, Baron J, Bergqvist A. 1997. Cancer risk after a hospital discharge diagnosis of endometriosis. *Am J Obstet Gynecol* **176:** 572–579. doi:10.1016/S0002-9378(97)70550-7

Carrick KS, Milvenan JS, Albores-Saavedra J. 2003. Serous tumor of low malignant potential arising in inguinal endosalpingiosis: report of a case. *Int J Gynecol Pathol* **22:** 412–415. doi:10.1097/01.pgp.0000092155.33490.52

Cheng W, Liu J, Yoshida H, Rosen D, Naora H. 2005. Lineage infidelity of epithelial ovarian cancers is controlled by HOX genes that specify regional identity in the reproductive tract. *Nat Med* **11:** 531–537. doi:10.1038/nm1230

Chiquoine AD. 1954. The identification, origin, and migration of the primordial germ cells in the mouse embryo. *Anat Rec* **118:** 135–146. doi:10.1002/ar.1091180202

Chui MH, Shih LM. 2020. Oncogenic *BRAF* and *KRAS* mutations in endosalpingiosis. *J Pathol* **250:** 148–158. doi:10.1002/path.5353

Colgan TJ, Murphy J, Cole DE, Narod S, Rosen B. 2001. Occult carcinoma in prophylactic oophorectomy specimens: prevalence and association with BRCA germline mutation status. *Am J Surg Pathol* **25:** 1283–1289. doi:10.1097/00000478-200110000-00009

Connolly DC, Bao R, Nikitin AY, Stephens KC, Poole TW, Hua X, Harris SS, Vanderhyden BC, Hamilton TC. 2003. Female mice chimeric for expression of the simian virus 40 TAg under control of the MISIIR promoter develop epithelial ovarian cancer. *Cancer Res* **63:** 1389–1397.

Crum CP, Drapkin R, Miron A, Ince TA, Muto M, Kindelberger DW, Lee Y. 2007. The distal fallopian tube: a new model for pelvic serous carcinogenesis. *Curr Opin Obstet Gynecol* **19:** 3–9. doi:10.1097/GCO.0b013e328011a21f

Dalrymple JC, Bannatyne P, Russell P, Solomon HJ, Tattersall MHN, Atkinson K, Carter J, Duval P, Elliott P, Friedlander M, et al. 1989. Extraovarian peritoneal serous papillary carcinoma. A clinicopathologic study of 31 cases. *Cancer* **64:** 110–115. doi:10.1002/1097-0142(19890701)64:1<110::AID-CNCR2820640120>3.0.CO;2-5

Dubeau L. 1999. The cell of origin of ovarian epithelial tumors and the ovarian surface epithelium dogma: does the emperor have no clothes? *Gynecol Oncol* **72:** 437–442. doi:10.1006/gyno.1998.5275

Dubeau L. 2008. The cell of origin of ovarian epithelial tumours. *Lancet Oncol* **9:** 1191–1197. doi:10.1016/S1470-2045(08)70308-5

Eggan K, Jurga S, Gosden R, Min IM, Wagers AJ. 2006. Ovulated oocytes in adult mice derive from non-circulating germ cells. *Nature* **441:** 1109–1114. doi:10.1038/nature04929

Esselen KM, Ng SK, Hua Y, White M, Jimenez CA, Welch WR, Drapkin R, Berkowitz RS, Ng SW. 2014. Endosalpingiosis as it relates to tubal, ovarian and serous neoplastic tissues: an immunohistochemical study of tubal and Müllerian antigens. *Gynecol Oncol* **132:** 316–321. doi:10.1016/j.ygyno.2013.12.007

Finn WF, Javert CT. 1949. Primary and metastatic cancer of the fallopian tube. *Cancer* **2:** 803–814. doi:10.1002/1097-0142(194909)2:5<803::AID-CNCR2820020510>3.0.CO;2-K

Flesken-Nikitin A, Hwang CI, Cheng CY, Michurina TV, Enikolopov G, Nikitin AY. 2013. Ovarian surface epithelium at the junction area contains a cancer-prone stem cell niche. *Nature* **495:** 241–245. doi:10.1038/nature11979

Friedrich G, Soriano P. 1991. Promoter traps in embryonic stem cells: a genetic screen to identify and mutate developmental genes in mice. *Genes Dev* **5:** 1513–1523. doi:10.1101/gad.5.9.1513

Fromm G-L, Gershenson DM, Silva EG. 1990. Papillary serous carcinoma of the peritoneum. *Obstet Gynecol* **75:** 89–95.

Fujino A, Arango NA, Zhan Y, Manganaro TF, Li X, MacLaughlin DT, Donahoe PK. 2009. Cell migration and activated PI3K/AKT-directed elongation in the developing rat Müllerian duct. *Dev Biol* **325:** 351–362. doi:10.1016/j.ydbio.2008.10.027

Gomperts M, Garcia-Castro M, Wylie C, Heasman J. 1994. Interactions between primordial germ cells play a role in their migration in mouse embryos. *Development* **120:** 135–141. doi:10.1242/dev.120.1.135

Grote D, Souabni A, Busslinger M, Bouchard M. 2006. Pax2/8-regulated Gata3 expression is necessary for morphogenesis and guidance of the nephric duct in the developing kidney. *Development* **133:** 53–61. doi:10.1242/dev.02184

Gruenwald P. 1941. The relationship of the growing Müllerian duct to the wolffian duct and its importance for the genesis of malformations. *Anat Rec* **81:** 1–19. doi:10.1002/ar.1090810102

Guioli S, Sekido R, Lovell-Badge R. 2007. The origin of the Müllerian duct in chick and mouse. *Dev Biol* **302:** 389–398. doi:10.1016/j.ydbio.2006.09.046

Hashimoto R. 2003. Development of the human Müllerian duct in the sexually undifferentiated stage. *Anat Rec* **272A:** 514–519. doi:10.1002/ar.a.10061

Heaps JM, Nieberg RK, Berek JS. 1990. Malignant neoplasms arising in endometriosis. *Obstet Gynecol* **75:** 1023–1028.

Herbst AL, Ulfelder H, Poskanzer DC. 1971. Adenocarcinoma of the vagina. Association of maternal stilbestrol therapy with tumor appearance in young women. *N Engl J Med* **284:** 878–881. doi:10.1056/NEJM197104222841604

Hummitzsch K, Irving-Rodgers HF, Hatzirodos N, Bonner W, Sabatier L, Reinhardt DP, Sado Y, Ninomiya Y, Wilhelm D, Rodgers RJ. 2013. A new model of development of the mammalian ovary and follicles. *PLoS ONE* **8:** e55578. doi:10.1371/journal.pone.0055578

Hummitzsch K, Anderson RA, Wilhelm D, Wu J, Telfer EE, Russell DL, Robertson SA, Rodgers RJ. 2015. Stem cells, progenitor cells, and lineage decisions in the ovary. *Endocrine Rev* **36:** 65–91. doi:10.1210/er.2014-1079

Johnson J, Canning J, Kaneko T, Pru JK, Tilly JL. 2004. Germline stem cells and follicular renewal in the postnatal mammalian ovary. *Nat Cell Biol* **428:** 145–150.

Johnson J, Bagley J, Skaznik-Wikiel M, Lee H-J, Adams GB, Niikura Y, Tschudy KS, Tilly JC, Cortes ML, Forkert R, et al. 2005. Oocyte generation in adult mammalian ovaries by putative germ cells in bone marrow and peripheral blood. *Cell* **122:** 303–315. doi:10.1016/j.cell.2005.06.031

Josso N, di Clemente N, Gouédard L. 2001. Anti-Müllerian hormone and its receptors. *Mol Cell Endocrinol* **179:** 25–32. doi:10.1016/S0303-7207(01)00467-1

Kadar N, Krumerman M. 1995. Possible metaplastic origin of lymph node "metastases" in serous ovarian tumor of low malignant potential (borderline serous tumor). *Gynecol Oncol* **59:** 394–397. doi:10.1006/gyno.1995.9955

Kobayashi A, Shawlot W, Kania A, Behringer RR. 2004. Requirement of *Lim1* for female reproductive tract development. *Development* **131:** 539–549. doi:10.1242/dev.00951

Koff AK. 1933. Development of the vagina in the human fetus. *Contrib Embryol* **24:** 59–91.

Kurita T. 2010. Developmental origin of vaginal epithelium. *Differentiation* **80:** 99–105. doi:10.1016/j.diff.2010.06.007

Lauchlan SC. 1994. The secondary müllerian system revisited. *Int J Gynecol Pathol* **13:** 73–79. doi:10.1097/00004347-199401000-00009

Lee HJ, Selesniemi K, Niikura Y, Niikura T, Klein R, Dombkowski DM, Tilly L. 2007a. Bone marrow transplantation generates immature oocytes and rescues longterm fertility in a preclinical mouse model of chemotherapy-induced premature ovarian failure. *J Clin Oncol* **25:** 3198–3204. doi:10.1200/JCO.2006.10.3028

Lee Y, Miron A, Drapkin R, Nucci MR, Medeiros F, Saleemuddin A, Garber J, Birch C, Mou H, Gordon RW, et al. 2007b. A candidate precursor to serous carcinoma that originates in the distal fallopian tube. *J Pathol* **211:** 26–35. doi:10.1002/path.2091

Liu Y, Yen HY, Austria T, Pettersson J, Peti-Peterdi J, Maxson R, Widschwendter M, Dubeau L. 2015. A mouse model that reproduces the developmental pathways and site specificity of the cancers associated with the human BRCA1 mutation carrier state. *EBioMed* **2:** 1318–1330. doi:10.1016/j.ebiom.2015.08.034

Lynch VJ, Roth JJ, Takahashi K, Dunn CW, Nonaka DF, Stopper GF, Wagner GP. 2004. Adaptive evolution of *HoxA-11* and *HoxA-13* at the origin of the uterus in mammals. *Proc Biol Sci* **271:** 2201–2207. doi:10.1098/rspb.2004.2848

McCoubrey A, Houghton O, McCallion K, McCluggage WG. 2005. Serous adenocarcinoma of the sigmoid mesentery arising in cystic endosalpingiosis. *J Clin Pathol* **58:** 1221–1223. doi:10.1136/jcp.2005.027946

Medeiros F, Muto MG, Lee Y, Elvin JA, Callahan MJ, Feltmate C, Garber JE, Cramer DW, Crum CP. 2006. The tubal fimbria is a preferred site for early adenocarcinoma in women with familial ovarian cancer syndrome. *Am J Surg Pathol* **30:** 230–236. doi:10.1097/01.pas.0000180854.28831.77

Mueller RF. 1994. The Denys–Drash syndrome. *J Med Genet* **31:** 471–477. doi:10.1136/jmg.31.6.471

Ness RB. 2003. Endometriosis and ovarian cancer: thoughts on shared pathophysiology. *Am J Obstet Gynecol* **189:** 280–294. doi:10.1067/mob.2003.408

Ness RB, Cottreau C. 1999. Possible role of ovarian epithelial inflammation in ovarian cancer. *J Natl Cancer Inst* **91:** 1459–1467. doi:10.1093/jnci/91.17.1459

Orthmann EG. 1886. Ein primäres carcinoma papillare tubae dextrae, verbunden mit ovarial-abscess. *Centrabl f Gynäk* **10:** 816–818.

Orvis GD, Behringer RR. 2007. Cellular mechanisms of Müllerian duct formation in the mouse. *Dev Biol* **306:** 493–504. doi:10.1016/j.ydbio.2007.03.027

Pacchiarotti J, Maki C, Ramos T, Marh J, Howerton K, Wong J, Pham J, Anorve S, Chow YC, Izadyar F. 2010. Differentiation potential of germ line stem cells derived from the postnatal mouse ovary. *Differentiation* **79:** 159–170. doi:10.1016/j.diff.2010.01.001

Piek JM, van Diest PJ, Zweemer RP, Jansen JW, Poort-Keesom RJ, Menko FH, Gille JJ, Jongsma AP, Pals G, Kenemans P, et al. 2001. Dysplastic changes in prophylactically removed fallopian tubes of women predisposed to developing ovarian cancer. *J Pathol* **195:** 451–456. doi:10.1002/path.1000

Prefumo F, Todeschini F, Fulcheri E, Venturini PL. 2002. Epithelial abnormalities in cystic ovarian endometriosis. *Gynecol Oncol* **84:** 280–284. doi:10.1006/gyno.2001.6529

Quddus MR, Sung CJ, Lauchlan C. 1999. Benign and malignant serous and endometrioid epithelium in the omentum. *Gynecol Oncol* **75:** 227–232. doi:10.1006/gyno.1999.5575

Reckelhoff JF, Maric C. 2010. Sex and gender differences in cardiovascular–renal physiology and pathophysiology. *Steroids* **75:** 745–746. doi:10.1016/j.steroids.2010.05.020

Rodgers RJ, Hummitzsch K. 2014. *New model of formation of the ovary.* Robinson Research Institute, Lower Hutt, New Zealand. https://www.youtube.com/watch?v=1O97DtAyaDc

Roly ZY, Backhouse B, Cutting A, Tan TY, Sinclair AH, Ayers KL, Major AT, Smith CA. 2018. The cell biology and molecular genetics of Müllerian duct development. *Wires Dev Biol* **7:** e310.

Saffman EE, Lasko P. 1999. Germline development in vertebrates and invertebrates. *Cell Molec Life Sci* **55:** 1141–1163. doi:10.1007/s000180050363

Sunde J, Wasickanin M, Katz TA, Wickersham EL, Steed DOE, Simper N. 2020. Prevalence of endosalpingiosis and other benign gynecologic lesions. *PLoS ONE* **15:** e0232487. doi:10.1371/journal.pone.0232487

Taylor HS, Vanden Heuvel GB, Igarashi P. 1997. A conserved Hox axis in the mouse and human female reproductive system: late establishment and persistent adult expression of the *Hoxa* cluster genes. *Biol Reprod* **57:** 1338–1345. doi:10.1095/biolreprod57.6.1338

Teixeira J, Maheswaran S, Donahoe PK. 2001. Müllerian inhibiting substance: an instructive developmental hormone with diagnostic and possible therapeutic applications. *Endocrinol Rev* **22:** 657–674.

Torres M, Gomez-Pardo E, Dressler GR, Gruss P. 1995. Pax-2 controls multiple steps of urogenital development. *Development* **121:** 4057–4065. doi:10.1242/dev.121.12.4057

Vignali M, Infantino M, Matrone R, Chiodo I, Somigliana E, Busacca M, Viganò P. 2002. Endometriosis: novel etiopathogenetic concepts and clinical perspectives. *Fertil Steril* **78:** 665–678. doi:10.1016/S0015-0282(02)03233-8

White YA, Woods DC, Takai Y, Ishihara O, Seki H, Tilly JL. 2012. Oocyte formation by mitotically active germ cells purified from ovaries of reproductive-age women. *Nature Med* **18:** 413–421. doi:10.1038/nm.2669

Young RH, Clement PB. 1996. Müllerianosis of the urinary bladder. *Mod Pathol* **9:** 731–737.

Zhang Y, Yang Z, Yang Y, Wang S, Shi L, Xie W, Sun K, Zou K, Wang L, Xiong J, et al. 2011. Production of transgenic mice by random recombination of targeted genes in female germline stem cells. *J Molec Cell Biol* **3:** 132–141. doi:10.1093/jmcb/mjq043

Zhou L, Wang L, Kang JX, Xie W, Li X, Wu C, Xu B, Wu J. 2014. Production of fat-1 transgenic rats using a postnatal female germline stem cell line. *Molec Hum Reprod* **20:** 271–281. doi:10.1093/molehr/gat081

Zorn KK, Bonome T, Gangi L, Chandramouli GV, Awtrey CS, Gardner GJ, Barrett JC, Boyd J, Birrer MJ. 2005. Gene expression profiles of serous, endometrioid, and clear cell subtypes of ovarian and endometrial cancer. *Clin Cancer Res* **11:** 6422–6430. doi:10.1158/1078-0432.CCR-05-0508

Zou K, Yuan Z, Yang Z, Luo H, Sun K, Zhou L, Xiang J, Shi L, Yu Q, Zhang Y, et al. 2009. Production of offspring from a germline stem cell line derived from neonatal ovaries. *Nature Cell Biol* **11:** 631–636. doi:10.1038/ncb1869

Rare Epithelial Ovarian Cancers: Low Grade Serous and Mucinous Carcinomas

Olivia Craig,[1,2,4] Abhimanyu Nigam,[1,2,4] Genevieve V. Dall,[3] and Kylie Gorringe[1,2]

[1]Department of Laboratory Research, Peter MacCallum Cancer Centre, Melbourne, VIC 3000, Australia
[2]The Sir Peter MacCallum Department of Oncology, University of Melbourne, Parkville, VIC 3010, Australia
[3]University of Melbourne, Parkville, VIC 3010, Australia
Correspondence: kylie.gorringe@petermac.org

The ovarian epithelial cancer histotypes can be divided into common and rare types. Common types include high-grade serous ovarian carcinomas and the endometriosis-associated cancers, endometrioid and clear-cell carcinomas. The less common histotypes are mucinous and low-grade serous, each comprising less than 10% of all epithelial carcinomas. Although histologically and epidemiologically distinct from each other, these histotypes share some genetic and natural history features that distinguish them from the more common types. In this review, we will consider the similarities and differences of these rare histological types, and the clinical challenges they pose.

Epithelial ovarian cancer (EOC) has long been recognized to comprise different histological subtypes. Currently, these are high-grade and low-grade serous, clear-cell, endometrioid, and mucinous carcinomas (Reid et al. 2017). Recent exploration of their biology has led to an increased understanding of the genetic, cellular, and epidemiological differences that underpin their histopathology, and subsequently informed more targeted clinical approaches. In this review, we focus on the two least common of these histotypes, mucinous ovarian carcinoma (MOC) and low-grade serous ovarian carcinoma (LGSC), comprising 3% and 5%–8% of all EOCs, respectively (Reid et al. 2017). We will consider their epidemiological risk factors, how these relate to putative cells of origin, their natural history via precursor tumors, and their pathological, genetic, and clinical features.

MUCINOUS OVARIAN CARCINOMA

MOC is characterized by the formation of large, mucin-containing tumors. Recent advances have revealed MOC is molecularly distinct from the more common epithelial malignancies, and should thus be recognized as a unique and separate entity.

Epidemiology

MOC is more likely to be diagnosed in younger women compared to other EOCs, with more than half aged under 55 at first presentation (Peres et al. 2019). In general, MOC does not

[4]These authors contributed equally to this work.

Cite this article as *Cold Spring Harb Perspect Med* doi: 10.1101/cshperspect.a038190

share risk factors with other EOCs, highlighting the need to regard it as an independent disease. In particular, hormonal factors known to influence the more common high-grade serous ovarian carcinoma (HGSC) are absent in MOC (Gates et al. 2010). Furthermore, there is a twofold increase in MOC development associated with a history of smoking (Collaborative Group on Epidemiological Studies of Ovarian Cancer et al. 2012; Santucci et al. 2019), a characteristic unique to this subtype of EOC. Recently, being overweight in childhood was shown to be associated with a higher risk of developing MOC (Aarestrup et al. 2019).

There is no association between family history and risk of MOC, and the *BRCA1* and *BRCA2* gene variants that are known to predispose to HGSC are not relevant for MOC (Risch et al. 2006). Large-scale genome-wide association studies show MOC to be genetically distinct from other EOCs. In 2015, Kelemen et al. (2015) found three single-nucleotide polymorphisms (SNPs) associated with MOC risk (2q13, 2q31, and 19q13). A later study added two further SNPs (3q22 and 9q31), additionally demonstrating that these were also shared by mucinous borderline tumors (Phelan et al. 2017). At present, only three loci have been identified showing a risk shared with other EOCs (9q34, 22q12, 2q13) (Kuchenbaecker et al. 2015). Although not always straightforward to identify the associated causative gene, functional studies supported *PAX8* (2q13) and *HOXD9* (2q31) as strong candidates (Kelemen et al. 2015).

Clinicopathological Features and Diagnosis

Mucinous ovarian tumors can be classified as benign, borderline, or malignant. According to the World Health Organization (WHO) diagnostic criteria, benign tumors usually present as cystadenomas comprising multinodal cysts and glands, with some cellular atypia but no stromal invasion. Borderline lesions also lack invasion, but demonstrate stratified gastrointestinal-type mucinous epithelium with papillae or pseudopapillae infoldings, mild-to-moderate nuclear atypia, and proliferation of >10% of the epithelial volume. Carcinoma is diagnosed when stromal invasion of >5 mm or >10 mm^2 is observed (Ledermann et al. 2014).

In 2014, the WHO introduced a new diagnostic classification, further segregating MOC into expansile or infiltrative subtypes (Kurman et al. 2014). Expansile carcinoma is defined by a confluent glandular growth pattern with absence of intervening normal ovarian parenchyma. This subtype is almost always found in early-stage disease, with 95% of expansile tumors identified at stage 1. As such, expansile MOC is associated with lower metastatic potential and overall better prognosis than infiltrative disease (Muyldermans et al. 2013). The latter is defined by small glands, nests, or individual cells infiltrating the stroma.

MOC is characterized by the development of very large tumors, commonly presenting as a multiloculated mucin-containing cystic mass exceeding 10 cm in size. MOC is unilateral in 79% of cases (Lee and Scully 2000) and is most often diagnosed at an early stage, with >80% of cases still confined to the ovary (Perren 2016). Patients typically present when symptoms arise due to the expansion of the large tumor mass and resultant pressure exerted on surrounding organs, with tumor presence confirmed by ultrasound, MRI, or PET/CT scans. However, this detection course is problematic, as until the tumor reaches such a size there are usually minimal symptoms, making early diagnosis difficult. The most commonly used serum marker for ovarian cancer, CA-125, is elevated in <70% of advanced-stage MOC (Zorn et al. 2009) and even less frequently in borderline tumors (Song et al. 2018). CEA and CA19-9 have also long been used for detection and prediction of malignancy (Lin et al. 2018; Lertkhachonsuk et al. 2020), and, recently, HE4 has emerged as a more ovarian cancer–specific alternative to CA-125 (Hamed et al. 2013); however, none of these biomarkers are MOC-specific. Thus, final diagnosis and whether a neoplasm is benign, borderline, or malignant is determined by histological analysis of tissue removed at surgical exploration or debulking.

Although now reported to comprise ~3% of all EOC diagnoses (Reid et al. 2017), the prevalence of MOC was initially thought to be as high as 12% (Seidman et al. 2003). This overestimate has since proven to be an artifact of the challenge in distinguishing primary MOC from misdiagnosed metastases of other sites of origin. The frequency of such an occurrence was demonstrated by Zaino et al. (2011), who found 61% of MOC patients in their study ($n = 44$) had metastases misdiagnosed as primary MOC. The most common origins for metastases confused with primary MOC are the stomach and gastrointestinal tract, pancreas, cervix, breast, and uterus (Seidman et al. 2003), with metastases from the appendix and biliary tract also seen (Lee and Scully 2000; Lee and Young 2003). Thorough investigation is therefore necessary to confidently diagnose a lesion as true primary MOC.

The knowledge that MOC typically presents as larger, predominantly unilateral tumors compared with metastases can aid in diagnosis. This was demonstrated by Seidman et al. (2003), who constructed an algorithm based on size and laterality to predict primary or metastatic origin with a significant success rate. Other factors that distinguish primary MOC from metastases are expansile patterns of invasion and presence of "other ovarian pathology," like mural nodules, Brenner tumors, or teratomas (Lee and Young 2003). The coexistence of benign and borderline areas within a single invasive tumor favors a diagnosis of primary MOC over one of metastatic origin. Such coexistence can also hinder classification, as dispersion of benign and invasive areas within such a large mass can make it difficult to accurately assess the malignancy of a tumor without sampling widely, as demonstrated by the reported rates of discordance between perioperative frozen and final pathological diagnosis (Park et al. 2019; Yoshida et al. 2021).

Immunohistochemistry analysis is another useful tool for distinguishing primary MOC from metastasis. Cytokeratin 7 (CK7) and cytokeratin 20 (CK20) are the most commonly used biomarkers in clinical practice (Vang et al. 2006). In particular, CK7 stains positively in MOC and negatively in metastatic colorectal cancer (McCluggage 2012). The utility of novel marker SATB2 in identifying primary MOC versus colorectal or appendiceal metastasis was recently demonstrated (Meagher et al. 2019). Promisingly, this study found combining SATB2 with CK7 distinguished gastrointestinal from primary ovarian tumors with >95% accuracy. Pathologists may also investigate established biomarkers known to be associated with certain metastatic sites to sequentially rule out potential extraovarian origins. Such pathological analysis can prompt further imaging or clinical investigations to identify metastatic origins. However, assessment based on these criteria is not infallible, and thus in the clinical context, diagnosis of metastatic versus primary origin can sometimes only be understood in retrospect, following patient outcomes. Thus, going forward, improved biomarkers are needed for earlier and more reliable diagnosis.

Natural History and Genetics

Currently, the cell of origin in MOC is unknown (Fig. 1). However, the prevalent theory suggests this disease may develop from the ovarian surface epithelium (OSE) through a continuum of progression from benign cystadenoma to malignancy, as areas of carcinoma are commonly found adjacent to or mixed with benign and borderline epithelium (Bell 2005). This morphological progression has been supported by genetic studies revealing shared key molecular events (Hunter et al. 2012; Cheasley et al. 2019). An alternative mechanism suggests the origin of MOC may lie in transitional cells or metaplasia of the fallopian tube–peritoneal junction (Seidman et al. 2011; Wong et al. 2011). Rarely, MOC can coexist with Brenner tumors or teratomas, and these have also been hypothesized to be precursor lesions to MOC (Seidman and Khedmati 2008). Recent genetic evidence supports a clonal relationship between primary MOC and nearby Brenner tumors (Simons et al. 2020). However, most primary MOCs do not have such associated tumors, and very few have haploid genomes suggestive of a germ cell origin (Kommoss et al. 2021).

Molecularly, MOC differs from that of other EOCs, exhibiting distinct genetic and gene-expression profiles (Heinzelmann-Schwarz et al.

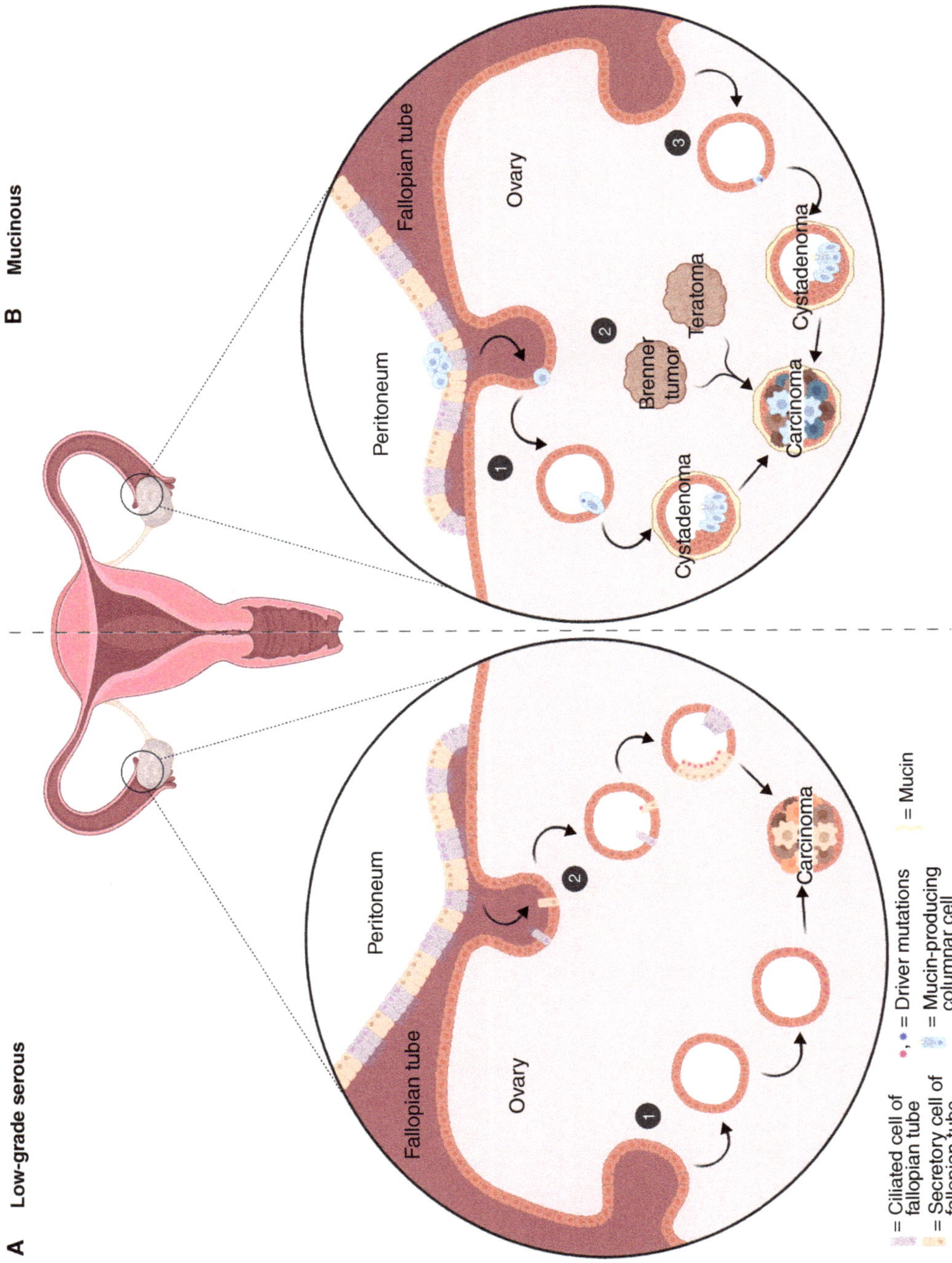

Figure 1. (*See following page for legend.*)

2006). *KRAS* is the most common and characteristic mutation of MOC, and is believed to represent an early founder event (Hunter et al. 2012; Mackenzie et al. 2015; Chang et al. 2016) with an incidence of 40%–65%. The most common mutation type is G12D (39%), followed by G12V (34%) (Cheasley et al. 2019). *TP53* mutations and *ERBB2* amplification can develop later in disease progression in 30%–64% and 20%–35% of cases, respectively (Anglesio et al. 2013a; Rechsteiner et al. 2013; Mackenzie et al. 2015; Cheasley et al. 2019). The presence of a *TP53* mutation in mucinous borderline tumors has been associated with an increased risk of recurrence with invasive carcinoma, supporting the role of this gene in driving invasive progression (Kang et al. 2021). The incidence of *ERBB2* amplification differs from that of other EOCs, as does *TP53*, which is much more frequently mutated in HGSC than MOC, but only rarely in endometrioid or clear-cell ovarian cancer (CCOC).

Regularly associated with MOC are homozygous deletions or mutations in *CDKN2A/B*, with aberrations reported in 20%–45% of cases (Mackenzie et al. 2015; Ryland et al. 2015; Cheasley et al. 2019). Less commonly, mutations are seen in *PI3KCA* (9%–13% incidence) and a collection of other genes including *RNF43*, *PTEN*, *ARID1A*, and *BRAF* at a frequency of >5% (Ryland et al. 2015; Meagher et al. 2018; Mueller et al. 2018; Cheasley et al. 2019). Although in the past microsatellite instability had been reported, recent studies with rigorous pathology review to exclude metastases have found few MOCs with microsatellite instability (Cheasley et al. 2019) or associated with Lynch syndrome (Chui et al. 2014; Rambau et al. 2016; Ryan et al. 2017). Additionally, MOC demonstrates a somatic mutational spectrum distinct from colorectal, appendiceal, gastric, and endometrial carcinomas (Cheasley et al. 2019).

Current Clinical Approach and Outcomes

Debulking surgery with the aim of complete resection is the principal approach for early- and late-stage MOC (Fig. 2). This typically consists of total hysterectomy and bilateral salpingo-oophorectomy, with appendectomy and lymphadenectomy often conducted in high-grade MOC. In instances of early-stage disease in which the tumor is confined to one ovary, unilateral salpingo-oophorectomy with uterus conservation is often preferred as a fertility preservation procedure for younger patients (Lee et al. 2015) with no detrimental effect on survival (Yoshihara et al. 2020).

In circumstances where MOC is diagnosed at early stages, the prognosis is better than that of other EOC types with a 5-year survival rate of >80% (Peres et al. 2019). Conversely, in the case of advanced MOC, the prognosis is poor and considerably worse compared to other EOCs, predominantly due to chemotherapy resistance. Hence, late-stage MOC exhibits a lower overall

Figure 1. Current theories of cell of origin and disease genesis in rare ovarian cancers. (*A*) Developmental models for low-grade serous ovarian carcinoma (LGSC). (1) The "incessant ovulation hypothesis." Frequent damage to the ovarian surface epithelium during ovulation results in the formation of ovarian epithelial neoplasms. During ovulation, the surface epithelium becomes enveloped by the stroma, forming an epithelial cell-inclusion cysts (EICs). EICs undergo rapid cell turnover, develop mutations, and form cystadenomas and cystadenofibromas, which then progress to serous borderline tumors (SBTs) and LGSCs. (2) The fallopian tube epithelium is the source of EICs. The fallopian tube mucosa consists of ciliated and secretory cells. As the EIC progresses toward an SBT and LGSC, the ratio of ciliated to secretory cells shifts toward a largely secretory mucosa (for SBT) or almost entirely secretory (LGSC). (*B*) Developmental models for mucinous ovarian carcinoma (MOC). (1) Metaplastic cells of the peritoneal–fallopian tube junction (or elsewhere in the Müllerian tract) with a mucin-producing cellular phenotype are incorporated into ovarian inclusion cysts. Over time, these cells gain driver mutations and contribute to the formation of a mucinous cystadenoma, which eventually progresses to carcinoma. (2) Brenner tumors and/or teratomas progress to a mucinous carcinoma. (3) Ovarian surface epithelium is incorporated into ovarian inclusion cysts, where a metaplastic change leads to a mucin-producing phenotype. The aberrant cell accumulates genetic changes facilitating neoplastic evolution. Over time, these cells contribute to the formation of a mucinous cystadenoma, which eventually progresses to carcinoma.

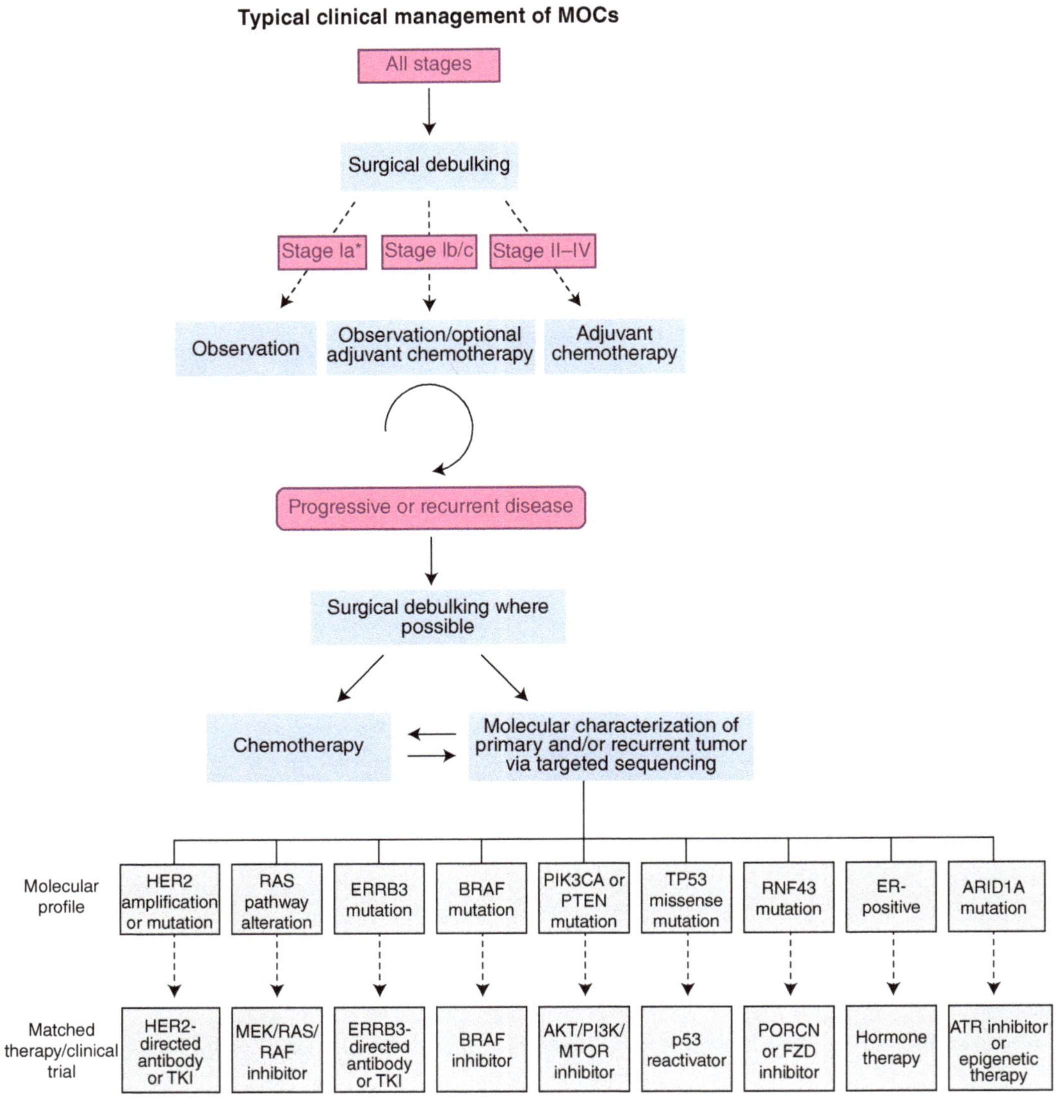

Figure 2. Typical clinical management of mucinous ovarian carcinomas (MOCs). Primary treatment for all stages involves surgical debulking of tumors. Further treatment is usually not necessary in stage 1a patients (adjuvant chemotherapy may be administered in high-grade cases). Adjuvant chemotherapy is offered to stage Ib and Ic patients, depending on grade, while it is routinely administered for stage II to IV cases. Upon disease progression or recurrence, second-round surgical debulking is performed when physically possible, usually combined with adjuvant chemotherapy. The increasing accessibility of tumor sequencing has recently yielded the use of tumor-specific management, in which therapies can be chosen to target distinct molecular profiles. (ER) Estrogen receptor, (MEK) mitogen-activated protein kinase, (FZD) frizzled.

survival, with median survival currently at 12–14 months for stage III or IV MOC (Hess et al. 2004; Zaino et al. 2011; Peres et al. 2019) compared with 37–42 months for HGSC.

Historically, chemotherapy treatment of MOC has been similar to other EOC types despite low representation of MOC in EOC clinical trials. The gold standard chemotherapy drugs for HGSC are still used for MOC despite documented differences in response patterns to platinum-based chemotherapy (Pectasides et al. 2005; Pisano et al. 2005; Shimada et al. 2009;

Alexandre et al. 2010; Schiavone et al. 2011). MOC cell lines exhibit platinum therapy resistance (Shimizu et al. 1998), reflecting the inferior response shown in patients. There have also been attempts to try neoadjuvant chemotherapy, but mucinous patient enrollment was insufficient to generate significant findings (Vergote et al. 2010; Kehoe et al. 2015). There are currently no definitive guidelines for chemotherapy in advanced primary MOC.

For recurrent MOC, data showing the efficacy of chemotherapy has proved even more arduous to obtain due to the rarity of these patients. Thus, most information has come from pooled trial data or retrospective reviews of cases (Ledermann et al. 2014). Currently, the sole published work investigating recurrent disease demonstrated that MOC had statistically significant lower response to second-line chemotherapy and shorter progression-free and overall survival than other ovarian cancer histotypes (Pignata et al. 2008).

With ineffective standard platinum-based chemotherapies, some clinicians administer therapeutics designed for gastrointestinal cancers; however, there is limited evidence to support their use (Ledermann et al. 2014). 5FU in combination with oxaliplatin (known as FOLFOX) had shown some promise in vitro and in vivo (Sato et al. 2009). Attempts such as the mEOC/GOG241 trial have been made to assess the efficacy of oxaliplatin and capecitabine for MOC (Gore et al. 2019). However, a nonsignificant benefit was reported in the oxaliplatin/capecitabine arm (hazard ratio [HR] 0.35, 95% confidence interval [CI] 0.08 = 1.41) and the trial was closed prematurely due to slow recruitment. A small 2019 retrospective study found adjuvant gastrointestinal-type chemotherapy improved survival in MOC patients; however, it is difficult to draw conclusions from such a limited sample size (Kurnit et al. 2019). There is also hope for combination gemcitabine and oxaliplatin (GEMOX), which has been tested in platinum-resistant pretreated patients but not MOC specifically (Vici et al. 2013; Yuan et al. 2013). Furthermore, some studies have shown promising results for irinotecan as MOC treatment (for review, see Xu et al. 2016). A recent retrospective analysis tried to investigate whether late-stage MOC patients benefited from receiving any chemotherapy regimens over those treated with surgery alone, and found a modest survival benefit. However, data were not available on which drugs were included, and pathology review was not performed, so it is likely that these results were skewed by inclusion of extraovarian metastases (Nasioudis et al. 2020).

Hyperthermic intraperitoneal chemotherapy (HIPEC) is an emerging treatment that has shown to be effective in other cancers such as colorectal and appendiceal, and the limited research on its benefit in MOC patients shows some promise (Zhang et al. 2020). However, these data are once again retrospective and involved only 54 participants. More clinical studies are needed to elucidate its true value.

LOW-GRADE SEROUS OVARIAN CARCINOMA

Of the EOC histotypes, serous ovarian carcinomas (SOCs) are the most common (Peres et al. 2019). Historically, SOC was thought to be a homogenous disease, but several clinicopathological, molecular, and genetic studies analyzing epithelial SOCs have generated a large body of evidence indicating that SOCs can be divided into high-grade (HGSC) and the rarer low-grade (LGSC) (Vang et al. 2009). This classification model, introduced in 2004, distinguishes HGSC and LGSC according to levels of nuclear atypia and mitotic count (Gershenson 2016). LGSCs now account for 5%–10% of patients diagnosed with ovarian, fallopian, and peritoneal carcinomas.

Epidemiology

Most epidemiological studies do not distinguish HGSC from LGSC; however, a recent analysis concluded that the majority of risk factors are shared between these histotypes (Wentzensen et al. 2016). These factors include age at menopause and use of hormone replacement therapy (HRT), where increased duration of ovulation or hormonal exposure is associated with a higher risk of disease. Disparity emerges with endometriosis (not significant for HGSC) and body mass index, parity, and oral contraceptive use, which were reported as weaker risk factors for LGSC. However, the study featured few cases of confirmed LGSC, limiting the power to detect the subtle hazard ratios observed in HGSC. LGSC is consistently diagnosed at a younger age than HGSC, and thus correlates with greater potential years of life lost (Chen et al. 2014; Gockley et al. 2017). Additionally, a particularly young age at diagnosis (<35) is a poor prognostic indicator for LGSC (Gershenson et al. 2015).

LGSC is not commonly associated with a family history or high-penetrance mutations in known ovarian cancer genes such as *BRCA1* or *BRCA2*. Several low-penetrance SNPs have been identified, including LGSC/serous borderline tumor (SBT)-specific loci on 3q28, 4q32.3, 8q21.11, 10q24.33, 18q11.2, and loci shared with HGSC such as 22q12, 2q13, 8q24.21, and 12q24.31 (Phelan et al. 2017). Associated genes include *PAX8* (2q13), *PVT1* and *MYC* (8q24.21), *HNF1A* (12q24.31), and *OBFC1* (10q24.33).

Clinicopathological Features and Diagnosis

LGSC tumors have histological features distinct from HGSC, and commonly demonstrate a clustered, micropapillary pattern of neoplastic cells invading the stroma (Vang et al. 2009). The mitotic index of LGSC is relatively low, and the cells tend to be uniform in size, with minimal nuclear atypia. Multiple microscopic bodies of calcium, known as psammoma bodies, are a frequent occurrence in LGSC (Vang et al. 2009).

LGSCs are thought to develop from noninvasive serous tumors. Benign serous ovarian tumors are comprised of cystadenomas, cystadenofibromas, and adenofibromas, which are mostly restricted to the ovaries (Longacre 2011). Cystadenomas have a smooth lining or protrusions and contain clear fluid that have similar viscosity to that of a mucinous tumor. Cystadenofibromas have similar features to the cystadenomas but contain fibrous stroma, while adenofibromas are more solid, firm, and typically contain more psammoma bodies than the other two subtypes (Longacre 2011).

SBTs are intermediate between benign tumors and malignant carcinomas (Hauptmann et al. 2017), with increased cellular proliferation compared with benign tumors and mild nuclear atypia without stromal invasion. SBTs present as single- or multicavity cystic tumors composed of ciliated epithelial cells (Hauptmann et al. 2017). Approximately 22% of SBT cases present with peritoneal implants featuring proliferating epithelial cells either on the surface of the peritoneum or in peritoneal invaginations, lacking subperitoneal invasion (du Bois et al. 2013).

LGSC patients suffer from rather diffuse symptoms akin to HGSC, rendering early diagnosis a challenge. As a result, more than half of LGSC patients are diagnosed at a late stage (stage III–IV) (Ricciardi et al. 2018). Common symptoms include abdominal pain and bowel impairment (Ricciardi et al. 2018), with diagnosis usually made on the basis of body imaging and physical examination along with serum biomarker assessment. CA-125 levels are high in only half of early-stage SOC cases, compared to >85% in patients with advanced stage disease (Fader et al. 2014). However, the clinical use of CA-125 has not been specifically assessed for LGSC.

Natural History and Genetics

Historically, "the incessant ovulation hypothesis" (Fathalla 1971) proposed that repeated damage to OSE cells during ovulation resulted in the generation of ovarian epithelial neoplasms. This model had support from the epidemiological risk factors seen in LGSC, as it suggested that the OSE was enveloped by the ovarian stroma during ovulation, generating epithelial cell-inclusion cysts (EICs; Fig. 1). These inclusion cysts were then thought to form benign cystadenomas or cystadenofibromas that subsequently progress to borderline and invasive LGSCs. This hypothesis was supported by an early gene-expression analysis (Bonome et al. 2005) that appeared to show SBTs and LGSCs clustering with the OSE rather than HGSC. However, the differences were mostly driven by proliferation and DNA damage gene sets.

More recent immunotyping of EIC cells suggests that the fallopian tube epithelium (FTE), rather than the OSE, might be the source of EIC via endosalpingiosis (Li et al. 2011). There are two types of epithelial cells that form the fallopian tube mucosa: ciliated and secretory. Both ciliated (α-tubulin$^+$) and secretory cells (PAX8$^+$) are present in EICs and serous cystadenomas, which have similar secretory cell/ciliated cell ratios. This ratio skews toward a greater abundance of secretory cells when the EIC progresses to an SBT and further to LGSCs, which are almost entirely composed of secretory cells. Analysis of 11 LGSC samples found that LGSC and FTE have very similar gene-expression profiles; furthermore, the gene-expression profiles of EIC, benign tumors, and SBT are more similar to that of the fallopian tube than the OSE (Qiu et al. 2017; Wang et al. 2019a). However, a study in mice expressing yellow fluorescent protein from an inducible oviductal (fallopian tube equivalent) promoter (OVGP1) showed inclusion cysts in mice before the onset of ovulation, which did not increase with age or number of ovulatory cycles (Wang et al. 2019b). This finding provides evidence against an ovulatory endosalpingiosis mechanism. Further support for a non-FTE origin of EIC comes from immunophenotyping, demonstrating that EIC is positive for both PAX8 and calretinin (a mesothelial cell marker), suggesting metaplasia of mesothelial cells (Park et al. 2018), although the inverse argument could also be made.

These contrasting studies highlight the challenges in determining cell of origin using gene-expression profiles alone. Regardless of the cell of origin, multiple studies have indicated a stepwise model for LGSC development, from benign cystadenoma/cystadenofibromas, through to SBT and eventually to LGSC (Li et al. 2011). Key evidence for this model is the early acquisition of shared key driver mutations in genes such as *BRAF* and *KRAS* (Hunter et al. 2011; Emmanuel et al. 2014).

The mutational profile of LGSC is also quite distinct from HGSC. The genomic landscape of HGSC includes mutations in *TP53*, *BRCA1*, and *BRCA2* (Cancer Genome Atlas Research Network [CGARN] 2011). Significantly fewer genomic studies have been conducted on LGSCs; however, mutations in the RAS/RAF signaling pathway (mostly *KRAS* [usually G12D and G12V], *NRAS* [Q61R and K61K], and *BRAF* [almost always V600E]) are found in approximately half of LGSC tumors and are largely mutually exclusive (Cheasley et al. 2021). Mutations in *TP53* are considerably rarer (Emmanuel et al. 2014; Hunter et al. 2015; Cheasley et al. 2021). Furthermore, a genetic study by Etemadmoghadam et al. (2017) identified frameshift mutations in *NF1*, encoding a negative regulator of the RAS pathway, in 9% of cases. Missense mutations in *EIF1AX* (5.6%–13%) and frameshift mutations in *USP9X* (11.3%–13%) are also observed in LGSC, with most *EIF1AX* mutations co-occurring with *NRAS* mutations (Hunter et al. 2015; Etemadmoghadam et al. 2017; Cheasley et al. 2021). *USP9X* appears to be a tumor suppressor gene that does not require a second hit, with frameshift mutations showing complete loss of protein despite retaining a normal copy and escaping silencing through X chromosome inactivation (Cheasley et al. 2021).

Compared to SBTs, LGSCs exhibit higher numbers of copy number aberrations, although they are more genetically stable than their high-grade counterparts (Hunter et al. 2015). The most common copy number events are loss of chromosomes 1p, 9, 16p, 18, 22, and X, and gains of 1q, 7, 8, and 12 (Hunter et al. 2015; Cheasley et al. 2021). In comparison to SBTs, loss of chromosomes 1p, 9q, 18q, and X were more common in LGSCs, while no loss of chromosome 22 or gain of 13 was observed in SBTs ($n = 57$) (Hunter et al. 2015). Nevertheless, in a study of paired borderline and invasive samples, copy number profiles were nearly identical, which provides evidence for a clonal relationship (Emmanuel et al. 2014). This study also found *NRAS* mutations to be associated with LGSCs but rare in SBTs lacking progression to invasion.

Current Clinical Approach and Outcomes

Cytoreductive surgery is standard for patients with primary LGSC (Fig. 3). It has been shown that patients with postoperative microscopic residual disease had significantly better overall survival than those with macroscopic disease

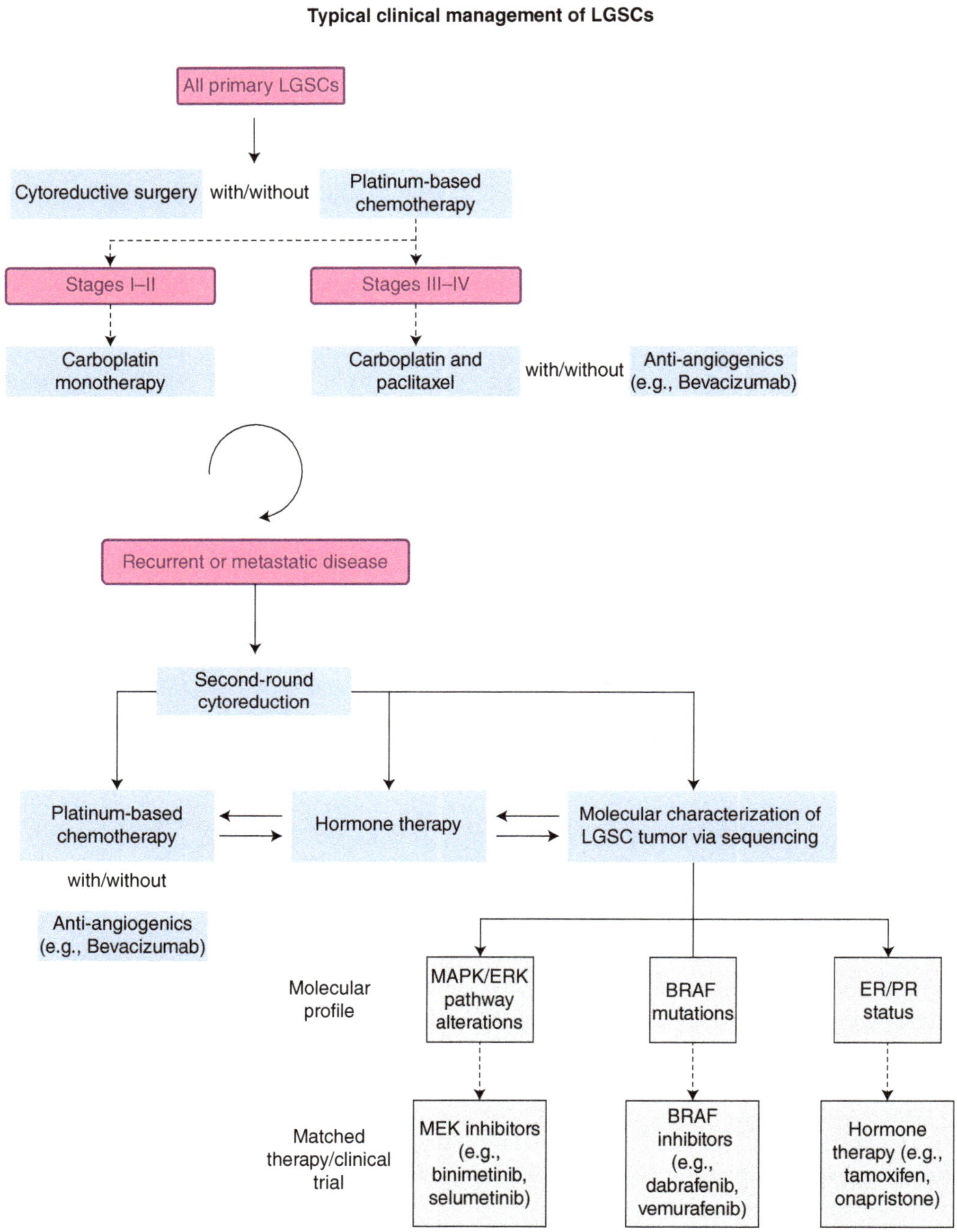

Figure 3. Typical clinical management of low-grade serous ovarian carcinomas (LGSCs). The primary treatment method for all LGSCs is cytoreductive surgery, possibly in combination with platinum-based chemotherapeutics; the type of chemotherapy administered is dependent on tumor stage. Patients with tumors that have recurred or progressed may receive a second round of cytoreductive surgery in conjunction with chemotherapeutics. Hormone therapy may be administered to patients with estrogen/progesterone receptor-positive (ER/PR-positive) tumors; patient tumors can also be sequenced to identify targetable mutations or pathway alterations, after which more personalized treatment strategies can be used.

(>1 cm) (97 mo vs. 35 mo, respectively) (Grabowski et al. 2016). Indeed, LGSC patients with macroscopic disease post-debulking exhibited similar progression-free and overall survival to HGSC patients with macroscopic disease (13 mo and 30 mo, respectively, for LGSC vs. 10 mo and 28 mo for HGSC [Chen et al. 2014]). In the relapse setting, a second round of cytoreduction has been proposed to be of a greater benefit (especially if no gross residual disease can be achieved) to patients with LGSC than for those with HGSC, in part due to the chemoresistant nature of LGSC (Moujaber et al. 2021).

In combination with surgery, platinum-based monotherapy is administered to patients with LGSC (Ledermann et al. 2013). However, with increased genetic stability and a lower proliferation rate than their high-grade counterpart, LGSCs are typically more resistant to standard chemotherapeutics (Gershenson et al. 2006, 2009). A study analyzing the efficacy of nonplatinum monotherapy in platinum-resistant HGSCs found the objective response rate (ORR) to treatment to be 19.7% (Gordon et al. 2001). By contrast, in a study of 58 LGSC patients with either platinum-sensitive or resistant tumors, who were treated with varying chemotherapy regimens (including hormonal therapy), ORRs were just 4.9% and 2.1%, respectively (Gershenson et al. 2009). The efficacy of neoadjuvant chemotherapy is equally low; in a study of 24 patients who underwent combined taxane and platinum-based therapy, only one had a complete response, with 21 patients experiencing stable disease and two patients progressing (Schmeler et al. 2008). Furthermore, a study of 36 LGSC patients found that only 11% had a partial response to neoadjuvant platinum-based chemotherapy; in sharp contrast, 75% of HGSC patients analyzed in the same study had a partial response to treatment (Cobb et al. 2020).

LGSC has a high recurrence rate; more than 80% of patients will experience relapse (Gershenson 2016). For some patients, second-round cytoreductive surgery may be advised. Again, the efficacy of surgery depends on the presence of macroscopic residual tumor postoperation. When no gross residual disease was present, patients experienced a roughly sixfold better progression-free survival than those that had macroscopic disease postsurgery for recurrent disease (Crane et al. 2015).

LGSC can exhibit a high expression of estrogen and progesterone receptors (ERs and PRs, respectively) (Sieh et al. 2013). Furthermore, patients with LGSC are diagnosed at a younger age and are likely to be premenopausal, thus implicating hormonal involvement in cancer progression. However, a study conducted by Sieh et al. (2013) found that there was no statistically significant correlation between ER/PR status and survival in LGSC patients. Retrospective studies by Gershenson et al. analyzed the efficacy of hormonal treatment regimens for LGSC patients with recurrent or stage II–IV disease. Clinical benefit from various hormonal therapies was observed in the recurrent population (Gershenson et al. 2012), and hormonal maintenance therapy was associated with improved progression-free survival (Gershenson et al. 2017). Almost all patients in these studies carried ER^+ tumors, and there was no difference in survival for ER^+/PR^+ cases compared to ER^+/PR^- in the maintenance setting, although numbers were small. Hormonal therapies are now an active area of clinical trial research, with at least two active trials listed evaluating combinations with letrozole in LGSC (NCT03673124 [clinicaltrials.gov/ct2/show/NCT03673124] with ribociclib and NCT04095364 [clinicaltrials.gov/ct2/show/NCT04095364] with/without carboplatin/paclitaxel). Another trial is underway to assess the efficacy of the antiprogesterone drug onapristone in treated patients with PR^+ LGSC (NCT03909152), and two others are evaluating fulvestrant either alone (NCT03926936 [clinicaltrials.gov/ct2/show/NCT03926936]) or in combination with the CDK4/6 inhibitor abemaciclib (NCT03531645).

TARGETED THERAPIES TO IMPROVE OUTCOMES OF RARE GYNECOLOGICAL CANCER SUBTYPES

For rare cancers such as MOC and LGSC, large clinical trial data sets are not available to direct clinical management strategies. As a result, treatment paradigms for rare cancers are undergoing a shift toward identifying and developing novel targeted therapy strategies for individual patients using multiomic sequencing approaches. Targeted therapies, aimed at aberrant genes/proteins detected by sequencing can then be tested for their efficacy, especially as combination therapies.

As mutations in the MAPK/ERK pathway are common in MOC and LGSC, inhibitors of mitogen-activated protein kinase (MEK inhibitors) are a potential therapy option for these patients (Miller et al. 2014). Indeed, at the cell line level, EOC cell growth was markedly reduced using the MEK inhibitor CI-1040. Recently, LGSC-specific cell lines have also been used to investigate various MEK inhibitors (Fernandez et al. 2016, 2019), with responses noted particularly in *KRAS*-mutated cell lines. A clinical trial testing the MEK inhibitor binimetinib was attempted in LGSC patients, but due to the small sample size no statistically significant effect on progression-free survival compared to chemotherapy was observed (Grisham et al. 2019). Nonetheless, individual durable responses were noted, particularly in patients with *KRAS* mutations. One case study reported a patient on this trial with recurrent, chemoresistant, and hormone therapy–resistant LGSC with a *KRAS* mutation who demonstrated partial response to MEKi, with an 81% reduction in tumor size during treatment (Han et al. 2018). While MOC patients were not included in this trial, given the high rate of *KRAS* mutations in this tumor subtype, there is also a strong rationale for binimetinib use in these patients. Another MEK inhibitor, selumetinib, has been tested on 52 LGSC patients (Farley et al. 2013; Miller et al. 2014). At the conclusion of this small trial, more than half of the patients had stable disease, while approximately 15% experienced complete or partial response to treatment. Median overall survival was 32.4 months. Patients were not selected for *RAS/RAF* mutations, and response was not related to the presence of such a mutation, with the caveat of a small sample size. Other current clinical trials of MEK inhibitors include evaluation of trametinib (NCT02101788 [clinicaltrials.gov/ct2/show/NCT02101788]), with preliminary outcomes reported suggesting improved progression-free survival and an objective tumor response rate of 26% (Gershenson et al. 2022).

A recent phase I clinical study using the RAF/MEK inhibitor VS-6766 and the FAK inhibitor defactinib to treat 25 patients with LGSC reported promising preliminary results; the ORR for all patients was 46%, increasing to 64% for patients with *KRAS* mutations (NCT03875820).

Mutations in *BRAF*, and in particular *BRAF*V600E, are a relatively common occurrence in LGSC and MOC (Moujaber et al. 2018). BRAF inhibitors are now successfully used in the treatment of metastatic melanoma (Hauschild et al. 2012). The efficacy of such treatment for MOC and LGSC has yet to be determined, although there are case reports of positive results from treatment. For example, a patient who had chemoresistant, recurrent LGSC underwent treatment with the BRAF inhibitor dabrafenib in combination with the MEK1/2 inhibitor trametinib; CA-125 levels declined over a 6-month treatment period (Mendivil et al. 2018). Similarly, a report by Stover et al. (2018) highlights the benefits of using targeted sequencing on two LGSC patients; for one patient with *BRAF*V600E, the BRAF inhibitor vemurafenib had considerable efficacy, marked by a decrease in CA-125 levels. Interestingly, the second patient who had progressive LGSC underwent hormonal therapy and responded to treatment, although a recurrent lesion harbored a mutation in *ESR1*, conferring resistance to antiestrogen therapy.

Bevacizumab, a monoclonal antibody that inhibits vascular endothelial growth factor, has been successfully implemented in colorectal carcinoma (Macedo et al. 2012). Subsequent studies have shown the benefit of Bevacizumab in EOC phase 3 trials, but limited MOC patient participation hindered collection of specific data for this subtype (Xu et al. 2016). The GOG241 trial also tested Bevacizumab in combination with carboplatin-paclitaxel or oxaliplatin-capecitabine, and showed no benefit from the addition of Bevacizumab, although only 18 confirmed MOC cases were available for analysis (Gore et al. 2019). Despite this, individual case reports have reported success with Bevacizumab monotherapy (Winer and Buckanovich 2010). Bevacizumab has also been tested in a small number of patients with LGSC with considerably greater success. In retrospective studies, Bevacizumab showed efficacy in patients for recurrent LGSC with response rates of 40%–47.5% and clinical benefit of 73%–78% (Grisham et al. 2014; Dalton et al. 2017). Bevacizumab was used alongside chemotherapy as a primary treatment strategy for patients in several randomized trials. Meta-analyses showed limited progression-free (but not overall) survival benefit, although LGSCs were not assessed separately from all serous or all low-grade carcinomas (Rossi et al. 2017).

Targeting of other growth factor receptors has been similarly considered although with much fewer samples. In cases of *ERBB2* amplification, anti-HER2 therapy using targeted antibodies or tyrosine kinase inhibitors has been successful in other cancers such as gastric and breast cancer. Given the relative frequency of HER2 overexpression in MOC, it is hoped such efforts might translate to this subtype. Evidence of efficacy has been provided by case studies of a few individual patients (McAlpine et al. 2009; Jain et al. 2012), but more robust data on larger sample sizes are lacking. The EGFR inhibitor cetuximab could be useful in treating *KRAS* wild-type MOC. Efficacy has been demonstrated successfully by Sato et al. (2012) in *KRAS* wild-type MOC cell lines and mice; again, however, there are currently no clinical data supporting its use.

Recently, other less frequent genetic events that occur in MOC patients were identified as having potential clinical utility, including *RNF43*, *ARID1A*, and *PIK3CA/PTEN* mutations (Gorringe et al. 2020). These events may be actionable using targeted agents currently used or being tested in other cancer types, potentially giving otherwise untreatable patients therapeutic options. Additionally, approximately 11% of MOC patients may be ER^+ and thus could benefit from hormonal therapy. By the same precision oncology paradigm, PARPi and immunotherapies were deemed unlikely to be useful in MOC treatment due to the rarity of homologous recombination deficiency (HRD) and mismatch repair deficiency (MRD). In LGSC, ~27% of cases recently analyzed had a genetic event that was predictive of benefit with an agent already in the clinic for another cancer type (Cheasley et al. 2021).

FUTURE DIRECTIONS

Overall, the major limitation of most clinical trials discussed above is their restricted sample size; due to the rarity of these diseases, recruiting patients with the given histotype as well as the specific mutation(s) being targeted is challenging. A further challenge is the paucity of patient-derived models to establish preclinical evidence for drug efficacy. Only a handful of cell lines and patient-derived xenografts are available for either MOC or LGSC (Table 1), and very recently a few novel tumor organoid models have been developed (Kopper et al. 2019). Older cell lines are relatively untrustworthy for studies as the subtype (especially LGSC) was often not recorded. Despite recent efforts to identify the origins of such cell lines using mutations and gene-expression data (Domcke et al. 2013; Barnes et al. 2021), it would generally be advisable to work with more recently derived models (Nelson et al. 2020; Shrestha et al. 2021).

In synergy with identifying appropriate targeted therapies, research should also focus on establishing markers of treatment response and resistance for MOC and LGSC. For example, Shrestha et al. (2021) combined genomic, transcriptomic, and proteomic methods to discover potential predictive markers of MEKi treatment response and new therapy combinations. Such studies can aid clinical trials in selecting patients who will likely have a better response to treatment. Sequencing approaches can also reveal novel driver mutations (either standalone or co-occurring), aiding in the identification of new treatment targets. *USP9X* and *EIF1AX* are two genes that have been recently identified as recurring mutations that may play a role in LGSC development (Hunter et al. 2015; Etemadmoghadam et al. 2017). In particular, the group of LGSC patients lacking the known RAS/RAF drivers remain to be fully explored for genetic drivers.

Table 1. Cell lines for use in mucinous ovarian carcinoma (MOC) and low-grade serous ovarian carcinoma (LGSC) research

Cell line	Original histological type	Likely histological type	Known mutations[a]	References
Plausible MOC cell lines				
MCAS	MOC	MOC	KRAS, TP53	Kidera et al. 1985; Anglesio et al. 2013b
RMUG-S	MOC	MOC	TP53	Sakayori et al. 1990
JHOM1	MOC	MOC (seromucinous?)	TP53, CDKN2A, PTEN	RIKEN cell bank
COV644	MOC	MOC	CDKN2A, MDM2 amplification	van den Berg-Bakker et al. 1993
Previous MOC cell lines that are likely to be non-MOC				
SW626	NK	Colorectal cancer ($CK20^+$)	APC, KRAS, TP53	Furlong et al. 1999
EFO27	MOC	Endometrioid/ endometrial	ARID1A, MSH2 (dMMR), PIK3CA, PTEN, TP53	Simon et al. 1983
JHOM2B	MOC	Colorectal cancer	TP53, BRAF, SMAD4	RIKEN cell bank
OMC-3	MOC	Pancreatic?	BRCA2, SMAD4, CDKN2A	Yamada et al. 1991; KL Gorringe, unpubl.
LGSC cell lines				
iOvCa241	LGSC	LGSC	KRAS	Shrestha et al. 2021
VOA-1312	LGSC	LGSC	KRAS	Shrestha et al. 2021
VOA-1056/VOA-3993	LGSC	LGSC	NRAS	Shrestha et al. 2021
VOA-3448/VOA-3723	LGSC	LGSC		Shrestha et al. 2021
VOA-4627/VOA-4698	LGSC	LGSC	TP53	Shrestha et al. 2021
VOA-6406	LGSC	LGSC	NRAS	Shrestha et al. 2021
VOA-8862	LGSC	LGSC	KRAS	Shrestha et al. 2021
VOA-9164	LGSC	LGSC	KRAS	Shrestha et al. 2021
CAISMOV24	LGSC	LGSC	KRAS	da Silva et al. 2017
PM-LGSC-01	LGSC	LGSC	KRAS	De Thaye et al. 2020
HeyA8	Moderately differentiated papillary cystadenocarcinoma	LGSC[b]	KRAS	Buick et al. 1985; Barnes et al. 2021
OVCAR8	NK	LGSC/HGSC[b]	TP53, KRAS, CTNNB1, ERBB2	Schilder et al. 1990; Barnes et al. 2021
TYK-nu	Undifferentiated	LGSC/HGSC[c]	NRAS, TP53	Yoshiya 1986; Barnes et al. 2021
OV7	Mixed	LGSC/HGSC[c]	KRAS, TP53	Boocock et al. 1995; Barnes et al. 2021

[a]From the *Cancer Cell Line Encyclopedia* unless otherwise stated (Ghandi et al. 2019).

[b]Original histology was nonspecific, the LGSC call is based on gene expression and mutations and therefore may be incorrect (Barnes et al. 2021).

[c]Described as poorly differentiated or undifferentiated. Do carry characteristic LGSC drivers, so potential progression to HGSC from an LGSC precursor.

Table 2. Characteristics of mucinous ovarian carcinoma (MOC) and low-grade serous ovarian carcinoma (LGSC)

	MOC	LGSC	References
Incidence	0.6/100,000	0.5/100,000	Howlader et al. 2017; Leary et al. 2017
Risk factors	Smoking	Number of children; age at menopause; endometriosis; oral contraceptive use; menopausal hormone therapy	Collaborative Group on Epidemiological Studies of Ovarian Cancer et al. 2012; Wentzensen et al. 2016
Cell of origin	Unknown—potentially ovarian surface epithelium, transitional cells of peritoneal junction, Brenner tumors, fallopian tube epithelium via endosalpingiosis, primordial germ cells	Unknown, possibly fallopian tube secretory cells or ovarian surface epithelium	Seidman and Khedmati 2008; Kurman et al. 2011; Chen et al. 2013; Qiu et al. 2017; Elias et al. 2018; Park et al. 2018; Wang et al. 2019b
Precursor tumors	Commonly, mucinous benign and borderline tumors; rarely, Brenner tumors, teratomas	Serous benign and borderline	Hunter et al. 2011, 2012; Emmanuel et al. 2014; Wang et al. 2015a,b; Cheasley et al. 2019
Stage distribution	Localized 48.2% Regional 25% Distant 26.7%	Localized 20.3% Regional 26.3% Distant 53.4%	Peres et al. 2019
Key genetic features (>25%)	*KRAS* (40%–65%), *TP53* (30%–64%), *ERRB2* (20%–35%), *CDK2NA* (20%–45%)	*NRAS* (25%), *BRAF* (14%), *KRAS* (20%), *EIF1AX* (13%), *USP9X* (13%)	McAlpine et al. 2009; Hunter et al. 2015; Mackenzie et al. 2015; Etemadmoghadam et al. 2017; Meagher et al. 2018; Moujaber et al. 2018; Mueller et al. 2018; Cheasley et al. 2019
IHC markers	$CK7^+$, $CK20^-$, $SATB2^-$	$WT1^+$, p53wt, $p16^-$/patchy	McCluggage 2012; Köbel et al. 2014; Sallum et al. 2018; Meagher et al. 2019
Response to platinum-based therapies (%)	26.3%–60%	4%–5%	Hess et al. 2004; Pectasides et al. 2005; Gershenson et al. 2006, 2009; Pignata et al. 2008; Schmeler et al. 2008; Alexandre et al. 2010
5-Year overall survival	Localized 83% Regional 70% Distant 14%	Localized 93% Regional 83% Distant 54%	Peres et al. 2019

Another application of a multiomics approach is to assist in elucidating the cell of origin for these rare cancers, which is still contentious for both histotypes. Using a combination of genomic, transcriptomic, methylation, and chromatin sequencing studies, further evidence can be obtained to either confirm or disprove the various theories (Li et al. 2011; Hao et al. 2017). Inducible animal model systems and lineage-tracing analysis could also be used to identify the correct cell type.

CONCLUDING REMARKS

Although MOC and LGSC are distinct from each other and the other ovarian histotypes, there are certain similarities, summarized in Table 2. The most notable similarity between these histotypes is not related to their biology, but simply their rarity, which confers profound clinical and research challenges. Both diseases are relatively chemoresistant, yet such rarity means that performing well-powered clinical trials in either subgroup is difficult. Hence, targeted agents for MOC and LGSC may best be tested using novel approaches such as registry trials, $n = 1$ trials, and basket trials in concert with other solid tumor types with similar genetic features. In addition, directed efforts must be made toward establishing relevant preclinical models to test the efficacy of targeted agents and combinations.

ACKNOWLEDGMENTS

K.G. is supported by a Victorian Cancer Agency Mid-Career Fellowship and the Peter MacCallum Foundation. A.N. is supported by a University of Melbourne International Research Scholarship. O.C. is supported by a University of Melbourne Graduate Research Scholarship. G.V.D. is supported by a Victorian Cancer Agency Early Career Fellowship.

REFERENCES

Aarestrup J, Trabert B, Ulrich LG, Wentzensen N, Sørensen TIA, Baker JL. 2019. Childhood overweight, tallness, and growth increase risks of ovarian cancer. *Cancer Epidemiol Biomarkers Prev* **28:** 183–188. doi:10.1158/1055-9965.EPI-18-0024

Alexandre J, Ray-Coquard I, Selle F, Floquet A, Cottu P, Weber B, Falandry C, Lebrun D, Pujade-Lauraine E; GINECO. 2010. Mucinous advanced epithelial ovarian carcinoma: clinical presentation and sensitivity to platinum-paclitaxel-based chemotherapy, the GINECO experience. *Ann Oncol* **21:** 2377–2381. doi:10.1093/annonc/mdq257

Anglesio MS, Kommoss S, Tolcher MC, Clarke B, Galletta L, Porter H, Damaraju S, Fereday S, Winterhoff BJ, Kalloger SE, et al. 2013a. Molecular characterization of mucinous ovarian tumours supports a stratified treatment approach with HER2 targeting in 19% of carcinomas. *J Pathol* **229:** 111–120. doi:10.1002/path.4088

Anglesio MS, Wiegand KC, Melnyk N, Chow C, Salamanca C, Prentice LM, Senz J, Yang W, Spillman MA, Cochrane DR, et al. 2013b. Type-specific cell line models for type-specific ovarian cancer research. *PLoS ONE* **8:** e72162. doi:10.1371/journal.pone.0072162

Barnes BM, Nelson L, Tighe A, Burghel GJ, Lin IH, Desai S, McGrail JC, Morgan RD, Taylor SS. 2021. Distinct transcriptional programs stratify ovarian cancer cell lines into the five major histological subtypes. *Genome Med* **13:** 140. doi:10.1186/s13073-021-00952-5

Bell DA. 2005. Origins and molecular pathology of ovarian cancer. *Mod Pathol* **18** (Suppl 2)**:** S19–S32. doi:10.1016/S0893-3952(22)04456-8

Bonome T, Lee JY, Park DC, Radonovich M, Pise-Masison C, Brady J, Gardner GJ, Hao K, Wong WH, Barrett JC, et al. 2005. Expression profiling of serous low malignant potential, low-grade, and high-grade tumors of the ovary. *Cancer Res* **65:** 10602–10612. doi:10.1158/0008-5472.CAN-05-2240

Boocock CA, Charnock-Jones DS, Sharkey AM, McLaren J, Barker PJ, Wright KA, Twentyman PR, Smith SK. 1995. Expression of vascular endothelial growth factor and its receptors flt and KDR in ovarian carcinoma. *J Natl Cancer Inst* **87:** 506–516. doi:10.1093/jnci/87.7.506

Buick RN, Pullano R, Trent JM. 1985. Comparative properties of five human ovarian adenocarcinoma cell lines. *Cancer Res* **45:** 3668–3676.

Cancer Genome Atlas Research Network (CGARN). 2011. Integrated genomic analyses of ovarian carcinoma. *Nature* **474:** 609–615. doi:10.1038/nature10166

Chang KL, Lee MY, Chao WR, Han CP. 2016. The status of *Her2* amplification and *Kras* mutations in mucinous ovarian carcinoma. *Hum Genomics* **10:** 40. doi:10.1186/s40246-016-0096-9

Cheasley D, Wakefield MJ, Ryland GL, Allan PE, Alsop K, Amarasinghe KC, Ananda S, Anglesio MS, Au-Yeung G, Böhm M, et al. 2019. The molecular origin and taxonomy of mucinous ovarian carcinoma. *Nat Commun* **10:** 3935. doi:10.1038/s41467-019-11862-x

Cheasley D, Nigam A, Zethoven M, Hunter S, Etemadmoghadam D, Semple T, Allan P, Carey MS, Fernandez ML, Dawson A, et al. 2021. Genomic analysis of low-grade serous ovarian carcinoma to identify key drivers and therapeutic vulnerabilities. *J Pathol* **253:** 41–54. doi:10.1002/path.5545

Chen C, Li J, Yao G, Chambers SK, Zheng W. 2013. Tubal origin of ovarian low-grade serous carcinoma. *Am J Clin Exp Obstet Gynecol* **1:** 13–36.

Chen M, Jin Y, Bi Y, Yin J, Wang Y, Pan L. 2014. A survival analysis comparing women with ovarian low-grade serous carcinoma to those with high-grade histology. *Onco Targets Ther* **7:** 1891–1899. doi:10.2147/OTT.S67812

Chui MH, Ryan P, Radigan J, Ferguson SE, Pollett A, Aronson M, Semotiuk K, Holter S, Sy K, Kwon JS, et al. 2014. The histomorphology of Lynch syndrome-associated ovarian carcinomas: toward a subtype-specific screening strategy. *Am J Surg Patho* **38:** 1173–1181. doi:10.1097/PAS.0000000000000298

Cobb LP, Sun CC, Iyer R, Nick AM, Fleming ND, Westin SN, Sood AK, Wong KK, Silva EG, Gershenson DM. 2020. The role of neoadjuvant chemotherapy in the management of low-grade serous carcinoma of the ovary and peritoneum: further evidence of relative chemoresistance. *Gynecol Oncol* **158:** 653–658. doi:10.1016/j.ygyno.2020.06.498

Collaborative Group on Epidemiological Studies of Ovarian Cancer; Beral V, Gaitskell K, Hermon C, Moser K, Reeves G, Peto R. 2012. Ovarian cancer and smoking: individual participant meta-analysis including 28,114 women with ovarian cancer from 51 epidemiological studies. *Lancet Oncol* **13:** 946–956. doi:10.1016/S1470-2045(12)70322-4

Crane EK, Sun CC, Ramirez PT, Schmeler KM, Malpica A, Gershenson DM. 2015. The role of secondary cytoreduction in low-grade serous ovarian cancer or peritoneal cancer. *Gynecol Oncol* **136:** 25–29. doi:10.1016/j.ygyno.2014.11.005

Dalton HJ, Fleming ND, Sun CC, Bhosale P, Schmeler KM, Gershenson DM. 2017. Activity of Bevacizumab-containing regimens in recurrent low-grade serous ovarian or peritoneal cancer: a single institution experience. *Gynecol Oncol* **145:** 37–40. doi:10.1016/j.ygyno.2017.01.027

da Silva RF, Cardozo DM, Rodrigues GOL, Souza-Araujo CN, Migita NA, Andrade L, Derchain S, Yunes JA, Guimarães F. 2017. CAISMOV24, a new human low-grade serous ovarian carcinoma cell line. *BMC Cancer* **17:** 756. doi:10.1186/s12885-017-3716-4

De Thaye E, Van de Vijver K, Van der Meulen J, Taminau J, Wagemans G, Denys H, Van Dorpe J, Berx G, Ceelen W, Van Bocxlaer J, et al. 2020. Establishment and characterization of a cell line and patient-derived xenograft (PDX) from peritoneal metastasis of low-grade serous ovarian carcinoma. *Sci Rep* **10:** 6688. doi:10.1038/s41598-020-63738-6

Domcke S, Sinha R, Levine DA, Sander C, Schultz N. 2013. Evaluating cell lines as tumour models by comparison of genomic profiles. *Nat Commun* **4:** 2126. doi:10.1038/ncomms3126

du Bois A, Ewald-Riegler N, de Gregorio N, Reuss A, Mahner S, Fotopoulou C, Kommoss F, Schmalfeldt B, Hilpert F, Fehm T, et al. 2013. Borderline tumours of the ovary: a cohort study of the Arbeitsgmeinschaft Gynakologische Onkologie (AGO) study group. *Eur J Cancer* **49:** 1905–1914. doi:10.1016/j.ejca.2013.01.035

Elias KM, Tsantoulis P, Tille JC, Vitonis A, Doyle LA, Hornick JL, Kaya G, Barnes L, Cramer DW, Puppa G, et al. 2018. Primordial germ cells as a potential shared cell of origin for mucinous cystic neoplasms of the pancreas and mucinous ovarian tumors. *J Pathol* **246:** 459–469. doi:10.1002/path.5161

Emmanuel C, Chiew YE, George J, Etemadmoghadam D, Anglesio MS, Sharma R, Russell P, Kennedy C, Fereday S, Hung J, et al. 2014. Genomic classification of serous ovarian cancer with adjacent borderline differentiates RAS pathway and *TP53*-mutant tumors and identifies *NRAS* as an oncogenic driver. *Clin Cancer Res* **20:** 6618–6630. doi:10.1158/1078-0432.CCR-14-1292

Etemadmoghadam D, Azar WJ, Lei Y, Moujaber T, Garsed DW, Kennedy CJ, Fereday S, Mitchell C, Chiew YE, Hendley J, et al. 2017. *EIF1AX* and *NRAS* mutations co-occur and cooperate in low-grade serous ovarian carcinomas. *Cancer Res* **77:** 4268–4278. doi:10.1158/0008-5472.CAN-16-2224

Fader AN, Java J, Krivak TC, Bristow RE, Tergas AI, Bookman MA, Armstrong DK, Tanner EJ, Gershenson DM. 2014. The prognostic significance of pre- and post-treatment CA-125 in grade 1 serous ovarian carcinoma: a Gynecologic Oncology Group study. *Gynecol Oncol* **132:** 560–565. doi:10.1016/j.ygyno.2013.11.016

Farley J, Brady WE, Vathipadiekal V, Lankes HA, Coleman R, Morgan MA, Mannel R, Yamada SD, Mutch D, Rodgers WH, et al. 2013. Selumetinib in women with recurrent low-grade serous carcinoma of the ovary or peritoneum: an open-label, single-arm, phase 2 study. *Lancet Oncol* **14:** 134–140. doi:10.1016/S1470-2045(12)70572-7

Fathalla MF. 1971. Incessant ovulation—a factor in ovarian neoplasia? *Lancet* **2:** 163. doi:10.1016/S0140-6736(71)92335-X

Fernandez ML, DiMattia GE, Dawson A, Bamford S, Anderson S, Hennessy BT, Anglesio MS, Shepherd TG, Salamanca C, Hoenisch J, et al. 2016. Differences in MEK inhibitor efficacy in molecularly characterized low-grade serous ovarian cancer cell lines. *Am J Cancer Res* **6:** 2235–2251.

Fernandez ML, Dawson A, Hoenisch J, Kim H, Bamford S, Salamanca C, DiMattia G, Shepherd T, Cremona M, Hennessy B, et al. 2019. Markers of MEK inhibitor resistance in low-grade serous ovarian cancer: EGFR is a potential therapeutic target. *Cancer Cell Int* **19:** 10. doi:10.1186/s12935-019-0725-1

Furlong MT, Hough CD, Sherman-Baust CA, Pizer ES, Morin PJ. 1999. Evidence for the colonic origin of ovarian cancer cell line SW626. *J Natl Cancer Inst* **91:** 1327–1328. doi:10.1093/jnci/91.15.1327

Gates MA, Rosner BA, Hecht JL, Tworoger SS. 2010. Risk factors for epithelial ovarian cancer by histologic subtype. *Am J Epidemiol* **171:** 45–53. doi:10.1093/aje/kwp314

Gershenson DM. 2016. Low-grade serous carcinoma of the ovary or peritoneum. *Ann Oncol* 27 (Suppl 1): i45–i49. doi:10.1093/annonc/mdw085

Gershenson DM, Sun CC, Lu KH, Coleman RL, Sood AK, Malpica A, Deavers MT, Silva EG, Bodurka DC. 2006. Clinical behavior of stage II-IV low-grade serous carcinoma of the ovary. *Obstet Gynecol* **108:** 361–368. doi:10.1097/01.AOG.0000227787.24587.d1

Gershenson DM, Sun CC, Bodurka D, Coleman RL, Lu KH, Sood AK, Deavers M, Malpica AL, Kavanagh JJ. 2009. Recurrent low-grade serous ovarian carcinoma is relatively chemoresistant. *Gynecol Oncol* **114:** 48–52. doi:10.1016/j.ygyno.2009.03.001

Gershenson DM, Sun CC, Iyer RB, Malpica AL, Kavanagh JJ, Bodurka DC, Schmeler K, Deavers M. 2012. Hormonal therapy for recurrent low-grade serous carcinoma of the ovary or peritoneum. *Gynecol Oncol* **125:** 661–666. doi:10.1016/j.ygyno.2012.02.037

Gershenson DM, Bodurka DC, Lu KH, Nathan LC, Milojevic L, Wong KK, Malpica A, Sun CC. 2015. Impact of age and primary disease site on outcome in women with low-grade serous carcinoma of the ovary or peritoneum: results of a large single-institution registry of a rare tumor. *J Clin Oncol* **33:** 2675–2682. doi:10.1200/JCO.2015.61.0873

Gershenson DM, Bodurka DC, Coleman RL, Lu KH, Malpica A, Sun CC. 2017. Hormonal maintenance therapy for women with low-grade serous cancer of the ovary or peritoneum. *J Clin Oncol* **35:** 1103–1111. doi:10.1200/JCO.2016.71.0632

Gershenson DM, Miller A, Brady WE, Paul J, Carty K, Rodgers W, Millan D, Coleman RL, Moore KN, Banerjee S, et al. 2022. Trametinib versus standard of care in patients with recurrent low-grade serous ovarian cancer (GOG 281/LOGS): an international, randomised, open-label, multicentre, phase 2/3 trial. *Lancet* **399:** 541–553. doi:10.1016/S0140-6736(21)02175-9

Ghandi M, Huang FW, Jané-Valbuena J, Kryukov GV, Lo CC, McDonald ER, Barretina J, Gelfand ET, Bielski CM, Li H, et al. 2019. Next-generation characterization of the *Cancer Cell Line Encyclopedia. Nature* **569:** 503–508. doi:10.1038/s41586-019-1186-3

Gockley A, Melamed A, Bregar AJ, Clemmer JT, Birrer M, Schorge JO, Del Carmen MG, Rauh-Hain JA. 2017. Outcomes of women with high-grade and low-grade advanced-stage serous epithelial ovarian cancer. *Obstet Gynecol* **129:** 439–447. doi:10.1097/AOG.0000000000001867

Gordon AN, Fleagle JT, Guthrie D, Parkin DE, Gore ME, Lacave AJ. 2001. Recurrent epithelial ovarian carcinoma: a randomized phase III study of pegylated liposomal doxorubicin versus topotecan. *J Clin Oncol* **19:** 3312–3322. doi:10.1200/JCO.2001.19.14.3312

Gore M, Hackshaw A, Brady WE, Penson RT, Zaino R, McCluggage WG, Ganesan R, Wilkinson N, Perren T, Montes A, et al. 2019. An international, phase III randomized trial in patients with mucinous epithelial ovarian cancer (mEOC/GOG 0241) with long-term follow-up: and experience of conducting a clinical trial in a rare gynecological tumor. *Gynecol Oncol* **153:** 541–548. doi:10.1016/j.ygyno.2019.03.256

Gorringe KL, Cheasley D, Wakefield MJ, Ryland GL, Allan PE, Alsop K, Amarasinghe KC, Ananda S, Bowtell DDL, Christie M, et al. 2020. Therapeutic options for mucinous ovarian carcinoma. *Gynecol Oncol* **156:** 552–560. doi:10.1016/j.ygyno.2019.12.015

Grabowski JP, Harter P, Heitz F, Pujade-Lauraine E, Reuss A, Kristensen G, Ray-Coquard I, Heitz J, Traut A, Pfisterer J, et al. 2016. Operability and chemotherapy responsiveness in advanced low-grade serous ovarian cancer. An analysis of the AGO Study Group metadatabase. *Gynecol Oncol* **140:** 457–462. doi:10.1016/j.ygyno.2016.01.022

Grisham RN, Iyer G, Sala E, Zhou Q, Iasonos A, DeLair D, Hyman DM, Aghajanian C. 2014. Bevacizumab shows activity in patients with low-grade serous ovarian and primary peritoneal cancer. *Int J Gynecol Cancer* **24:** 1010–1014. doi:10.1097/IGC.0000000000000190

Grisham R, Monk JB, Banerjee S, Coleman LR, Oza MA, Oehler KM, Kalbacher E, Mirza Raza M, del Campo MJ, Marth C, et al. 2019. 1 MILO/ENGOT-OV11: phase-3 study of binimetinib versus physician's choice chemotherapy (PCC) in recurrent or persistent low-grade serous carcinomas of the ovary, fallopian tube, or primary peritoneum. *Int J Gynecol Cancer* **29:** A1. doi:10.1136/ijgc-2019-IGCS.1

Hamed EO, Ahmed H, Sedeek OB, Mohammed AM, Abd-Alla AA, Abdel Ghaffar HM. 2013. Significance of HE4 estimation in comparison with CA125 in diagnosis of ovarian cancer and assessment of treatment response. *Diagn Pathol* **8:** 11. doi:10.1186/1746-1596-8-11

Han C, Bellone S, Zammataro L, Schwartz PE, Santin AD. 2018. Binimetinib (MEK162) in recurrent low-grade serous ovarian cancer resistant to chemotherapy and hormonal treatment. *Gynecol Oncol Rep* **25:** 41–44. doi:10.1016/j.gore.2018.05.011

Hao D, Li J, Jia S, Meng Y, Zhang C, Wang L, Di LJ. 2017. Integrated analysis reveals tubal- and ovarian-originated serous ovarian cancer and predicts differential therapeutic responses. *Clin Cancer Res* **23:** 7400–7411. doi:10.1158/1078-0432.CCR-17-0638

Hauptmann S, Friedrich K, Redline R, Avril S. 2017. Ovarian borderline tumors in the 2014 WHO classification: evolving concepts and diagnostic criteria. *Virchows Arch* **470:** 125–142. doi:10.1007/s00428-016-2040-8

Hauschild A, Grob JJ, Demidov LV, Jouary T, Gutzmer R, Millward M, Rutkowski P, Blank CU, Miller WH, Kaempgen E, et al. 2012. Dabrafenib in BRAF-mutated metastatic melanoma: a multicentre, open-label, phase 3 randomised controlled trial. *Lancet* **380:** 358–365. doi:10.1016/S0140-6736(12)60868-X

Heinzelmann-Schwarz VA, Gardiner-Garden M, Henshall SM, Scurry JP, Scolyer RA, Smith AN, Bali A, Vanden Bergh P, Baron-Hay S, Scott C, et al. 2006. A distinct molecular profile associated with mucinous epithelial ovarian cancer. *Br J Cancer* **94:** 904–913. doi:10.1038/sj.bjc.6603003

Hess V, A'Hern R, Nasiri N, King DM, Blake PR, Barton DP, Shepherd JH, Ind T, Bridges J, Harrington K, et al. 2004. Mucinous epithelial ovarian cancer: a separate entity requiring specific treatment. *J Clin Oncol* **22:** 1040–1044. doi:10.1200/JCO.2004.08.078

Howlader N, Noone A, Krapcho M, Miller D, Bishop K, Kosary C, Yu M, Ruhl J, Tatalovich Z, Mariotto A, et al. 2017. *SEER cancer statistics review 1975–2014*. National Cancer Institute, Bethesda, MD.

Hunter SM, Anglesio MS, Sharma R, Gilks CB, Melnyk N, Chiew YE, deFazio A, Longacre TA, Huntsman DG, Gorringe KL, et al. 2011. Copy number aberrations in benign serous ovarian tumors: a case for reclassification? *Clin Cancer Res* **17:** 7273–7282. doi:10.1158/1078-0432.CCR-11-2080

Hunter SM, Gorringe KL, Christie M, Rowley SM, Bowtell DD, Australian Ovarian Cancer Study G, Campbell IG. 2012. Pre-invasive ovarian mucinous tumors are characterized by *CDKN2A* and *RAS* pathway aberrations. *Clin Cancer Res* **18:** 5267–5277. doi:10.1158/1078-0432.CCR-12-1103

Hunter SM, Anglesio MS, Ryland GL, Sharma R, Chiew YE, Rowley SM, Doyle MA, Li J, Gilks CB, Moss P, et al. 2015. Molecular profiling of low grade serous ovarian tumours identifies novel candidate driver genes. *Oncotarget* **6:** 37663–37677. doi:10.18632/oncotarget.5438

Jain A, Ryan PD, Seiden MV. 2012. Metastatic mucinous ovarian cancer and treatment decisions based on histology and molecular markers rather than the primary location. *J Natl Compr Canc Netw* **10:** 1076–1080. doi:10.6004/jnccn.2012.0113

Kang EY, Cheasley D, LePage C, Wakefield MJ, da Cunha Torres M, Rowley S, Salazar C, Xing Z, Allan P, Bowtell DDL, et al. 2021. Refined cut-off for TP53 immunohistochemistry improves prediction of TP53 mutation status in ovarian mucinous tumors: implications for outcome analyses. *Mod Pathol* **34:** 194–206. doi:10.1038/s41379-020-0618-9

Kehoe S, Hook J, Nankivell M, Jayson GC, Kitchener H, Lopes T, Luesley D, Perren T, Bannoo S, Mascarenhas M, et al. 2015. Primary chemotherapy versus primary surgery for newly diagnosed advanced ovarian cancer (CHORUS): an open-label, randomised, controlled, non-inferiority trial. *Lancet* **386:** 249–257. doi:10.1016/S0140-6736(14)62223-6

Kelemen LE, Lawrenson K, Tyrer J, Li Q, Lee JM, Seo JH, Phelan CM, Beesley J, Chen X, Spindler TJ, et al. 2015. Genome-wide significant risk associations for mucinous ovarian carcinoma. *Nat Genet* **47:** 888–897. doi:10.1038/ng.3336

Kidera Y, Yoshimura T, Ohkuma Y, Iwasaka T, Sugimori H. 1985. Establishment and characterization of a cell line derived from mucinous cystadenocarcinoma of human ovary. *Nippon Sanka Fujinka Gakkai Zasshi* **37:** 1820–1824.

Köbel M, Bak J, Bertelsen BI, Carpen O, Grove A, Hansen ES, Levin Jakobsen AM, Lidang M, Masback A, Tolf A, et al. 2014. Ovarian carcinoma histotype determination is highly reproducible, and is improved through the use of immunohistochemistry. *Histopathology* **64:** 1004–1013. doi:10.1111/his.12349

Kommoss FKF, Cheasley D, Wakefield MJ, Scott CL, Campbell IG, Gilks CB, Gorringe K. 2021. Primary mucinous ovarian neoplasms rarely show germ cell histogenesis. *Histopathology* **78:** 640–642. doi:10.1111/his.14297

Kopper O, de Witte CJ, Lohmussaar K, Valle-Inclan JE, Hami N, Kester L, Balgobind AV, Korving J, Proost N, Begthel H, et al. 2019. An organoid platform for ovarian cancer captures intra- and interpatient heterogeneity. *Nat Med* **25:** 838–849. doi:10.1038/s41591-019-0422-6

Kuchenbaecker KB, Ramus SJ, Tyrer J, Lee A, Shen HC, Beesley J, Lawrenson K, McGuffog L, Healey S, Lee JM, et al. 2015. Identification of six new susceptibility loci for invasive epithelial ovarian cancer. *Nat Genet* **47:** 164–171. doi:10.1038/ng.3185

Kurman RJ, Vang R, Junge J, Hannibal CG, Kjaer SK, Shih Ie M. 2011. Papillary tubal hyperplasia: the putative precursor of ovarian atypical proliferative (borderline) serous tumors, noninvasive implants, and endosalpingiosis. *Am J Surg Pathol* **35:** 1605–1614. doi:10.1097/PAS.0b013e318229449f

Kurman RJ, Carcangiu ML, Herrington CS, Young RH. 2014. *WHO classification of tumours of female reproductive organs*. IARC, Lyon, France.

Kurnit KC, Sinno AK, Fellman BM, Varghese A, Stone R, Sood AK, Gershenson DM, Schmeler KM, Malpica A, Fader AN, et al. 2019. Effects of gastrointestinal-type chemotherapy in women with ovarian mucinous carcinoma. *Obstet Gynecol* **134:** 1253–1259. doi:10.1097/AOG.0000000000003579

Leary AF, Quinn M, Fujiwara K, Coleman RL, Kohn E, Sugiyama T, Glasspool R, Ray-Coquard I, Colombo N, Bacon M, et al. 2017. Fifth Ovarian Cancer Consensus Conference of the Gynecologic Cancer Intergroup (GCIG): clinical trial design for rare ovarian tumours. *Ann Oncol* **28:** 718–726. doi:10.1093/annonc/mdw662

Ledermann JA, Raja FA, Fotopoulou C, Gonzalez-Martin A, Colombo N, Sessa C; ESMO Guidelines Working Group. 2013. Newly diagnosed and relapsed epithelial ovarian carcinoma: ESMO Clinical Practice Guidelines for diagnosis, treatment and follow-up. *Ann Oncol* **24** (Suppl 6): vi24–vi32. doi:10.1093/annonc/mdt333

Ledermann JA, Luvero D, Shafer A, O'Connor D, Mangili G, Friedlander M, Pfisterer J, Mirza MR, Kim JW, Alexandre J, et al. 2014. Gynecologic Cancer Intergroup (GCIG) consensus review for mucinous ovarian carcinoma. *Int J Gynecol Cancer* **24:** S14–S19. doi:10.1097/IGC.0000000000000296

Lee KR, Scully RE. 2000. Mucinous tumors of the ovary: a clinicopathologic study of 196 borderline tumors (of intestinal type) and carcinomas, including an evaluation of 11 cases with "pseudomyxoma peritonei." *Am J Surg Pathol* **24:** 1447–1464. doi:10.1097/00000478-200011000-00001

Lee KR, Young RH. 2003. The distinction between primary and metastatic mucinous carcinomas of the ovary: gross and histologic findings in 50 cases. *Am J Surg Pathol* **27:** 281–292. doi:10.1097/00000478-200303000-00001

Lee JY, Jo YR, Kim TH, Kim HS, Kim MA, Kim JW, Park NH, Song YS. 2015. Safety of fertility-sparing surgery in primary mucinous carcinoma of the ovary. *Cancer Res Treat* **47:** 290–297. doi:10.4143/crt.2014.004

Lertkhachonsuk AA, Buranawongtrakoon S, Lekskul N, Rermluk N, Wee-Stekly WW, Charakorn C. 2020. Serum CA19-9, CA-125 and CEA as tumor markers for mucinous ovarian tumors. *J Obstet Gynaecol Res* **46:** 2287–2291. doi:10.1111/jog.14427

Li J, Abushahin N, Pang S, Xiang L, Chambers SK, Fadare O, Kong B, Zheng W. 2011. Tubal origin of "ovarian" low-grade serous carcinoma. *Mod Pathol* **24:** 1488–1499. doi:10.1038/modpathol.2011.106

Lin W, Cao D, Shen K. 2018. Prognostic significance of preoperative serum CEA in primary mucinous ovarian carcinoma: a retrospective cohort study. *Cancer Manag Res* **10:** 6913–6920. doi:10.2147/CMAR.S186258

Longacre TA. 2011. Benign and low grade serous epithelial tumors: recent developments and diagnostic problems. *Surg Pathol Clin* **4:** 331–373. doi:10.1016/j.path.2010.12.011

Macedo LT, da Costa Lima AB, Sasse AD. 2012. Addition of Bevacizumab to first-line chemotherapy in advanced colorectal cancer: a systematic review and meta-analysis, with emphasis on chemotherapy subgroups. *BMC Cancer* **12:** 89. doi:10.1186/1471-2407-12-89

Mackenzie R, Kommoss S, Winterhoff BJ, Kipp BR, Garcia JJ, Voss J, Halling K, Karnezis A, Senz J, Yang W, et al. 2015. Targeted deep sequencing of mucinous ovarian tumors reveals multiple overlapping RAS-pathway activating mutations in borderline and cancerous neoplasms. *BMC Cancer* **15:** 415. doi:10.1186/s12885-015-1421-8

McAlpine JN, Wiegand KC, Vang R, Ronnett BM, Adamiak A, Köbel M, Kalloger SE, Swenerton KD, Huntsman DG, Gilks CB, et al. 2009. HER2 overexpression and amplification is present in a subset of ovarian mucinous carcinomas and can be targeted with trastuzumab therapy. *BMC Cancer* **9:** 433. doi:10.1186/1471-2407-9-433

McCluggage WG. 2012. Immunohistochemistry in the distinction between primary and metastatic ovarian mucinous neoplasms. *J Clin Pathol* **65:** 596–600. doi:10.1136/jcp.2010.085688

Meagher NS, Schuster K, Voss A, Budden T, Pang CNI, deFazio A, Ramus SJ, Friedlander ML. 2018. Does the primary site really matter? Profiling mucinous ovarian cancers of uncertain primary origin (MO-CUP) to personalise treatment and inform the design of clinical trials. *Gynecol Oncol* **150:** 527–533. doi:10.1016/j.ygyno.2018.07.013

Meagher NS, Wang L, Rambau PF, Intermaggio MP, Huntsman DG, Wilkens LR, El-Bahrawy MA, Ness RB, Odunsi K, Steed H, et al. 2019. A combination of the immunohistochemical markers CK7 and SATB2 is highly sensitive and specific for distinguishing primary ovarian mucinous tumors from colorectal and appendiceal metastases. *Mod Pathol* **32:** 1834–1846. doi:10.1038/s41379-019-0302-0

Mendivil AA, Tung PK, Bohart R, Bechtol K, Goldstein BH. 2018. Dramatic clinical response following dabrafenib and trametinib therapy in a heavily pretreated low grade serous ovarian carcinoma patient with a BRAF V600E mutation. *Gynecol Oncol Rep* **26:** 41–44. doi:10.1016/j.gore.2018.09.002

Miller CR, Oliver KE, Farley JH. 2014. MEK1/2 inhibitors in the treatment of gynecologic malignancies. *Gynecol Oncol* **133:** 128–137. doi:10.1016/j.ygyno.2014.01.008

Moujaber T, Etemadmoghadam D, Kennedy CJ, Chiew YE, Balleine RL, Saunders C, Wain GV, Gao B, Hogg R, Srirangan S, et al. 2018. *BRAF* mutations in low-grade serous ovarian cancer and response to BRAF inhibition. *JCO Precis Oncol* 1–14. doi:10.1200/PO.17.00221

Moujaber T, Balleine RL, Gao B, Madsen I, Harnett PR, DeFazio A. 2021. New therapeutic opportunities for women with low-grade serous ovarian cancer. *Endocr Relat Cancer* **29:** R1–R16. doi:10.1530/ERC-21-0191

Mueller JJ, Schlappe BA, Kumar R, Olvera N, Dao F, Abu-Rustum N, Aghajanian C, DeLair D, Hussein YR, Soslow RA, et al. 2018. Massively parallel sequencing analysis of mucinous ovarian carcinomas: genomic profiling and differential diagnoses. *Gynecol Oncol* **150:** 127–135. doi:10.1016/j.ygyno.2018.05.008

Muyldermans K, Moerman P, Amant F, Leunen K, Neven P, Vergote I. 2013. Primary invasive mucinous ovarian carcinoma of the intestinal type: importance of the expansile versus infiltrative type in predicting recurrence and lymph node metastases. *Eur J Cancer* **49:** 1600–1608. doi:10.1016/j.ejca.2012.12.004

Nasioudis D, Albright BB, Ko EM, Haggerty AF, Giuntoli RL II, Burger RA, Morgan MA, Latif NA. 2020. Advanced stage primary mucinous ovarian carcinoma. Where do we stand? *Arch Gynecol Obstet* **301:** 1047–1054. doi:10.1007/s00404-020-05489-3

Nelson L, Tighe A, Golder A, Littler S, Bakker B, Moralli D, Murtuza Baker S, Donaldson IJ, Spierings DCJ, Wardenaar R, et al. 2020. A living biobank of ovarian cancer ex vivo models reveals profound mitotic heterogeneity. *Nat Commun* **11:** 822. doi:10.1038/s41467-020-14551-2

Park KJ, Patel P, Linkov I, Jotwani A, Kauff N, Pike MC. 2018. Observations on the origin of ovarian cortical inclusion cysts in women undergoing risk-reducing salpingo-oophorectomy. *Histopathology* **72:** 766–776. doi:10.1111/his.13444

Park JY, Lee SH, Kim KR, Kim YT, Nam JH. 2019. Accuracy of frozen section diagnosis and factors associated with final pathological diagnosis upgrade of mucinous ovarian tumors. *J Gynecol Oncol* **30:** e95. doi:10.3802/jgo.2019.30.e95

Pectasides D, Fountzilas G, Aravantinos G, Kalofonos HP, Efstathiou E, Salamalekis E, Farmakis D, Skarlos D, Briasoulis E, Economopoulos T, et al. 2005. Advanced stage mucinous epithelial ovarian cancer: The Hellenic Cooperative Oncology Group experience. *Gynecol Oncol* **97:** 436–441. doi:10.1016/j.ygyno.2004.12.056

Peres LC, Cushing-Haugen KL, Köbel M, Harris HR, Berchuck A, Rossing MA, Schildkraut JM, Doherty JA. 2019. Invasive epithelial ovarian cancer survival by histotype and disease stage. *J Natl Cancer Inst* **111:** 60–68. doi:10.1093/jnci/djy071

Perren TJ. 2016. Mucinous epithelial ovarian carcinoma. *Ann Oncol* **27:** i53–i57. doi:10.1093/annonc/mdw087

Phelan CM, Kuchenbaecker KB, Tyrer JP, Kar SP, Lawrenson K, Winham SJ, Dennis J, Pirie A, Riggan MJ, Chornokur G, et al. 2017. Identification of 12 new susceptibility loci for different histotypes of epithelial ovarian cancer. *Nat Genet* **49:** 680–691. doi:10.1038/ng.3826

Pignata S, Ferrandina G, Scarfone G, Scollo P, Odicino F, Cormio G, Katsaros D, Villa A, Mereu L, Ghezzi F, et al. 2008. Activity of chemotherapy in mucinous ovarian cancer with a recurrence free interval of more than 6 months: results from the SOCRATES retrospective study. *BMC Cancer* **8:** 252. doi:10.1186/1471-2407-8-252

Pisano C, Greggi S, Tambaro R, Losito S, Iodice F, Di Maio M, Ferrari E, Falanga M, Formato R, Iaffaioli VR, et al. 2005. Activity of chemotherapy in mucinous epithelial ovarian cancer: a retrospective study. *Anticancer Res* **25:** 3501–3505.

Qiu C, Lu N, Wang X, Zhang Q, Yuan C, Yan S, Dongol S, Li Y, Sun X, Sun C, et al. 2017. Gene expression profiles of ovarian low-grade serous carcinoma resemble those of fallopian tube epithelium. *Gynecol Oncol* **147:** 634–641. doi:10.1016/j.ygyno.2017.09.029

Rambau PF, Duggan MA, Ghatage P, Warfa K, Steed H, Perrier R, Kelemen LE, Köbel M. 2016. Significant frequency of MSH2/MSH6 abnormality in ovarian endometrioid carcinoma supports histotype-specific Lynch syndrome screening in ovarian carcinomas. *Histopathology* **69:** 288–297. doi:10.1111/his.12934

Rechsteiner M, Zimmermann AK, Wild PJ, Caduff R, von Teichman A, Fink D, Moch H, Noske A. 2013. TP53 mutations are common in all subtypes of epithelial ovarian cancer and occur concomitantly with KRAS mutations in the mucinous type. *Exp Mol Pathol* **95:** 235–241. doi:10.1016/j.yexmp.2013.08.004

Reid BM, Permuth JB, Sellers TA. 2017. Epidemiology of ovarian cancer: A review. *Cancer Biol Med* **14:** 9–32. doi:10.20892/j.issn.2095-3941.2016.0084

Ricciardi E, Baert T, Ataseven B, Heitz F, Prader S, Bommert M, Schneider S, du Bois A, Harter P. 2018. Low-grade serous ovarian carcinoma. *Geburtshilfe Frauenheilkd* **78:** 972–976. doi:10.1055/a-0717-5411

Risch HA, McLaughlin JR, Cole DE, Rosen B, Bradley L, Fan I, Tang J, Li S, Zhang S, Shaw PA, et al. 2006. Population BRCA1 and BRCA2 mutation frequencies and cancer penetrances: a kin-cohort study in Ontario, Canada. *J Natl Cancer Inst* **98:** 1694–1706. doi:10.1093/jnci/djj465

Rossi L, Verrico M, Zaccarelli E, Papa A, Colonna M, Strudel M, Vici P, Bianco V, Tomao F. 2017. Bevacizumab in ovarian cancer: a critical review of phase III studies. *Oncotarget* **8:** 12389–12405. doi:10.18632/oncotarget.13310

Ryan NAJ, Evans DG, Green K, Crosbie EJ. 2017. Pathological features and clinical behavior of Lynch syndrome-associated ovarian cancer. *Gynecol Oncol* **144:** 491–495. doi:10.1016/j.ygyno.2017.01.005

Ryland GL, Hunter SM, Doyle MA, Caramia F, Li J, Rowley SM, Christie M, Allan PE, Stephens AN, Bowtell DD, et al. 2015. Mutational landscape of mucinous ovarian carcinoma and its neoplastic precursors. *Genome Med* **7:** 87. doi:10.1186/s13073-015-0210-y

Sakayori M, Nozawa S, Udagawa Y, Chin K, Lee SG, Sakuma T, Iizuka R, Wada Y, Yoshida S, Takeda Y. 1990. Biological properties of two newly established cell lines (RMUG-S, RMUG-L) from a human ovarian mucinous cystadenocarcinoma. *Hum Cell* **3:** 52–56.

Sallum LF, Andrade L, Ramalho S, Ferracini AC, de Andrade Natal R, Brito ABC, Sarian LO, Derchain S. 2018. WT1, p53 and p16 expression in the diagnosis of low- and high-grade serous ovarian carcinomas and their relation to prognosis. *Oncotarget* **9:** 15818–15827. doi:10.18632/oncotarget.24530

Santucci C, Bosetti C, Peveri G, Liu X, Bagnardi V, Specchia C, Gallus S, Lugo A. 2019. Dose-risk relationships between cigarette smoking and ovarian cancer histotypes: a comprehensive meta-analysis. *Cancer Causes Control* **30:** 1023–1032. doi:10.1007/s10552-019-01198-8

Sato S, Itamochi H, Kigawa J, Oishi T, Shimada M, Naniwa J, Uegaki K, Nonaka M, Terakawa N. 2009. Combination chemotherapy of oxaliplatin and 5-fluorouracil may be an effective regimen for mucinous adenocarcinoma of the ovary: a potential treatment strategy. *Cancer Sci* **100:** 546–551. doi:10.1111/j.1349-7006.2008.01065.x

Sato N, Saga Y, Mizukami H, Wang D, Fujiwara H, Takei Y, Machida S, Ozawa K, Suzuki M. 2012. Cetuximab inhibits the growth of mucinous ovarian carcinoma tumor cells lacking KRAS gene mutations. *Oncol Rep* **27:** 1336–1340. doi:10.3892/or.2012.1626

Schiavone MB, Herzog TJ, Lewin SN, Deutsch I, Sun X, Burke WM, Wright JD. 2011. Natural history and outcome of mucinous carcinoma of the ovary. *Am J Obstet Gynecol* **205:** 480 e481–488. doi:10.1016/j.ajog.2011.06.049

Schilder RJ, Hall L, Monks A, Handel LM, Fornace AJ Jr, Ozols RF, Fojo AT, Hamilton TC. 1990. Metallothionein gene expression and resistance to cisplatin in human ovarian cancer. *Int J Cancer* **45:** 416–422. doi:10.1002/ijc.2910450306

Schmeler KM, Sun CC, Bodurka DC, Deavers MT, Malpica A, Coleman RL, Ramirez PT, Gershenson DM. 2008. Neoadjuvant chemotherapy for low-grade serous carcinoma of the ovary or peritoneum. *Gynecol Oncol* **108:** 510–514. doi:10.1016/j.ygyno.2007.11.013

Seidman JD, Khedmati F. 2008. Exploring the histogenesis of ovarian mucinous and transitional cell (Brenner) neoplasms and their relationship with Walthard cell nests: a study of 120 tumors. *Arch Pathol Lab Med* **132:** 1753–1760. doi:10.5858/132.11.1753

Seidman JD, Kurman RJ, Ronnett BM. 2003. Primary and metastatic mucinous adenocarcinomas in the ovaries: incidence in routine practice with a new approach to improve intraoperative diagnosis. *Am J Surg Pathol* **27:** 985–993. doi:10.1097/00000478-200307000-00014

Seidman JD, Yemelyanova A, Zaino RJ, Kurman RJ. 2011. The fallopian tube-peritoneal junction: a potential site of carcinogenesis. *Int J Gynecol Pathol* **30:** 4–11. doi:10.1097/PGP.0b013e3181f29d2a

Shimada M, Kigawa J, Ohishi Y, Yasuda M, Suzuki M, Hiura M, Nishimura R, Tabata T, Sugiyama T, Kaku T. 2009. Clinicopathological characteristics of mucinous adenocarcinoma of the ovary. *Gynecol Oncol* **113:** 331–334. doi:10.1016/j.ygyno.2009.02.010

Shimizu Y, Nagata H, Kikuchi Y, Umezawa S, Hasumi K, Yokokura T. 1998. Cytotoxic agents active against mucinous adenocarcinoma of the ovary. *Oncol Rep* **5:** 99–101. doi:10.3892/or.5.1.99

Shrestha R, Llaurado Fernandez M, Dawson A, Hoenisch J, Volik S, Lin YY, Anderson S, Kim H, Haegert AM, Colborne S, et al. 2021. Multiomics characterization of low-grade serous ovarian carcinoma identifies potential biomarkers of MEK inhibitor sensitivity and therapeutic vulnerability. *Cancer Res* **81:** 1681–1694. doi:10.1158/0008-5472.CAN-20-2222

Sieh W, Köbel M, Longacre TA, Bowtell DD, deFazio A, Goodman MT, Hogdall E, Deen S, Wentzensen N, Moysich KB, et al. 2013. Hormone-receptor expression and ovarian cancer survival: An Ovarian Tumor Tissue Analysis consortium study. *Lancet Oncol* **14:** 853–862. doi:10.1016/S1470-2045(13)70253-5

Simon WE, Albrecht M, Hansel M, Dietel M, Holzel F. 1983. Cell lines derived from human ovarian carcinomas: growth stimulation by gonadotropic and steroid hormones. *J Natl Cancer Inst* **70:** 839–845.

Simons M, Simmer F, Bulten J, Ligtenberg MJ, Hollema H, van Vliet S, de Voer RM, Kamping EJ, van Essen DF, Ylstra B, et al. 2020. Two types of primary mucinous ovarian tumors can be distinguished based on their origin. *Mod Pathol* **33:** 722–733. doi:10.1038/s41379-019-0401-y

Song T, Lee DH, Jung YW, Yun BS, Seong SJ, Choi CH, Lee JW, Bae DS, Kim BG. 2018. Elevated preoperative CA125 or CA19-9 in borderline ovarian tumors: could it be suggestive of advanced stage or a poor prognosis? *Gynecol Obstet Invest* **83:** 45–51. doi:10.1159/000475817

Stover EH, Feltmate C, Berkowitz RS, Lindeman NI, Matulonis UA, Konstantinopoulos PA. 2018. Targeted next-generation sequencing reveals clinically actionable BRAF and ESR1 mutations in low-grade serous ovarian carcinoma. *JCO Precis Oncol* **2018:** PO.18.00135. doi:10.1200/PO.18.00135

van den Berg-Bakker CA, Hagemeijer A, Franken-Postma EM, Smit VT, Kuppen PJ, van Ravenswaay Claasen HH, Cornelisse CJ, Schrier PI. 1993. Establishment and characterization of 7 ovarian carcinoma cell lines and one granulosa tumor cell line: growth features and cytogenetics. *Int J Cancer* **53:** 613–620. doi:10.1002/ijc.2910530415

Vang R, Gown AM, Barry TS, Wheeler DT, Yemelyanova A, Seidman JD, Ronnett BM. 2006. Cytokeratins 7 and 20 in primary and secondary mucinous tumors of the ovary: analysis of coordinate immunohistochemical expression profiles and staining distribution in 179 cases. *Am J Surg Pathol* **30:** 1130–1139. doi:10.1097/01.pas.0000213281.43036.bb

Vang R, Shih Ie M, Kurman RJ. 2009. Ovarian low-grade and high-grade serous carcinoma: pathogenesis, clinicopathologic and molecular biologic features, and diagnostic problems. *Adv Anat Pathol* **16:** 267–282. doi:10.1097/PAP.0b013e3181b4fffa

Vergote I, Tropé CG, Amant F, Kristensen GB, Ehlen T, Johnson N, Verheijen RH, van der Burg ME, Lacave AJ, Panici PB, et al. 2010. Neoadjuvant chemotherapy or primary surgery in stage IIIC or IV ovarian cancer. *N Engl J Med* **363:** 943–953. doi:10.1056/NEJMoa0908806

Vici P, Sergi D, Pizzuti L, Mariani L, Arena MG, Barba M, Maugeri-Sacca M, Vincenzoni C, Vizza E, Corrado G, et al. 2013. Gemcitabine-oxaliplatin (GEMOX) as salvage treatment in pretreated epithelial ovarian cancer patients. *J Exp Clin Cancer Res* **32:** 49. doi:10.1186/1756-9966-32-49

Wang Y, Schwartz LE, Anderson D, Lin MT, Haley L, Wu RC, Vang R, Shih Ie M, Kurman RJ. 2015a. Molecular analysis of ovarian mucinous carcinoma reveals different cell of origins. *Oncotarget* **6:** 22949–22958. doi:10.18632/oncotarget.5146

Wang Y, Wu RC, Shwartz LE, Haley L, Lin MT, Shih Ie M, Kurman RJ. 2015b. Clonality analysis of combined Brenner and mucinous tumours of the ovary reveals their monoclonal origin. *J Pathol* **237:** 146–151. doi:10.1002/path.4572

Wang Y, Hong S, Mu J, Wang Y, Lea J, Kong B, Zheng W. 2019a. Tubal origin of "ovarian" low-grade serous carcinoma: a gene expression profile study. *J Oncol* **2019:** 8659754. doi:10.1155/2019/8659754

Wang Y, Sessine MS, Zhai Y, Tipton C, McCool K, Kuick R, Connolly DC, Fearon ER, Cho KR. 2019b. Lineage tracing suggests that ovarian endosalpingiosis does not result from escape of oviductal epithelium. *J Pathol* **249:** 206–214. doi:10.1002/path.5308

Wentzensen N, Poole EM, Trabert B, White E, Arslan AA, Patel AV, Setiawan VW, Visvanathan K, Weiderpass E, Adami HO, et al. 2016. Ovarian cancer risk factors by histologic subtype: an analysis from the Ovarian Cancer Cohort Consortium. *J Clin Oncol* **34:** 2888–2898. doi:10.1200/JCO.2016.66.8178

Winer I, Buckanovich RJ. 2010. A case of progressive mucinous ovarian cancer of low malignant potential responsive to biologic therapy with Bevacizumab. *Gynecol Oncol* **116:** 578–579. doi:10.1016/j.ygyno.2009.10.068

Wong AK, Seidman JD, Barbuto DA, McPhaul LW, Silva EG. 2011. Mucinous metaplasia of the fallopian tube: a diagnostic pitfall mimicking metastasis. *Int J Gynecol Pathol* **30:** 36–40. doi:10.1097/PGP.0b013e3181f45f28

Xu W, Rush J, Rickett K, Coward JI. 2016. Mucinous ovarian cancer: a therapeutic review. *Crit Rev Oncol Hematol* **102:** 26–36. doi:10.1016/j.critrevonc.2016.03.015

Yamada T, Ueda M, Otsuki Y, Ueki M, Sugimoto O. 1991. Establishment and characterization of a cell line (OMC-3) originating from a human mucinous cystadenocarcinoma of the ovary. *Gynecol Oncol* **40:** 118–128. doi:10.1016/0090-8258(91)90102-B

Yoshida H, Tanaka H, Tsukada T, Abeto N, Kobayashi-Kato M, Tanase Y, Uno M, Ishikawa M, Kato T. 2021. Diagnostic discordance in intraoperative frozen section diagnosis of ovarian tumors: a literature review and analysis of 871 cases treated at a Japanese cancer center. *Int J Surg Pathol* **29:** 30–38. doi:10.1177/1066896920960518

Yoshihara M, Kajiyama H, Tamauchi S, Iyoshi S, Yokoi A, Suzuki S, Kawai M, Nagasaka T, Takahashi K, Matsui S, et al. 2020. Impact of uterus-preserving surgery on stage I primary mucinous epithelial ovarian carcinoma: a multi-institutional study with propensity score-weighted analysis. *Int J Gynaecol Obstet* **150:** 177–183. doi:10.1002/ijgo.13244

Yoshiya N. 1986. Establishment of a cell line from human ovarian cancer (undifferentiated carcinoma of FIGO classification) and analysis of its cell-biological characteristics and sensitivity to anticancer drugs. *Nippon Sanka Fujinka Gakkai Zasshi* **38:** 1747–1753.

Yuan SF, Zhang LP, Zhu LJ, Chen WJ, Zheng WE, Xiong JP. 2013. Phase II clinical study on the GEMOX regimen as second-line therapy for advanced ovarian cancer. *Asian Pac J Cancer Prev* **14:** 3949–3953. doi:10.7314/APJCP.2013.14.6.3949

Zaino RJ, Brady MF, Lele SM, Michael H, Greer B, Bookman MA. 2011. Advanced stage mucinous adenocarcinoma of the ovary is both rare and highly lethal: a gynecologic oncology group study. *Cancer* **117:** 554–562. doi:10.1002/cncr.25460

Zhang Y, Li C, Luo S, Su Y, Gang X, Chu P, Zhang J, Wu H, Liu G. 2020. Retrospective study of the epidemiology, pathology, and therapeutic management in patients with mucinous ovarian tumors. *Technol Cancer Res Treat* **19:** 1533033820946423. doi:10.1177/1533033820946423

Zorn KK, Tian C, McGuire WP, Hoskins WJ, Markman M, Muggia FM, Rose PG, Ozols RF, Spriggs D, Armstrong DK. 2009. The prognostic value of pretreatment CA 125 in patients with advanced ovarian carcinoma: a gynecologic oncology group study. *Cancer* **115:** 1028–1035. doi:10.1002/cncr.24084

Ovarian Clear Cell Carcinoma: An Endometriosis-Associated Cancer with Therapeutic Challenges

Ruby Yun-Ju Huang[1,2,3,4] **and Jimmy Jin-Che Lin**[4]

[1]School of Medicine, College of Medicine, National Taiwan University, Taipei 10051, Taiwan

[2]Graduate Institute of Oncology, College of Medicine, National Taiwan University, Taipei 10051, Taiwan

[3]Department of Obstetrics and Gynaecology, Yong Loo Lin School of Medicine, National University of Singapore, Singapore 117597, Singapore

[4]Master's Program in Smart Medicine and Health Informatics, International College, National Taiwan University, Taipei 10051, Taiwan

Correspondence: rubyhuang@ntu.edu.tw

Ovarian clear cell carcinoma (OCCC) is a histological subtype of epithelial ovarian cancer with distinct pathological features, molecular profiles, and biological functions. OCCC has high incidence rates in East Asia compared to the Western hemisphere and Europe and is associated with endometriosis. With its relative resistance to conventional treatment regimens and the worst stage-adjusted prognosis among ovarian cancer subtypes, there is an urgent need to optimize therapeutic options and to improve patient outcomes. To achieve this goal, better patient stratification strategies are required. These strategies could derive from comprehensive and in-depth multidimensional analysis of tumor heterogeneity. Understanding intertumor heterogeneity could assist us in stratifying OCCC patients based on features that are prognostic or predictive. Recent genomic, epigenomic, and transcriptomic profiling analyses allow us to provide an integrative perspective on the diverse heterogeneity in OCCC that could pave the way for novel translational research and clinical development in the future.

Modern cancer treatment has evolved to become a paradigmatic example of precision medicine. As a result, the questions of *Who, What, When,* and *How* to treat have never been so relevant. Answers to these questions are often a result of new research breakthroughs and technological innovations, but some diseases have benefited from these advancements more than others. For instance, epithelial ovarian cancer (EOC) treatment has been reshaped into a precision management strategy based on *BRCA* mutations or homologous recombination deficiency (HRD) status, which determines the efficacy of poly(ADP-ribose) polymerase (PARP) inhibitors. Innovative diagnostic tools toward these molecular features have been developed to stratify patients accordingly, and novel therapeutic strategies are now being implemented in the clinic. A similar paradigm shift is expected for other cancer types, where there is a significant unmet therapeutic need.

Cite this article as *Cold Spring Harb Perspect Med* doi: 10.1101/cshperspect.a041315

Ovarian clear cell carcinoma (OCCC) is a disease that needs such a paradigm shift. OCCC is a histological subtype of EOC that has its own distinct epidemiology among populations, pathological features, and molecular characteristics (Iida et al. 2021). The prevalence of OCCC varies worldwide and among different ethnicities; it is particularly high in East Asian countries when compared with those in the West. In Europe and North America, OCCC accounts for 3%–12% of EOC (Köbel et al. 2010; Mackay et al. 2010; Anglesio et al. 2011), while in East Asia, rates approach 25% (Okamoto et al. 2014; Yamagami and Aoki 2015). However, OCCC is still considered rare by several medical organizations, such as the European Society of Gynaecological Oncology (ESGO) and the Gynecologic Cancer Intergroup (GCIG), with an annual incidence of <6 per 100,000 (Okamoto et al. 2014; Colombo et al. 2019). In contrast, the most common subtype of EOC—the serous subtype—accounts for between 49% (Chan et al. 2008; based on the Surveillance, Epidemiology, and End Results Program between 1988 and 2001) and 70% (Prat 2014), and its incidence is highest in Scandinavian populations (Parkin et al. 2002). One possible explanation for these discrepancies in epidemiology is OCCC's association with endometriosis.

OCCC is an endometriosis-related subtype of EOC. A study of the British Columbia Cancer Agency's database showed that 51% of OCCC pathological diagnoses showed coexisting endometriosis (Stamp et al. 2016). Thus, one hypothesis for the pathogenesis of OCCC is the neoplastic transformation of deposits from retrograde menstruation. This hypothesis is further supported by cohort studies from Japan and Taiwan that have shown that women with endometriosis are at higher risk of developing OCCC later in life (Kobayashi et al. 2007; Wang et al. 2014; Khalique et al. 2020). Strategies to identify endometriosis patients who are at risk of developing OCCC have not yet been developed.

Furthermore, the treatment strategy for OCCC has not drastically changed in the last few decades. The specific treatment of OCCC largely follows the consensus recommendations for EOC made by the European Society for Medical Oncology and European Society of Gynaecological Oncology (ESMO–ESGO) (Colombo et al. 2019) and GCIG (Vergote et al. 2022). Surgery plus platinum/paclitaxel-based chemotherapy is still the backbone of the management of EOC in general and OCCC specifically. The one exception is for patients in the earliest stages of OCCC (IA–IC1, as defined by the International Federation of Gynecology and Obstetrics [FIGO]) who have already received fully staged surgery; for these patients, the benefit of adjuvant chemotherapy is uncertain and is thus recommended only on an individual basis. The literature emphasizes the necessity for complete surgical resection in advanced-stage EOC; however, in advanced-stage cases where primary debulking surgery is not feasible, neoadjuvant chemotherapy is recommended, to be followed by interval debulking, if possible. In OCCC, the poorer response to chemotherapy makes this therapeutic choice in the advanced-stage settings trickier, so this option should be carefully assessed (Gadducci et al. 2021). The lower 5-year overall survival (OS) of stage III and IV OCCC versus high-grade serous cancer (HGSC, the most common form of EOC [17.5% vs. 22.2%]) can also probably be explained by the former's poor response to chemotherapy. This is even more challenging in cases of recurrent OCCC. The recurrence rate for early-stage patients is 29% (Hemman and Rattanaburi 2022) and 67% for advanced-stage patients (Hogen et al. 2019; Hemman and Rattanaburi 2022). Second-line treatment of OCCC follows the guidelines for HGSC, which is based on platinum sensitivity (Colombo et al. 2019). There is little evidence in the literature regarding the effectiveness of second-line treatment for OCCC (Gadducci et al. 2021).

Similarly, targeted therapy, which has shown some benefit for HGSC patients, is of limited use in OCCC. For example, while concomitant or maintenance bevacizumab has been indicated for high-risk EOC patients (Oza et al. 2015; Colombo et al. 2019; Gadducci et al. 2021), the role of bevacizumab in OCCC is less clear. Recent studies from Japanese centers suggest that including bevacizumab in first-line chemotherapy improves the progression-free survival (PFS) of advanced OCCC patients (Tate et al. 2021; Seki et al.

2022). Maintenance treatment with PARP inhibitors is another targeted therapy for HGSC (Vergote et al. 2022) but is of limited use in OCCC. PARP inhibitors are primarily effective against HGSC, which is platinum-sensitive and associated with *BRCA1/2* mutations or with HRD, mutations which are detected in only 6% of OCCC (Gadducci et al. 2021; Giannini et al. 2023).

In sum, OCCC management has yet to benefit from advances in precision medicine. Significant gaps remain in our understanding of endometriosis and its presumed progression to OCCC. We only have partial knowledge as to which OCCC patients are at risk for disease relapse or recurrence and whether they would benefit from additional treatments either in the adjuvant setting or in the maintenance scenario. We also do not know for certain which therapeutic targets might serve as an Achilles heel for OCCC. To answer these questions, we need to understand the nature and extent of tumor heterogeneity within OCCC, which will help the development of preclinical, translational, and clinical research. Herein, we discuss tumor heterogeneity in OCCC from genomic, epigenomic, transcriptomic, and integrated perspectives to shed some light on the disease and help chart the path forward.

GENOMIC HETEROGENEITY OF OCCC

Around 50% of OCCC tumors have loss-of-function mutations in the tumor suppressor gene *ARID1A*, which encodes BRG1-associated factor 250a protein (BAF250a), a subunit of the SWI/SNF chromatin-remodeling complex (Jones et al. 2010; Wiegand et al. 2010). BAF250a regulates transcription by directly regulating chromatin remodeling or indirectly affecting histone modifications. OCCC has also been shown to feature perturbations in the PI3K/AKT pathway, with 50% of OCCC tumors acquiring *PIK3CA* mutations (Iida et al. 2021). A recent large-scale genomic profiling study of 421 OCCC tumors confirmed that *ARID1A* and *PIK3A* are each mutated in ~49% of tumors, with 21% of *ARID1A* mutations having no coexisting *PIK3CA* mutations (Bolton et al. 2022).

Exploring the value of *ARID1A* mutation as a prognostic marker for OCCC has been one key area of research. Many studies have directly sequenced the *ARID1A* gene or used immunohistochemical (IHC) staining for BAF250a to detect its loss, both in OCCC and endometriosis. These studies have shown conflicting results, which cannot be attributed to differences in cohort sizes. Katagiri et al. (2012) (cohort = 60) and Itamochi et al. (2015) (cohort = 112) suggested that loss of *ARID1A* expression in OCCC negatively impacts survival. However, Maeda et al. (2010) (cohort = 149) and Heinze et al. (2022) (cohort = 545) did not observe this trend and showed no difference in survival. A nonsignificant trend toward better survival for patients with *ARID1A* mutations compared with those with *ARID1A*-wild-type/*TP53*-mutated tumors was reported by Bolton et al. (2022) (cohort = 421). Therefore, stratifying patients based on *ARID1A* mutation status to identify high-risk groups might not have high clinical relevance in the real-world setting. Similarly, it is not clear whether *ARID1A* mutations could be used to identify endometriosis patients who are at risk for OCCC. An IHC study showed loss of expression of BAF250a in human endometriomas when compared with normal endometrium. Another study showed that knocking down *ARID1A* in an endometriotic cell line was sufficient to drive neoplastic transformation (Lakshminarasimhan et al. 2017). These data suggest that *ARID1A* is an early driver of endometriosis. However, not every endometriotic lesion is equal in terms of pathogenic risks. Wiegand et al. (2010) found *ARID1A* mutations and loss of BAF250a expression in endometriotic lesions adjacent to OCCC but not in distant ones. In deep-infiltrating endometriosis lesions not associated with malignant risk, Anglesio et al. (2017) found mutations in *KRAS*, not *ARID1A*.

Mutations of the telomerase reverse transcriptase (*TERT*) promoter have been found in 16%–22% of OCCC tumors (Wu et al. 2014; Huang et al. 2015; Bolton et al. 2022; Kobayashi et al. 2023) and tend to be mutually exclusive with *ARID1A*/*PIK3CA*. In early-stage I or II OCCC patients, *TERT* promoter mutation is an independent prognostic factor and correlates with worse survival (Huang et al. 2015). However, Bolton et al.'s large-scale genomic profiling study did not find an association between *TERT* mutation with survival (Bolton et al. 2022). It also has been reported that *TERT* promoter mutations could result in different functional consequences. Kobayashi et al. (2023) found *TERT* mutations of the suppressor (i.e., inhibitor) type in 8.6% of total OCCC and a recurrence rate of 62.5% in OCCC with the same mutations (contrasted with recurrence rates of 20.8% with the unaffected type and only 7.7% with the enhancer, i.e., promoter, type). The transcriptional effects of *TERT* promoter mutations in OCCC might thus be diverse and have yet to be elucidated. Therefore, their prognostic value for identifying high-risk patients warrants further investigation.

Several studies have proposed OCCC classification schemes based on the genomic landscape. Choi et al. (2017) proposed subtyping OCCC based on *ARID1A* positivity as demonstrated by BAF250a IHC staining. In a Danish study, OCCC patients were further stratified into four different molecular subgroups: *PIK3CA*, *ARID1A*, *PIK3CA-ARID1A*, and undetermined (Oliveira et al. 2021). Seven genomic clusters were identified in a 2022 large-scale study (Bolton et al. 2022): four were characterized by the presence of an *ARID1A* mutation, two clusters were *ARID1A* wild-type, and one had mutations in *SMARCA4*. Nevertheless, it has become clear that these genomic clusters might not be the most robust tool to help identify at-risk OCCC patients. There appear to be additional heterogeneities at play, among which may be stronger determining factors.

EPIGENETIC HETEROGENEITY OF OCCC

The importance of *ARID1A* in the maintenance of epigenetic landscapes has been established in many cancer types. BAF250a targets SWI/SNF complexes to enhancers, where it works with transcription factors to facilitate gene activation that may play a role in colorectal cancer and neuroblastoma (Mathur et al. 2017; Shi et al. 2020). It has also been shown to regulate chromatin accessibility and positioning of the transcriptional activator BRG1 (another SWI/SNF subunit, encoded by *SMARCA4*) in both the normal endometrium and in endometrial cancer (Suryo Rahmanto et al. 2020). In endometriosis cells, down-regulation of *ARID1A* alters the distribution of histone modifications and significantly affects gene expression, concomitant with the induction of potentially oncogenic cellular transformation ability in vitro (e.g., anchorage independence and invasion) (Lakshminarasimhan et al. 2017). In breast cancer cells, loss of *ARID1A* profoundly alters histone modifications and the transcriptome (Guo et al. 2018). As *ARID1A* mutations appear to be an important driver for OCCC, these findings suggest that regulation of the epigenetic/chromatin machinery might be crucial. BAF250a regulates chromatin accessibility at both IFN-γ and IFN-γ-responsive genes and interacts directly with EZH2 to reshape immune-related gene clusters in OCCC (Li et al. 2020). This may in part explain the preferential response to immune checkpoint blockade seen in selected OCCC cases (Sia et al. 2022).

How the transcriptional machinery and the resulting transcriptome is shaped by *ARID1A* mutations in OCCC, particularly in the context of disease refractoriness, and whether the plasticity of the epigenetic landscape ever reaches a therapeutically nonresponsive state are yet to be determined. This will be particularly important to establish when it comes to considering the use of epigenetic modifiers to target *ARID1A*-mutated classes of OCCC. Potential targets that would result in synthetic lethality in the presence of *ARID1A* mutations, including EZH2, HDAC2, HDAC6, and BRD2, have recently been proposed (Caumanns et al. 2018). Conceivably, inhibitors of these targets could benefit select OCCC patients. It will be crucial to further elucidate the roles these epigenetic factors play in different transcriptomic backgrounds given the heterogeneity observed and its influence on OCCC outcomes.

TRANSCRIPTOMIC HETEROGENEITY OF OCCC

OCCC-specific gene signatures that distinguish this disease from nonclear cell subtypes have been described (Yamaguchi et al. 2010; Yanaihara et al. 2012). A transcriptomic meta-analysis study of all EOC histotypes identified at least five gene-expression-based molecular subtypes (GEMS) (Table 1; Tan et al. 2013). These GEMS are very robust and display high concordance with findings from Tothill's Australian cohort and the TCGA (Tothill et al. 2008; The Cancer Genome Atlas Research Network 2011). Within the GEMS classification scheme, OCCC was assigned to the Stem-B subtype, along with other non-high-grade serous (mucinous, endometrioid) tumors. The exercise clearly demonstrated that the non-high-grade serous tumors, including OCCC, form a distinct group at the transcriptomic level.

By clustering OCCC independently, Tan et al. were able to identify transcriptomic subtypes. Specifically, aggregated analysis of 222 OCCC gene expression profiles identified two OCCC GEMS: EpiCC (epithelial-like), which is associated with early-stage disease, has a higher rate of mutations in the SWI/SNF complex, and exhibits higher expression of genes related to metabolic and metallothionein-binding pathways; and MesCC (mesenchymal-like), which is associated with late-stage disease and enrichment of genes involved in immune-related pathways and stromal signals (Tan et al. 2019). The features of MesCC correlate well with epithelial–mesenchymal transition (EMT), a crucial process during cancer metastasis (Nieto et al. 2016). Therefore, as OCCC progresses from the early to the advanced stage, it is plausible that there may exist a switch in the transcriptomic landscape from EpiCC to MesCC; however, more experimental evidence is required to establish a causal relationship. A large-scale profiling study (Bolton et al. 2022) of 212 OCCC tumors by RNA sequencing produced results consistent with these findings. Two expression clusters were identified: classic and high-grade serous-like. Parallels between the classic and EpiCC subtypes and the high-grade serous-like and MesCC can be seen, despite the lack of a head-to-head comparison. Classic OCCC showed enrichment of transcripts encoding proteins involved in metabolic pathways and was associated with early-stage disease and a history of endometriosis. In contrast, the high-grade serous-like subtype showed enrichment for transcripts encoding proteins involved in extracellular matrix (ECM) organization and was associated with significantly increased mortality. Both studies (Tan et al. 2019; Bolton et al. 2022) clearly demonstrate the existence of a critical switch during OCCC progression from early- to late-stage disease, which might be driven by mechanisms such as EMT and metabolic reprogramming.

These transcriptomic subtypes provide us with a rather straightforward path to a stratification scheme for high-risk patients based on clinical staging. For early-stage OCCC (FIGO I and II), although the majority of patients have favorable long-term survival, cancer recurs in some after a short disease-free period. This is particularly true for OCCC with stage IC2 ("capsule ruptured before surgery or tumor on the surface of the ovary or fallopian tube"), stage IC3 ("malignant cells in ascitic fluid or in peritoneal washings"), and stage II ("tumor involving one or both ovaries or fallopian tubes with pelvic extension or peritoneal cancer") disease, in which the recurrence rate can be as high as 22%–29.1% (Berek et al. 2021; Gadducci et al. 2021; Hemman and Rattanaburi 2022; Huang et al. 2023). Therefore, it is crucial to further dissect the heterogeneity of early-stage OCCC to precisely identify patients who are at risk. Molecular features derived from these transcriptomic subtypes could provide a basis for stratification. For advanced-stage OCCC (FIGO III and IV), since the general survival outcome is poorer, the priority should be to identify reasonable therapeutic options for residual disease based on the transcriptomic profiles.

Several lines of evidence have suggested that immune features within transcriptomic profiles are pivotal factors for determining OCCC prognosis. EpiCC and MesCC display differential enrichment of immune signals indicative of the presence of different immune cells *in silico* (Tan et al. 2019). Signals for regulatory T cells (Tregs) and activated dendritic cells are enriched in EpiCC, while signals for $CD4^+$ memory and γδT cells are enriched in MesCC. Hence, there is a shift of the immune landscape during the transition from early- to advanced-stage OCCC. In a study of 50 OCCCs across all clinical stages, Ye et al. identified immune and nonimmune transcriptomic subtypes. The immune subtype was associated with enrichment of PD-1 and PI3K-AKT-mTOR signaling and poor clinical

Table 1. Ovarian clear cell carcinoma (OCCC) molecular subtypes

References	Subtypes	EpiCC	MesCC
Tan et al. 2019	Clinical associations	Early-stage disease	Late-stage disease
		Better PFS[a]	Worse PFS[a]
	Enriched immune signals	Activated dendritic cells	$CD4^+$ memory cells
		Treg	γδT cell
	Transcriptomic character	Higher rate of SWI/SNF mutations	Enrichment of immune-related pathways and stromal signal genes
		More expression of metabolic pathway genes	
References	**Subtypes**	**Classic**	**High-grade-serous-like**
Bolton et al. 2022	Clinical associations	Early-stage disease	Advanced-stage disease
		History of endometriosis	Poorer survival
	Transcriptomic enrichment	Metabolic pathway proteins	ECM
			Mesenchymal differentiation
References	**Subtypes**	**Nonimmune**	**Immune**
Ye et al. 2022	Clinical associations	Better PFS and OS	Worse PFS and OS
			Recurrent disease
	Transcriptomic enrichment	Metabolic pathways	Apoptosis and angiogenesis
			Epithelial-mesenchymal transition
			PI3K-AKT-mTOR and *KRAS* signaling
			Immune cells ($CD8^+$ T cells, Treg, macrophages M1, monocyte, and dendritic cells)

Continued

Table 1. *Continued*

References	Subtypes	ProA and AP	PD1-high and CTLA4-high
Heong et al. 2021	Clinical associations	Better DFS (AP only)	Worse DFS and OS (both subtypes)
		Better OS (both subtypes)	DFS and OS benefit from adjuvant chemotherapy (both subtypes)
	Gene overexpression	ProA: stromal markers, ECM production/ remodeling	PD1-high: T-cell regulation, cell migration, and homing CTLA4-high: adaptive immune responses
		AP: cell–cell adhesion, T-cell regulation	
References	**Subtypes**	**Immune-cold**	**Immune-hot**
Huang et al. 2023	Clinical associations	Stage I tumors	Stage II tumors
		Nonrecurrent disease	Recurrent disease
			Worse PFS
	irGES[b]	ProA	PD1-high and CTLA4-high (in tumors with recurrence)
	MesCC score[c]	Lower	Higher
	Immune cell enrichment		$CD45^+$ total TILs
			Bevacizumab response
			$CD8^+$ vs. Treg

(PFS) Progression-free survival, (Treg) regulatory T cells, (ECM) extracellular matrix, (OS) overall survival, (ProA) pro-angiogenic, (AP) antigen-presenting, (DFS) disease-free survival, (irGES) immune-related gene expression signatures, (TIL) tumor-infiltrating lymphocytes.

[a]Data from Ye et al. (2022).

[b]Data based on Heong et al. (2021).

[c]Data based on Tan et al. (2019).

outcome. Interestingly, the immune and nonimmune subtypes also corresponded to mesenchymal and epithelial subtypes, respectively (Ye et al. 2022). These data collectively suggest that an immune-cold landscape might produce better outcomes in OCCC (Huang et al. 2023). Indeed, in early-stage OCCC, evidence from immune transcript profiling of 44 OCCC tumors indicates that an immune-cold landscape predominates during stages IA ("tumor limited to one ovary [capsule intact] or fallopian tube") and IB ("tumor limited to one or both ovaries [capsule intact] or fallopian tubes") disease (Berek et al. 2021), and the tumor shifts to an immune-hot landscape in stage IC2/IC3/II disease. The immune landscape significantly impacts survival (Huang et al. 2023). The features of the immune response that underlie this might vary. Many immune-hot tumors with poor prognoses are CTLA-4 high or PD-1 high subtypes (Heong et al. 2021) or are enriched in infiltrating $CD8^+$ T cells (Ye et al. 2022). The molecular stratification studies described above point to a new way to predict early-stage OCCC patients at risk of recurrence following first-line treatment. However, we are yet to explore how the immune landscape in OCCC is altered during the transition to advanced disease. It will be critical to elucidate how metabolic and EMT reprogramming reshapes the tumor immune microenvironment (TIME) during OCCC progression and relapse.

AN INTEGRATIVE VIEW OF OCCC HETEROGENEITY

Integrating the genomic and transcriptomic data yields a more in-depth view of the molecular heterogeneity of OCCC. Some molecular features show clear correlations between genomic and transcriptomic findings, but others do not. The EpiCC and MesCC subtypes share some molecular features (Tan et al. 2019); both exhibit high rates of *ARID1A* and *PIK3CA* mutations, low rates of *TP53* and *BRCA1/2* mutations, high rates of *ZNF217* amplification, and higher scores for the two OCCC-specific gene signatures (Yamaguchi et al. 2010; Yanaihara et al. 2012). However, EpiCC has a higher frequency of mutations in components of the SWI/SNF complex. These results suggest that EpiCC and MesCC have different epigenetic profiles and echo the finding that classic OCCC tumors harbor single or coexisting *ARID1A* mutations while high-grade serous-like OCCC tumors are dominated by *TP53* mutations with wild-type *ARID1A* (Bolton et al. 2022). Therefore, it is plausible that the epithelial and mesenchymal subtypes of OCCC could be used to stratify patients with alterations in *ARID1A*-related pathways. Several lines of evidence suggest that the epithelial and mesenchymal phenotypes link to the *ARID1A/BRG1* axis. Loss of *ARID1A* has been shown to promote EMT and sensitizes tumors to proteotoxic stress in pancreatic cancer (Tomihara et al. 2021). In neuroblastomas, *ARID1A* loss promotes the adrenergic-to-mesenchymal transition by influencing the activity of enhancers (Shi et al. 2020). Depletion of *BRG1* has also been shown to induce spontaneous EMT in human mammary epithelial cells via defective DNA repair (Wang et al. 2016). All these mechanisms lead to potential avenues for *ARID1A*-specific therapeutic stratification via epithelial/mesenchymal transcriptomic subtyping—for example, targeting DNA repair pathways in OCCC patients with *AR1DA* mutations according to GEMS. However, more evidence needs to be generated from preclinical models designed to specifically address these novel therapeutic strategies.

The differences in the immune landscape described above, however, seem not to correlate to genomic features but rather to epithelial/mesenchymal transcriptomic subtypes. For example, the transcriptomic immune and nonimmune subtypes described by Ye et al. (2022) do not clearly correlate with particular genomic alterations but do with the expression of genes involved in EMT. The lack of correlation between genomic alterations and immune landscape in tumors is in contrast to what has been suggested by the preclinical models (e.g., the loss of *ARID1A* in an OCCC cell line resulted in decreased chromatin accessibility around IFN-γ-responsive genes leading to the decreased expression) (Li et al. 2020). Thus, real-world evidence from different cohorts seems to suggest that the immune landscapes in different genomic backgrounds (e.g., *ARID1A* mutation) are more complicated than the data obtained in preclinical settings. This needs to be taken into consideration when designing clinical trials, testing the idea that there may be an *ARID1A*-specific vulnerability to immunotherapy. Nevertheless, deep whole-genome sequencing (WGS) should be applied to explore whether more complex genomic alterations could be the source of these transcriptomic and immune phenotypes in OCCC. Alterations other than single-nucleotide variants, such as fusion transcripts, might be another possibility. Indeed, from capture RNA-seq profiling of 105 OCCC tumors, Stružinská et al. (2023) found a relatively high frequency of fusion transcripts, up to 13%, with several novel fusion transcripts of unknown function identified. The role of such transcripts in tumorigenesis merits future investigation. Alternatively, the disconnect between genomic alterations and transcriptomic/immune subtypes might reflect the existence of different cells of origin.

The transcriptomic subtypes of OCCC—such as the EpiCC/MesCC subtypes proposed by Tan et al. (2019) and the immune/not-immune subtypes proposed by Ye et al. (2022)—are clearly correlated with metabolic pathways. One unique metabolic feature of OCCC cells is their clear cytoplasm loaded with glycogen particles. Cytoplasmic glycogen accumulation is mainly driven by expression of the transcription factor hepatocyte nuclear factor 1β (HNF1β) (Ji et al. 2018). This unique feature suggests that OCCC cells deploy different molecular mechanisms for regulation of their metabolic requirements compared with other histological subtypes of EOC. It has been demonstrated that OCCC cells critically depend on cysteine for survival and are metabolically heterogeneous. Cysteine deprivation can target both glycolytic and respiring OCCC cells by elevating oxidative stress and energy exhaustion and causes lethality (Novera et al. 2020). Indeed, preclinical data have shown that depletion of the antioxidant glutathione (GSH) and the glutamate-cysteine ligase synthetase catalytic subunit (GCLC, a rate-limiting enzyme for GSH synthesis) could be a strategy for achieving synthetic lethality in *ARID1A*-deficient cancers (Ogiwara et al. 2019). Therefore, *ARID1A*-mutated classic EpiCC could be the OCCC subtype against which to test metabolic agents.

FUTURE DIRECTIONS

OCCC remains underinvestigated, compared with the more common high-grade serous carcinoma. The standard of care for most patients remains adjuvant platinum/taxane chemotherapy following debulking surgery. The benefit of adjuvant chemotherapy varies between early versus advanced-stage OCCC. In early-stage OCCC, adjuvant chemotherapy benefits people with stage IC/II disease (Bogani et al. 2020), but recurrence is still expected for high-risk patients (Huang et al. 2023).

There are neither active clinical agents nor trials of treatments aimed at high-risk early-stage OCCC, however. For advanced-stage OCCC, stage-specific survival outcome is still worse than high-grade serous carcinoma following standard-of-care (Chan et al. 2008). These late-stage patients are usually included in the histotype-agnostic clinical trials being developed for high-grade serous carcinoma, both in front-line settings and in recurrence. The slowly emerging OCCC-specific clinical trials are also mainly for the recurrence setting. Therefore, there is a subset of OCCC patients who have been left out in therapeutic development. Investment to plug this gap thus requires more sophisticated translational research designed to incorporate the concept of OCCC heterogeneity.

To achieve this goal, the transformation of omics-based profiling methods into clinically compatible assays will be crucial. The ovarian cancer field has gained rich experience into how biomarker-driven clinical trials could be run from the development of HRD assays in high-grade serous carcinoma. However, the validity, utility, and regulatory path of these novel assays to encompass the genomic, gene expression, and immune features specific to OCCC would need to be mapped carefully.

The existence of intratumoral heterogeneity (ITH) should not be overlooked. Multiomic signals in OCCC should be analyzed in a spatial profiling context to unravel the complexity of the tumor microenvironment (TME) (Wang et al. 2021; Tai et al. 2023). Although Ye et al.'s immune subtype and Huang et al.'s immune-hot subtype show that adverse tumor biology and immune features are consistently related, whether they stem from the infiltration of immune cells or from the immune mimicry of tumor cells remains unclear (Ye et al. 2022; Huang et al. 2023). Tai et al.'s spatially resolved analysis of said infiltration of immune cells and the immune mimicry of neighboring tumor cells showed that both play crucial roles in shaping the immune subtype in OCCC (Tai et al. 2023). In addition, it will be crucial to understand how immune features differ between primary and recurrent tumors in both classic and high-grade serous-like OCCC. It is unclear whether the immune landscape of recurrent tumors with different transcriptomic backgrounds have consistent patterns or features. Posttreatment changes in OCCC TME should also be explored by spatial analysis.

Another interesting area for future exploration is disease prevention for OCCC. OCCC is an endometriosis-related EOC subtype that arises from neoplastic transformation of deposits from retrograde menstruation. One study in Taiwan using the National Health Insurance Database has clearly demonstrated that women with a history of endometriosis have significantly higher risks of developing EOC (hazard ratio of 7.36) (Wang et al. 2014). Although endometriosis is now regarded as a potential precursor lesion leading to the development of OCCC and endometrioid carcinoma, the carcinogenic process seems to follow pathogenic *ARID1A* driver mutations in endometriotic lesions, not *KRAS* (Anglesio et al. 2017; Suda et al. 2018). This could suggest OCCC preventative measures to identify at-risk endometriosis patients. Also, it remains an open question whether any genetic predispositions lead endometriosis lesions toward the disparate mutagenic paths of either *ARID1A* or *KRAS*, culminating in different risks for OCCC.

Intriguingly, since classic OCCC is more likely to be associated with prior history of endometriosis (Bolton et al. 2022), high-grade serous-like OCCC might be a completely different disease with its own carcinogenesis path and cell of origin. The enzyme responsible for cysteine production, cystathionase (CTH)/cystathionine-γ-lyase, has been shown to be preferentially expressed in OCCC compared with other histotypes and is a lineage marker for OCCC (Cochrane et al. 2017). The cells of origin for OCCC are ciliated cells of the endometrium that highly express CTH rather than the secretory endometrium. Since the MesCC subtype expresses relatively high levels of CTH (Tan et al. 2019), it is highly plausible that the nonclassic OCCC subtype originates from the same ciliated cells but undergoes a different carcinogenesis pathway, triggered by other driver mutations such as *TP53*. A recent study suggests that while OCCC and endometrioid ovarian carcinoma arise from the same cell type (both are associated with endometriosis), in the former, DNA methylation at the promoter of the estrogen receptor gene (*ESR1*) is enriched, potentially locking cells into a state that leads to its particular histotype (Beddows et al. 2024). However, Müllerian metaplasia—implanted coelomic epithelial and mesenchymal cells that have *trans*-differentiated or transformed into malignant Müllerian-directed epithelium and stroma—might be an alternative mechanism to explain the carcinogenesis for nonclassic OCCC tumors, possibly from endometriotic lesions (Kurman and Shih 2010; Li et al. 2012; Sourial et al. 2014). Therefore, the cell state of origin model and Müllerian metaplasia might provide other research avenues to explore preventive measures for OCCC.

COMPETING INTEREST STATEMENT

The authors state that no potential or actual conflict of interest, whether of a financial or other nature, is involved in this submission.

ACKNOWLEDGMENTS

This study was supported by NTU Core Consortiums (NTU-CC-113L892603) and National Science and Technology Council (NSTC 112-2314-B-002-050) to R.Y.-J.H. R.Y.-J.H. is currently supported by the Yushan Fellow Program by the Ministry of Education (MOE), Taiwan (NTU-113V2007-1). R.Y.-J.H. wrote the manuscript. J.J.-C.L. cowrote and edited the manuscript.

REFERENCES

Anglesio MS, Carey MS, Köbel M, Mackay H, Huntsman DG. 2011. Clear cell carcinoma of the ovary: a report from the first ovarian clear cell symposium, June 24th, 2010. *Gynecol Oncol* **121:** 407–415. doi:10.1016/j.ygyno.2011.01.005

Anglesio MS, Papadopoulos N, Ayhan A, Nazeran TM, Noë M, Horlings HM, Lum A, Jones S, Senz J, Seckin T, et al. 2017. Cancer-associated mutations in endometriosis without cancer. *N Engl J Med* **376:** 1835–1848. doi:10.1056/NEJMoa1614814

Beddows I, Fan H, Heinze K, Johnson BK, Leonova A, Senz J, Djirackor S, Cho KR, Pearce CL, Huntsman DG, et al. 2024. Cell state of origin impacts development of distinct endometriosis-related ovarian carcinoma histotypes. *Cancer Res* **84:** 26–38. doi:10.1158/0008-5472.CAN-23-1362

Berek JS, Renz M, Kehoe S, Kumar L, Friedlander M. 2021. Cancer of the ovary, fallopian tube, and peritoneum: 2021 update. *Int J Gynaecol Obstet* **155**(Suppl. 1)**:** 61–85. doi:10.1002/ijgo.13878

Bogani G, Ditto A, Lopez S, Bertolina F, Murgia F, Pinelli C, Chiappa V, Raspagliesi F. 2020. Adjuvant chemotherapy vs. observation in stage I clear cell ovarian carcinoma: a systematic review and meta-analysis. *Gynecol Oncol* **157:** 293–298. doi:10.1016/j.ygyno.2019.12.045

Bolton KL, Chen D, Corona de la Fuente R, Fu Z, Murali R, Köbel M, Tazi Y, Cunningham JM, Chan ICC, Wiley BJ, et al. 2022. Molecular subclasses of clear cell ovarian carcinoma and their impact on disease behavior and outcomes. *Clin Cancer Res* **28:** 4947–4956. doi:10.1158/1078-0432.CCR-21-3817

Caumanns JJ, Wisman GBA, Berns K, van der Zee AGJ, de Jong S. 2018. ARID1A mutant ovarian clear cell carcinoma: a clear target for synthetic lethal strategies. *Biochim Biophys Acta Rev Cancer* **1870:** 176–184. doi:10.1016/j.bbcan.2018.07.005

Chan JK, Teoh D, Hu JM, Shin JY, Osann K, Kapp DS. 2008. Do clear cell ovarian carcinomas have poorer prognosis compared to other epithelial cell types? A study of 1411 clear cell ovarian cancers. *Gynecol Oncol* **109:** 370–376. doi:10.1016/j.ygyno.2008.02.006

Choi JY, Han HH, Kim YT, Lee JH, Kim BG, Kang S, Cho NH. 2017. Ovarian clear cell carcinoma sub-typing by ARID1A expression. *Yonsei Med J* **58:** 59–66. doi:10.3349/ymj.2017.58.1.59

Cochrane DR, Tessier-Cloutier B, Lawrence KM, Nazeran T, Karnezis AN, Salamanca C, Cheng AS, McAlpine JN, Hoang LN, Gilks CB, et al. 2017. Clear cell and endometrioid carcinomas: are their differences attributable to distinct cells of origin? *J Pathol* **243:** 26–36. doi:10.1002/path.4934

Colombo N, Sessa C, du Bois A, Ledermann J, McCluggage WG, McNeish I, Morice P, Pignata S, Ray-Coquard I, Vergote I, et al. 2019. ESMO–ESGO consensus conference recommendations on ovarian cancer: pathology and molecular biology, early and advanced stages, borderline tumours and recurrent disease. *Ann Oncol* **30:** 672–705. doi:10.1093/annonc/mdz062

Gadducci A, Multinu F, Cosio S, Carinelli S, Ghioni M, Aletti GD. 2021. Clear cell carcinoma of the ovary: epidemiology, pathological and biological features, treatment options and clinical outcomes. *Gynecol Oncol* **162:** 741–750. doi:10.1016/j.ygyno.2021.06.033

Giannini A, Di Dio C, Di Donato V, D'oria O, Salerno MG, Capalbo G, Cuccu I, Perniola G, Muzii L, Bogani G. 2023. PARP inhibitors in newly diagnosed and recurrent ovarian cancer. *Am J Clin Oncol* **46:** 414–419. doi:10.1097/COC.0000000000001024

Guo X, Zhang Y, Mayakonda A, Madan V, Ding LW, Lin LH, Zia S, Gery S, Tyner JW, Zhou W, et al. 2018. ARID1A and CEBPα cooperatively inhibit UCA1 transcription in breast cancer. *Oncogene* **37:** 5939–5951. doi:10.1038/s41388-018-0371-4

Heinze K, Nazeran TM, Lee S, Krämer P, Cairns ES, Chiu DS, Leung SC, Kang EY, Meagher NS, Kennedy CJ, et al. 2022. Validated biomarker assays confirm that ARID1A loss is confounded with MMR deficiency, $CD8^+$ TIL infiltration, and provides no independent prognostic value in endometriosis-associated ovarian carcinomas. *J Pathol* **256:** 388–401. doi:10.1002/path.5849

Hemman W, Rattanaburi A. 2022. Incidence and predictive factors for recurrent clear cell ovarian carcinoma: results from a single center in Thailand. *Obstet Gynecol Sci* **65:** 188–196. doi:10.5468/ogs.21313

Heong V, Tan TZ, Miwa M, Ye J, Lim D, Herrington CS, Iida Y, Yano M, Yasuda M, Ngoi NY, et al. 2021. A multiethnic analysis of immune-related gene expression signatures in patients with ovarian clear cell carcinoma. *J Pathol* **255:** 285–295. doi:10.1002/path.5769

Hogen L, Vicus D, Ferguson SE, Gien LT, Nofech-Mozes S, Lennox GK, Bernardini MQ. 2019. Patterns of recurrence and impact on survival in patients with clear cell ovarian carcinoma. *Int J Gynecol Cancer* **29:** 1164–1169. doi:10.1136/ijgc-2019-000287

Huang HN, Chiang YC, Cheng WF, Chen CA, Lin MC, Kuo KT. 2015. Molecular alterations in endometrial and ovarian clear cell carcinomas: clinical impacts of telomerase reverse transcriptase promoter mutation. *Mod Pathol* **28:** 303–311. doi:10.1038/modpathol.2014.93

Huang RY, Huang KJ, Chen KC, Hsiao SM, Tan TZ, Wu CJ, Hsu C, Chang WC, Pan CY, Sheu BC, et al. 2023. Immune-hot tumor features associated with recurrence in early-stage ovarian clear cell carcinoma. *Int J Cancer* **152:** 2174–2185. doi:10.1002/ijc.34428

Iida Y, Okamoto A, Hollis RL, Gourley C, Herrington CS. 2021. Clear cell carcinoma of the ovary: a clinical and molecular perspective. *Int J Gynecol Cancer* **31:** 605–616. doi:10.1136/ijgc-2020-001656

Itamochi H, Oumi N, Oishi T, Shoji T, Fujiwara H, Sugiyama T, Suzuki M, Kigawa J, Harada T. 2015. Loss of ARID1A expression is associated with poor prognosis in patients with stage I/II clear cell carcinoma of the ovary. *Int J Clin Oncol* **20:** 967–973. doi:10.1007/s10147-015-0811-x

Ji JX, Wang YK, Cochrane DR, Huntsman DG. 2018. Clear cell carcinomas of the ovary and kidney: clarity through genomics. *J Pathol* **244:** 550–564. doi:10.1002/path.5037

Jones S, Wang TL, Shih IM, Mao TL, Nakayama K, Roden R, Glas R, Slamon D, Diaz LA, Vogelstein B, et al. 2010. Frequent mutations of chromatin remodeling gene *ARID1A* in ovarian clear cell carcinoma. *Science* **330:** 228–231. doi:10.1126/science.1196333

Katagiri A, Nakayama K, Rahman MT, Rahman M, Katagiri H, Nakayama N, Ishikawa M, Ishibashi T, Iida K, Kobayashi H, et al. 2012. Loss of ARID1A expression is related to shorter progression-free survival and chemoresistance in ovarian clear cell carcinoma. *Mod Pathol* **25:** 282–288. doi:10.1038/modpathol.2011.161

Khalique S, Lord CJ, Banerjee S, Natrajan R. 2020. Translational genomics of ovarian clear cell carcinoma. *Semin Cancer Biol* **61:** 121–131. doi:10.1016/j.semcancer.2019.10.025

Kobayashi H, Sumimoto K, Moniwa N, Imai M, Takakura K, Kuromaki T, Morioka E, Arisawa K, Terao T. 2007. Risk of developing ovarian cancer among women with ovarian endometrioma: a cohort study in Shizuoka, Japan. *Int J Gynecol Cancer* **17:** 37–43. doi:10.1111/j.1525-1438.2006.00754.x

Kobayashi T, Nishikimi K, Mitsuhashi A, Piao H, Matsuoka A, Otsuka S, Tate S, Shozu M, Usui H. 2023. Suppressor-type *TERT* mutations associated with recurrence in ovarian clear cell carcinoma. *Genes Chromosomes Cancer* **62:** 471–476. doi:10.1002/gcc.23129

Köbel M, Kalloger SE, Huntsman DG, Santos JL, Swenerton KD, Seidman JD, Gilks CB; Cheryl Brown Ovarian Cancer Outcomes Unit of the British Columbia Cancer Agency Vancouver BC. 2010. Differences in tumor type in low-stage versus high-stage ovarian carcinomas. *Int J Gynecol Pathol* **29:** 203–211. doi:10.1097/PGP.0b013e3181c042b6

Kurman RJ, Shih LM. 2010. The origin and pathogenesis of epithelial ovarian cancer: a proposed unifying theory. *Am J Surg Pathol* **34:** 433–443. doi:10.1097/PAS.0b013e3181cf3d79

Lakshminarasimhan R, Andreu-Vieyra C, Lawrenson K, Duymich CE, Gayther SA, Liang G, Jones PA. 2017. Down-regulation of ARID1A is sufficient to initiate neoplastic transformation along with epigenetic reprogramming in non-tumorigenic endometriotic cells. *Cancer Lett* **401:** 11–19. doi:10.1016/j.canlet.2017.04.040

Li J, Fadare O, Xiang L, Kong B, Zheng W. 2012. Ovarian serous carcinoma: recent concepts on its origin and carcinogenesis. *J Hematol Oncol* **5:** 8. doi:10.1186/1756-8722-5-8

Li J, Wang W, Zhang Y, Cieślik M, Guo J, Tan M, Green MD, Wang W, Lin H, Li W, et al. 2020. Epigenetic driver mutations in ARID1A shape cancer immune phenotype and immunotherapy. *J Clin Invest* **130:** 2712–2726. doi:10.1172/JCI134402

Mackay HJ, Brady MF, Oza AM, Reuss A, Pujade-Lauraine E, Swart AM, Siddiqui N, Colombo N, Bookman MA, Pfisterer J, et al. 2010. Prognostic relevance of uncommon ovarian histology in women with stage III/IV epithelial ovarian cancer. *Int J Gynecol Cancer* **20:** 945–952. doi:10.1111/IGC.0b013e3181dd0110

Maeda D, Mao TL, Fukayama M, Nakagawa S, Yano T, Taketani Y, Shih IM. 2010. Clinicopathological significance of loss of ARID1A immunoreactivity in ovarian clear cell carcinoma. *Int J Mol Sci* **11:** 5120–5128. doi:10.3390/ijms11125120

Mathur R, Alver BH, San Roman AK, Wilson BG, Wang X, Agoston AT, Park PJ, Shivdasani RA, Roberts CW. 2017. ARID1A loss impairs enhancer-mediated gene regulation and drives colon cancer in mice. *Nat Genet* **49:** 296–302. doi:10.1038/ng.3744

Nieto MA, Huang RY-J, Jackson RA, Thiery JP. 2016. EMT: 2016. *Cell* **166:** 21–45. doi:10.1016/j.cell.2016.06.028

Novera W, Lee ZW, Nin DS, Dai MZ, Binte Idres S, Wu H, Damen JMA, Tan TZ, Sim AYL, Long YC, et al. 2020. Cysteine deprivation targets ovarian clear cell carcinoma *via* oxidative stress and iron-sulfur cluster biogenesis deficit. *Antioxid Redox Signal* **33:** 1191–1208. doi:10.1089/ars.2019.7850

Ogiwara H, Takahashi K, Sasaki M, Kuroda T, Yoshida H, Watanabe R, Maruyama A, Makinoshima H, Chiwaki F, Sasaki H, et al. 2019. Targeting the vulnerability of glutathione metabolism in ARID1A-deficient cancers. *Cancer Cell* **35:** 177–190.e8. doi:10.1016/j.ccell.2018.12.009

Okamoto A, Glasspool RM, Mabuchi S, Matsumura N, Nomura H, Itamochi H, Takano M, Takano T, Susumu N, Aoki D, et al. 2014. Gynecologic Cancer InterGroup (GCIG) consensus review for clear cell carcinoma of the ovary. *Int J Gynecol Cancer* **24**(Suppl. 3)**:** S20–S25. doi:10.1097/IGC.0000000000000289

Oliveira DVNP, Schnack TH, Poulsen TS, Christiansen AP, Høgdall CK, Høgdall EV. 2021. Genomic sub-classification of ovarian clear cell carcinoma revealed by distinct mutational signatures. *Cancers (Basel)* **13:** 5242. doi:10.3390/cancers13205242

Oza AM, Cook AD, Pfisterer J, Embleton A, Ledermann JA, Pujade-Lauraine E, Kristensen G, Carey MS, Beale P, Cervantes A, et al. 2015. Standard chemotherapy with or without bevacizumab for women with newly diagnosed ovarian cancer (ICON7): overall survival results of a phase 3 randomised trial. *Lancet Oncol* **16:** 928–936. doi:10.1016/S1470-2045(15)00086-8

Parkin DM, Whelan SL, Ferlay J, Teppo L, Thomas DB. 2002. *Cancer incidence in five continents, Vol. VIII*. IARC Scientific Publications, Lyon, France.

Prat J. 2014. Staging classification for cancer of the ovary, fallopian tube, and peritoneum. *Int J Gynaecol Obstet* **124:** 1–5. doi:10.1016/j.ijgo.2013.10.001

Seki T, Tate S, Nishikimi K, Unno Y, Itoi M, Ikeda S, Yoshikawa N, Akashi H, Suzuki E, Tanaka N, et al. 2022. Bevacizumab in first-line chemotherapy to improve the survival outcome for advanced ovarian clear cell carcinoma: a multicenter, retrospective analysis. *J Clin Oncol* **40:** 5502–5502. doi:10.1200/JCO.2022.40.16_suppl.5502

Shi H, Tao T, Abraham BJ, Durbin AD, Zimmerman MW, Kadoch C, Look AT. 2020. ARID1A loss in neuroblastoma promotes the adrenergic-to-mesenchymal transition by regulating enhancer-mediated gene expression. *Sci Adv* **6:** eaaz3440. doi:10.1126/sciadv.aaz3440

Sia TY, Manning-Geist B, Gordhandas S, Murali R, Marra A, Liu YL, Friedman CF, Hollmann TJ, Zivanovic O, Chi DS, et al. 2022. Treatment of ovarian clear cell carcinoma with immune checkpoint blockade: a case series. *Int J Gynecol Cancer* **32:** 1017–1024. doi:10.1136/ijgc-2022-003430

Sourial S, Tempest N, Hapangama DK. 2014. Theories on the pathogenesis of endometriosis. *Int J Reprod Med* **2014:** 179515. doi:10.1155/2014/179515

Stamp JP, Gilks CB, Wesseling M, Eshragh S, Ceballos K, Anglesio MS, Kwon JS, Tone A, Huntsman DG, Carey MS. 2016. BAF250a expression in atypical endometriosis and endometriosis-associated ovarian cancer. *Int J Gynecol Cancer* **26:** 825–832. doi:10.1097/IGC.0000000000000698

Stružinská I, Hájková N, Hojný J, Krkavcová E, Michálková R, Dvořák J, Němejcová K, Matěj R, Laco J, Drozenová J, et al. 2023. A comprehensive molecular analysis of 113 primary ovarian clear cell carcinomas reveals common therapeutically significant aberrations. *Diagn Pathol* **18:** 72. doi:10.1186/s13000-023-01358-0

Suda K, Nakaoka H, Yoshihara K, Ishiguro T, Tamura R, Mori Y, Yamawaki K, Adachi S, Takahashi T, Kase H, et al. 2018. Clonal expansion and diversification of cancer-associated mutations in endometriosis and normal endometrium. *Cell Rep* **24:** 1777–1789. doi:10.1016/j.celrep.2018.07.037

Suryo Rahmanto Y, Shen W, Shi X, Chen X, Yu Y, Yu Z-C, Miyamoto T, Lee M-H, Singh V, Asaka R, et al. 2020. Inactivation of Arid1a in the endometrium is associated with endometrioid tumorigenesis through transcriptional reprogramming. *Nat Commun* **11:** 2717. doi:10.1038/s41467-020-16416-0

Tai Y-T, Lin W-C, Wang DY-T, Ye J, Tan TZ, Wei L-H, Huang RY-J. 2023. Spatial profiling of ovarian clear cell carcinoma reveals immune-hot features. bioRxiv doi:10.1101/2023.07.27.550775

Tan TZ, Miow QH, Huang RY-J, Wong MK, Ye J, Lau JA, Wu MC, Bin Abdul Hadi LH, Soong R, Choolani M, et al. 2013. Functional genomics identifies five distinct molecular subtypes with clinical relevance and pathways for growth control in epithelial ovarian cancer. *EMBO Mol Med* **5:** 1051–1066. doi:10.1002/emmm.201201823

Tan TZ, Ye J, Yee CV, Lim D, Ngoi NYL, Tan DSP, Huang RY-J. 2019. Analysis of gene expression signatures identifies prognostic and functionally distinct ovarian clear cell carcinoma subtypes. *EBioMedicine* **50:** 203–210. doi:10.1016/j.ebiom.2019.11.017

Tate S, Nishikimi K, Matsuoka A, Otsuka S, Shiko Y, Ozawa Y, Kawasaki Y, Shozu M. 2021. Bevacizumab in first-line chemotherapy improves progression-free survival for advanced ovarian clear cell carcinoma. *Cancers (Basel)* **13:** 3177. doi:10.3390/cancers13133177

The Cancer Genome Atlas Research Network. 2011. Integrated genomic analyses of ovarian carcinoma. *Nature* **474:** 609–615. doi:10.1038/nature10166

Tomihara H, Carbone F, Perelli L, Huang JK, Soeung M, Rose JL, Robinson FS, Deribe YL, Feng N, Takeda M, et al. 2021. Loss of ARID1A promotes epithelial-mesenchymal transition and sensitizes pancreatic tumors to proteotoxic stress. *Cancer Res* **81:** 332–343. doi:10.1158/0008-5472.CAN-19-3922

Tothill RW, Tinker AV, George J, Brown R, Fox SB, Lade S, Johnson DS, Trivett MK, Etemadmoghadam D, Locandro B, et al. 2008. Novel molecular subtypes of serous and endometrioid ovarian cancer linked to clinical outcome. *Clin Cancer Res* **14:** 5198–5208. doi:10.1158/1078-0432.CCR-08-0196

Vergote I, Gonzalez-Martin A, Lorusso D, Gourley C, Mirza MR, Kurtz J-E, Okamoto A, Moore K, Kridelka F, McNeish I, et al. 2022. Clinical research in ovarian cancer: consensus recommendations from the gynecologic cancer InterGroup. *Lancet Oncol* **23:** e374–e384. doi:10.1016/S1470-2045(22)00139-5

Wang KC, Chang WH, Lee WL, Huang N, Huang HY, Yen MS, Guo CY, Wang PH. 2014. An increased risk of epithelial ovarian cancer in Taiwanese women with a new surgico-pathological diagnosis of endometriosis. *BMC Cancer* **14:** 831. doi:10.1186/1471-2407-14-831

Wang H, Bierie B, Li AG, Pathania S, Toomire K, Dimitrov SD, Liu B, Gelman R, Giobbie-Hurder A, Feunteun J, et al. 2016. BRCA1/FANCD2/BRG1-driven DNA repair stabilizes the differentiation state of human mammary epithelial cells. *Mol Cell* **63:** 277–292. doi:10.1016/j.molcel.2016.05.038

Wang DY-T, Tan TZ, Tai Y-T, Ye J, Lin W-C, Wei L-H, Huang RY-J. 2021. Case study: digital spatial profiling of metastatic clear cell carcinoma reveals intra-tumor heterogeneity in epithelial-mesenchymal gradient. bioRxiv doi:10.1101/2021.05.27.445912

Wiegand KC, Shah SP, Al-Agha OM, Zhao Y, Tse K, Zeng T, Senz J, McConechy MK, Anglesio MS, Kalloger SE, et al. 2010. *ARID1A* mutations in endometriosis-associated ovarian carcinomas. *N Engl J Med* **363:** 1532–1543. doi:10.1056/NEJMoa1008433

Wu RC, Ayhan A, Maeda D, Kim KR, Clarke BA, Shaw P, Chui MH, Rosen B, Shih IM, Wang TL. 2014. Frequent somatic mutations of the telomerase reverse transcriptase promoter in ovarian clear cell carcinoma but not in other major types of gynaecological malignancy. *J Pathol* **232:** 473–481. doi:10.1002/path.4315

Yamagami W, Aoki D. 2015. Annual Report of the Committee on Gynecologic Oncology, the Japan Society of Obstetrics and Gynecology. *J Obstet Gynaecol Res* **41:** 167–177. doi:10.1111/jog.12596

Yamaguchi K, Mandai M, Oura T, Matsumura N, Hamanishi J, Baba T, Matsui S, Murphy SK, Konishi I. 2010. Identification of an ovarian clear cell carcinoma gene signature that reflects inherent disease biology and the carcinogenic processes. *Oncogene* **29:** 1741–1752. doi:10.1038/onc.2009.470

Yanaihara N, Anglesio MS, Ochiai K, Hirata Y, Saito M, Nagata C, Iida Y, Takakura S, Yamada K, Tanaka T, et al. 2012. Cytokine gene expression signature in ovarian clear cell carcinoma. *Int J Oncol* **41:** 1094–1100. doi:10.3892/ijo.2012.1533

Ye S, Li Q, Wu Y, Jiang W, Zhou S, Zhou X, Yang W, Tu X, Shan B, Huang S, et al. 2022. Integrative genomic and transcriptomic analysis reveals immune subtypes and prognostic markers in ovarian clear cell carcinoma. *Br J Cancer* **126:** 1215–1223. doi:10.1038/s41416-022-01705-w

Models of High-Grade Serous Ovarian Carcinoma

Oscar J. Pundel and Benjamin G. Neel

Perlmutter Cancer Center, NYU Grossman School of Medicine, New York, New York 10016, USA

Correspondence: benjamin.neel@nyulangone.org

High-grade serous ovarian carcinoma (HGSC) remains an incompletely understood, highly lethal disease. Historically, a lack of fidelitous in vitro and in vivo models representing HGSC biology and therapy response has been a major barrier to progress. As we discuss below, multiple (if not most) early studies used—and some investigators continue to use—human "ovarian cancer cell lines" that lack key genomic/genetic features of HGSC, rendering their conclusions questionable. The frequently deployed ID8 syngeneic mouse model is similarly suspect, as it derives from ovarian surface epithelium (OSE) and is *Trp53* wild-type. In contrast, most, if not all, HGSC arises in fallopian tube epithelium (FTE), and bona fide HGSC is universally *TP53* mutant or silenced. Over the past 10 years, attempts have been made to rectify these historical deficiencies, including careful assessment of the genetic composition of standard ovarian cancer cell lines and the development of mouse and human organoids, genetically engineered mouse models (GEMMs), and patient-derived xenografts (PDXs). In this review, we discuss these advances, exploring their differences, strengths, and weaknesses. We also describe "next-generation" approaches to more faithfully model HGSC cells in the context of a more realistic tumor microenvironment.

HISTORICAL HGSC CELL LINE MODELS

As is the case for several other malignancies, it is difficult to pinpoint the first high-grade serous ovarian carcinoma (HGSC) cell line derived and maintained successfully. Most literature points to work by Jorgen Fogh and Germain Trempe in 1975, who developed CAOV-1 and SKOV-3 cells (Fogh and Trempe 1975). SKOV-3 was derived from the ascitic fluid of a patient with ovarian adenocarcinoma at the Sloan Kettering Institute for Cancer Research (now Memorial Sloan Kettering Cancer Center), while CAOV-1was derived from a human ovarian tumor obtained from a patient at the M.D. Anderson Hospital and Tumor Institute (currently M. D. Anderson Cancer Center). Fogh and Trempe also mention a cell line called RPMI-13, generated by Ishihara et al. (1962), but this line has since disappeared from publications.

These early models were followed quickly by the generation of OVCA420 by the group of Robert Knapp in 1981 (Bast et al. 1981) and OVCAR-3, developed by the group of Robert Ozols in 1983 (Hamilton et al. 1983). These and the earlier lines, some of which remain in wide use, contributed to foundational studies of HGSC pathobiology. For example, OVCA420

Cite this article as *Cold Spring Harb Perspect Med* doi: 10.1101/cshperspect.a041949

advanced the then new field of cancer-associated antigens by revealing the biomarker CA125 (Bast et al. 1981), whose blood levels are used for monitoring HGSC in patients (Bast et al. 1983). The first description of OVCAR-3 pointed to its potential as a model for cisplatin resistance and for studying the role of estrogens/androgens in tumor biology. Several conventional ovarian cancer cell lines also can generate tumors (cell-derived xenografts [CDXs]) in immune-incompetent mice (Fogh et al. 1977). This capacity facilitated early studies of host–tumor interactions, although this work could not assess the critical role of the adaptive immune system. Moreover, as we explore further below, many early models were wrongly classified as HGSC, and their histopathologic origin remains unclear. Consequently, some results obtained using these models might have misled ovarian cancer researchers.

Conventional Human-Derived Cell Culture Models

Conventional two-dimensional (2D) ovarian cancer cell lines are derived from primary tumors or ascites, and their morphological, genetic, and molecular features have been characterized to varying extents (Fig. 1, top panel; Table 1). Their ease of use, low cost, and widespread availability made them prominent in HGSC research. These cells are immortalized, typically grow quickly, and usually can be single-cell cloned. Today, they are most useful for molecular genetic studies aimed at uncovering signaling pathways in HGSC cells, including drug resistance mechanisms, as well as for large-scale genetic screens (e.g., using short hairpin RNA [shRNA] or clustered regularly interspaced short palindromic repeats [CRISPR]/CRISPR-associated protein 9 [Cas9] deletion or editing approaches). However, it is also critical that researchers be aware of the limitations of these lines for probing *HGSC* pathogenesis.

For example, researchers should be aware that many lines annotated as "high-grade serous ovarian cancer" are wrongly characterized. Virtually all (>95%) cases of HGSC feature defects in *TP53*, mostly point mutations or deletions, as the initial step in disease development (Ahmed et al. 2010; The Cancer Genome Atlas Research Network et al. 2011; Kurman 2013; Hoadley et al. 2014). Additional genetic alterations follow rapidly, most often copy number variations (CNVs), including amplifications or deletions. *KRAS*, *PIK3CA*, *MYC*, *MECOM*, *CCNE1*, and/or *EMSY* are often amplified; *PTEN*, *BRCA1*, and/or *BRCA2* are often deleted. Germline *BRCA1/2* mutations contribute to 15%–20% of HGSC. However, somatic point mutations in *KRAS*, *BRAF*, *CTNNB1*, *ARID1A*, or *ERBB2* (HER2), as well as HER2 amplification, which are found in other ovarian cancer subtypes, are rare in HGSC. Although HGSC presents with multiple chromosomal defects, once these are established, tumor genetics remains relatively stable (Kandoth et al. 2013; Cheng et al. 2022).

These fundamental genetic features can provide clues to the origin of conventional ovarian cancer cell lines. Indeed, several groups analyzed the genetics of ovarian cancer cell lines to assess the likelihood that they represent HGSC (Korch et al. 2012; Anglesio et al. 2013; Domcke et al. 2013; Beaufort et al. 2014). Domcke et al. compared CNV and mutational landscapes in 47 "ovarian cancer" cell lines to those in actual tumors. Beaufort et al. used a similar approach, while including protein profiling, to address the same issues. Both found that many lines had been classified incorrectly. For example, SKOV-3 and A2780 cells are more likely to be of clear cell or endometrioid ovarian cancer origin rather than representative of HGSC. These findings were particularly troubling, as these lines are the most used models of "HGSC," contributing to >3000 publications. A few lines, less well known at the time (e.g., Kuramochi, JHOS4, OVCAR4), were genetically much closer to actual HGSC. Subsequently, Fleury et al. (2015) generated six new HGSC cell lines, including one with a germline *BRCA1* and another with a germline *BRCA2* mutation. These cells were characterized for morphology, growth properties, platinum sensitivity, and ability to grow under anchorage-independent conditions, migration, and tumorigenicity. More recently, Papp et al. (2018) reported an integrated genomic, epigenomic, and expression analysis of

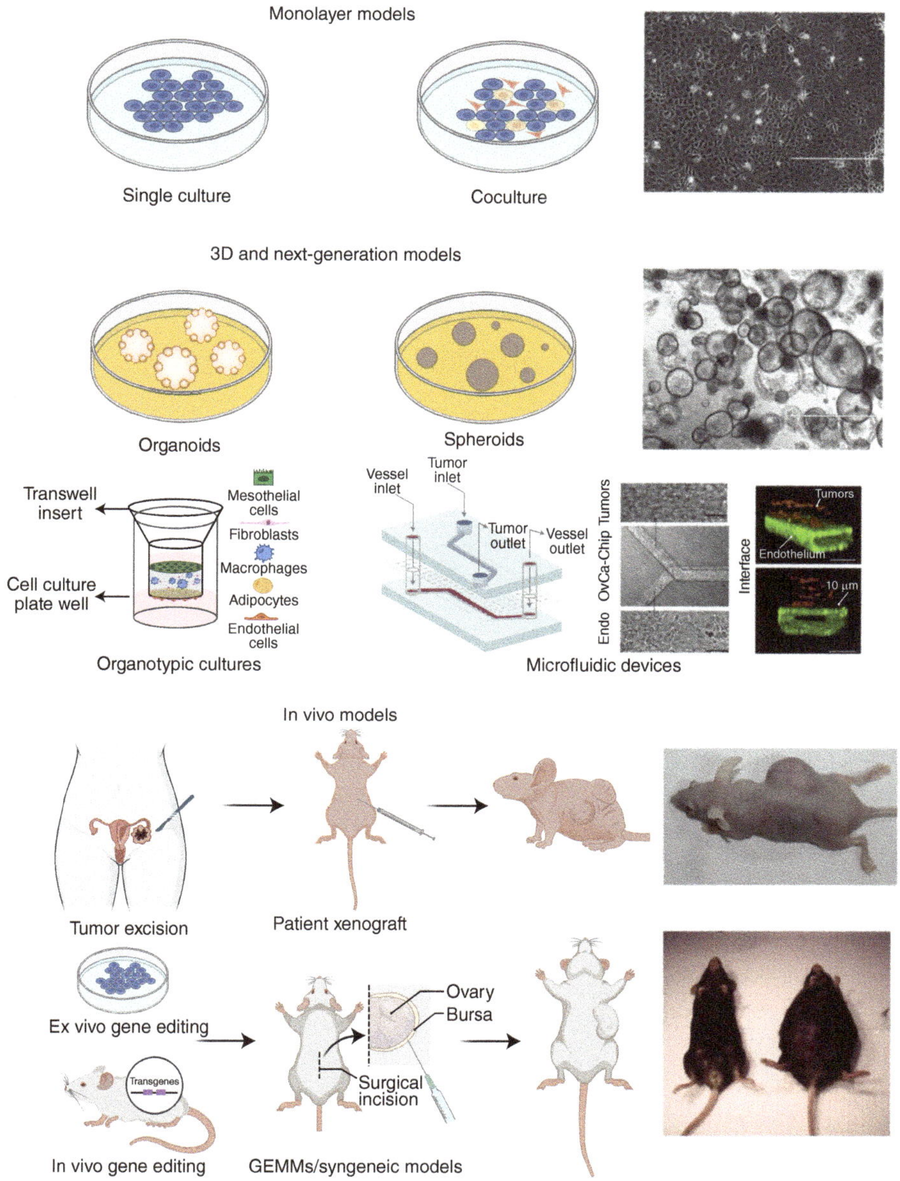

Figure 1. Representative models of high-grade serous ovarian carcinoma (HGSC). (*Top right* panel) *Trp53*$^{-/-}$;*Ccne1*^{OE};*Myc*^{OE} fallopian tube epithelial (FTE) cells growing in monolayer culture in a Petri dish. Scale bar, 400 μm. (*Middle* panel, *top right*) *Trp53*$^{-/-}$;*Ccne1*^{OE};*Akt2*^{OE} FTE cells growing as organoids. Scale bar, 1 mm. (*Middle* panel, *bottom left*) Schematic representation of an organotypic "pentaculture" model including mesothelial cells, fibroblasts, macrophages, adipocytes, and endothelial cells. (Figure reprinted from Estermann et al. 2023 under the terms of the Creative Commons CC-BY license.) (*Middle* panel, *bottom right*) OvCa-Chip, based on Saha et al. (2021), showing sequentially the schematic computer-aided design, microscopy pictures of OvCa-Chip (*center*) with A2780 human ovarian endometroid adenocarcinoma cells cultured on the upper microchannel (*top*) and a human primary endothelial cell–formed vessel inside the lower channel (*bottom*), and a confocal fluorescence micrograph of a cross section of the OvCa-Chip, with spheroidal A2780 cells (red) cocultured with primary endothelial cells (green). Scale bar, 100 μm. (*Bottom* panel, *top right*) Nude mouse with OVCAR3 xenograft. (*Bottom* panel, *right*) C57BL6 mice with or without ID8 syngeneic tumor. (Figure based on Cho et al. 2019 and created with BioRender.com.)

Table 1. Commonly used ovarian cancer cell lines

Name	Origin	Mutational landscape	Notable observations	References
KURAMOCHI	Ascites from patient with metastatic adenocarcinoma	*TP53*^{D281Y}, *MYC* and *KRAS* amplification, *BRCA2*^{R2318}		Motoyama 1981
COV362	Pleural effusion from HGSC patient	*TP53*^{Y220C}, *BRCA1*^{F872}, *RB1* deletion, *MYC* amplification		van den Berg-Bakker et al. 1993
COV318	Ascites from high-grade serous ovarian adenocarcinoma patient	*TP53*^{I195F}, *CCNE1* amplification		van den Berg-Bakker et al. 1993
TYK-nu	Derived from serially transplanted tumor in nude mice originally from an undifferentiated carcinoma of the ovary	*TP53*^{R175H}, *NRAS*^{G12D}, *NRAS*^{Q61K}	Cisplatin sensitive	Yoshiya 1986
OVKATE	High-grade serous ovarian adenocarcinoma from metastatic site	*TP53*^{R282W}, *MTOR*^{DeltaT1834T1837TAAT}	Cisplatin and paclitaxel resistant; dogs can smell this cell line	Yanagibashi et al. 1997; Ohta 2001; Murarka et al. 2019
CaOV-4	High-grade serous ovarian adenocarcinoma from subserosa of fallopian tube	*TP53*^{V147D}, *MYC* amplification		Wright et al. 1981; Langland et al. 2010
CaOV-3	High-grade serous ovarian adenocarcinoma	*TP53*^{G136X}, *EGFR*^{R255Q}		Buick et al. 1985
OVCAR-3	Ascites of ovarian adenocarcinoma after combination chemotherapy with cyclophosphamide, adriamycin, and cisplatin	*TP53*^{R248G}, *PIK3R1* and *CCNE1* amplification	Cisplatin, adriamycin, and melphalan resistant	Hamilton et al. 1983; Ikediobi et al. 2006
ES-2	Originally classified as ovarian clear cell adenocarcinoma	*TP53*^{S241F}, *BRAF*^{V600G}, *PALB2*^{M296}, *TERT*$^{242\_243CC>TT}$	Cisplatin, etoposide, doxorubicin, and bleomycin sensitive	Lau et al. 1991; Devor and Bender 2021
SNU-8	Ovarian serous cystadenocarcinoma from ascites	*KRAS*^{G12D}, *TP53*^{P142}, *CCNE1* amplification	CA125 producing	Yuan et al. 1997; Ku and Park 2005; Domcke et al. 2013
OVCAR-8	High-grade serous ovarian adenocarcinoma	*TP53*^{T126}, *KRAS*^{P121H}, *CTNNB1*^{Q26R}, *ERBB2*^{G776V}	Cisplatin resistant	Alley et al. 1988; Schilder et al. 1990: Ikediobi et al. 2006

Continued

Table 1. *Continued*

Name	Origin	Mutational landscape	Notable observations	References
SNU-840	Malignant ovarian Brenner tumor	*PIK3CA*^{H1047R}	CA125 producing	Yuan et al. 1997
HEY	High-grade ovarian serous adenocarcinoma from ascites, but likely misclassified	*BRAF*^{G464E}, *KRAS*^{G12D}		Buick et al. 1985; Langland et al. 2010; Domcke et al. 2013
OVCA420	Ovarian serous adenocarcinoma	*TP53*^{R273H}	CA125 producing	Bast et al. 1981
SKOV-3	Adenocarcinoma from ascites, now believed to be of endometrial/clear cell origin	*TP53*^{S90}, *PIK3CA*^{H1047R}, *FBXW7*^{R505L}, *APC* deletion, *ARID1A*^{G586}, *KRAS* amplification	Cisplatin refractory, docetaxel and doxorubicin sensitive	Fogh and Trempe 1975; Ikediobi et al. 2006; Domcke et al. 2013; Beaufort et al. 2014
A2780	Ovarian endometroid adenocarcinoma in an untreated patient	*PTEN* catalytic domain deletion, *ATM*^{P604S}, *BRAF*^{V226M}, *ARID1A*^{R1721}, *PIK3CA*^{G365L}	Drug sensitive, but drug-resistant variants are readily available	Westin et al. 1982; Louie et al. 1985
TOV-21G	Ovarian clear cell adenocarcinoma	*KRAS*^{G12C}, *PIK3CA*^{H1047Y}, *PTEN*^{G143}, *CTNNB1*^{K292N}, *ARID1A*^{Y551}, hypermutated with low CNA		Provencher et al. 2000; Domcke et al. 2013

Green: likely HGSC. Orange: possibly HGSC. Red: unlikely HGSC, as annotated by Domcke et al. (2013).
(HGSC) High-grade serous ovarian carcinoma, (CNA) copy number alteration.

45 ovarian cancer cell lines, 19 of which were classified as HGSC. These investigators also tested the sensitivity of these lines to various targeted agents. Any researcher wishing to use established cell lines to study HGSC should consult these seminal reports to ensure that their choice of cell system is appropriate (Table 1).

Researchers should also consider how the genetics of conventional cell lines align with the current clinicopathological classification of HGSC, which is based on homologous recombination (HR) status (Konstantinopoulos et al. 2015). HR-deficient (HRD) lines feature mutations/loss of *BRCA1/2*, *RB1*, Fanconi anemia (FA) genes, or genes involved in sensing double-stranded breaks. HGSCs with EMSY amplification or PTEN loss are considered "possibly HRD," while HR-proficient (HRP) lines include those with *CCNE1* amplification. HRD cell lines/tumors respond better than their HRP counterparts to poly(ADP ribose) polymerase inhibitors (PARPi) and thus are more relevant to studies of PARPi action/resistance (Kortmann et al. 2011; AlHilli et al. 2016).

Although useful for many types of experiments, even "correct" 2D HGSC cell line models have several limitations/drawbacks. First, the basal growth medium used for conventional cell lines (typically Dulbecco's modified Eagle medium [DMEM] or Roswell Park Memorial Institute [RPMI]) differs considerably from what HGSC cells experience in the tumor microenvironment (TME). Media composition is optimized to allow investigators to exchange media every 2–3 days and therefore contains much higher concentrations of nutrients (e.g., glucose and amino acids) than cells encounter in vivo. For example, the concentration of glucose in standard, "high-glucose" DMEM (400 mg/dL) resembles that in a patient with uncontrolled diabetes. Cells in tumors are exposed to nutrient gradients and can be nutrient limited in some regions; in contrast, nutrient concentrations are more uniform in cell culture. Cell lines are typically maintained in supraphysiologic oxygen concentrations (20%, compared with ~7% in capillaries and much less in tumor cores), and their pH is buffered in the physiologic range (as opposed to the often-acidic TME). In concert (or even individually), these differences can have major effects on cancer cell biology including drug resistance (Muir and Vander Heiden 2018) and metastatic potential (Natarajan et al. 2019).

Furthermore, conventional cell line models are almost always established with—and typically are maintained in—serum-containing growth media, which imposes strong selective pressure on ovarian (and other types of) tumor cells. Serum contains growth factors, other secretory proteins/hormones, and small molecules (e.g., vitamins, nucleoside precursors) that promote cell growth, but also has components (e.g., pre–transforming growth factor β [TGF-β], which can be liberated by cancer cell proteases) that potently inhibit epithelial cells (Xu et al. 2009; Moses et al. 2016; Janus et al. 2024). The requirement that cell lines grow on tissue culture plastic, which is much stiffer than the typical ovarian TME (e.g., metastases growing on the pliable, adipocyte-rich omentum) imposes additional selective pressure on primary tumor cells. Stiff substrates can cause DNA damage (Cho et al. 2019), which could result in "genetic drift" upon continued passaging (Quevedo et al. 2020), and also trigger signaling pathways (e.g., integrins, Hippo/YAP) that can affect cell fate (Engler et al. 2006; Connelly et al. 2010; Dasgupta and McCollum 2019) and drug response (Kalli et al. 2023; Mai et al. 2024).

Cells grown in tissue culture plates typically attach to extracellular matrix (ECM) proteins, such as collagens, fibronectin, or proteoglycans, which can come from serum and/or be produced by the cancer cells themselves. In tumors, in contrast, ECM is produced predominantly by cancer-associated fibroblasts (CAFs) or other cells in the TME. Interactions with integrins trigger complex intracellular signaling pathways (Cooper and Giancotti 2019; Li et al. 2023); hence, if the cell culture ECM differs from ECM in the tumor, cell behavior can be altered. For example, Pietilä et al. demonstrated that HGSC dynamically changes the collagen subtypes and accumulation in the TME. Cell lines treated with platinum compounds secreted more collagen 6, which potentiated platinum resistance (Pietilä et al. 2021). Some of these drawbacks can be overcome by coating tissue culture plastic with tumor-derived ECM or by using hydrogels engineered to display ECM-like motifs (discussed later in this work), but these approaches still imperfectly replicate in vivo setting.

Another major difference between 2D cultures and tumors, of course, is that the former lack the interactions between cancer cells and other cell types in the TME. The interplay between these populations is complex, yet their implications are profound for tumor biology, with clear effects on proliferation, metastasis, and therapy response (Izar et al. 2020; Vázquez-García et al. 2022). Coculture methods have existed for decades, with the earliest examples of application to ovarian cancer dating back to the 1980s. Yet, cocultures are limited by how long they can be maintained and by the variable survival of different TME cell populations. Newer technologies, discussed below, can enable more realistic studies of a more diverse TME in the laboratory.

In summary, established ovarian cancer cell lines have provided valuable insights into HGSC biology, drug resistance, and therapeutic targets. However, the conclusions of the many earlier studies using SKOV3 and A2780 cells (as well as other lines unlikely to represent HGSC) must be viewed with caution if one wishes to make inferences about HGSC pathobiology. Moreover, even bona fide HGSC-like lines fail to represent tumor heterogeneity, complexity, and microenvironment.

Spheroids

Spheroids predate organoids as a 3D model of cancer. Indeed, Sutherland et al. first reported spheroids as a model of nodular carcinoma in

1971, while the first (mammary) organoid model was reported by Li et al. in 1987 (Sutherland et al. 1971; Li et al. 1987). Many HGSC cell lines, as well as primary tumor cells, can be maintained as spheroids (Yee et al. 2022; Tomas and Shepherd 2023). In such cultures, cancer cells are placed in low adhesive plates (e.g., bacterial or poly-HEMA-coated plates) or in "hanging drop" cultures and aggregate into clusters ("spheroids") that better mimic several features of tumors than conventional 2D cultures (Fig. 1, middle panel, top). For example, spheroids might better maintain tumor-initiating cells (often misleadingly termed "cancer stem cells") than 2D cultures (Liao et al. 2014). Compared with the latter, spheroids also exhibit distinct cell–cell and cell–ECM interactions, lower rigidity/stretch, and more realistic nutrient and oxygen gradients (Tadić et al. 2024). In concert, these result in a mixture of proliferating, outer-layer cells and hypoxic, quiescent, and/or dead cells in the spheroid core. Consequently, spheroids and standard 2D cultures differ in signaling pathways, gene expression, drug response, tumor-initiating capability, and genetic vulnerabilities (e.g., CRISPR-Cas9 screens). Unlike organoids, however, cells in spheroids grow on top of each other in a nonstructured way. In this context, spheroid cultures might be particularly relevant mimics of HGSC ascites, which contains tumor cells aggregated into similar clusters, although often admixed with other cell types that can influence their phenotype (Shield et al. 2009; Flörkemeier et al. 2024).

Although the development of organoids and more complex approaches have made spheroids less popular 3D models of HGSC tumors, they can be helpful for investigating HGSC metastasis and drug responses. Readers interested in such approaches can consult the several recent reviews covering the use of spheroid cultures in general (Fang and Eglen 2017) and specifically for ovarian cancer research (Han et al. 2021; Yee et al. 2022).

Primary 2D Cultures and Organoids

The shortcomings of conventional cell lines discussed above prompted investigators to develop primary cell models of HGSC. Early efforts used 2D cultures of human or mouse fallopian tube epithelial (FTE) cells (the primary cell-of-origin for HGSC) or ovarian surface epithelium (OSE), which were transformed with large T antigen or human telomerase reverse transcriptase (hTERT), followed by the introduction of other HGSC genetic defects. For example, Karst et al. (2011) immortalized primary FTE cells with hTERT, depleted *TP53* using shRNA, and expressed an activated mutant of CDK4 (R24X) to inhibit the retinoblastoma protein (RB) pathway. Subsequent depletion of PP2A and MYC overexpression conferred tumorigenicity. These early studies showed that transformation of FTE cells could result in HGSC, providing important evidence in support of the "FTE cell-of-origin model." However, the specific genetic manipulations used are not common in bona fide HGSC, limiting the relevance of this model.

Ince et al. (2015) formulated a complex, serum-free, chemically defined media, termed "OCMI," which they used to isolate and characterize 25 new ovarian cancer lines. These lines retained the histopathology, molecular profiles (gene and protein expression), and genomic landscape of the cognate primary tumors. At least five (and possibly seven) of the lines they derived are likely HGSC based on mutation status and gene and protein expression data. Nelson et al. (2020) subsequently used OCMI to establish a "living biobank" of ex vivo ovarian cancer cultures from 76 primary tumors and ascites samples. These authors concluded that such cultures can be obtained "routinely," although long-term cultures were generated from only 76/290 samples attempted (26%), a much lower frequency than reported by Ince et al. Of the 76 cultures established, Nelson et al. characterized 15 in detail, 10 from HGSC cases. These expressed standard HGSC markers (PAX8, WT1), had *TP53* mutations, exhibited extensive chromosomal instability (CIN), and retained drug responses like their cognate parental tumors. OCMI media is now commercially available, which will allow its utility to be tested more broadly.

More recently, 3D organoid systems have been developed both to culture primary HGSC cells and to engineer HGSC from normal FTE organoids by introducing relevant genetic defects. Organoids are self-organized 3D tissue mimics, often generated from tissue stem cells, which can recreate aspects of the early structural and functional complexity of an organ in the Petri dish (Fig. 1, middle panel, top). Methods to embed primary cells or cell lines in artificial or tumor-derived ECM have been around since the 1980s (Kleinman et al. 1986), but widespread application of these models to cancer research is relatively new, with most advances occurring in the last decade. Typically, single cells or small tissue explants are suspended within a biological scaffold, such as Matrigel or hydrogels (discussed below). Matrigel is an ECM preparation from the Engelbreth–Holm–Swarm (EHS) mouse sarcoma, first described in 1977 (Orkin et al. 1977), which contains a variety of ECM proteins including laminins, collagen IV, entactin, proteoglycans, and others. As noted above, these proteins are more faithful mimics of tumor ECM and have more realistic stiffness compared with plastic. However, the elastic modulus (a measure of stiffness) of Matrigel is ~400–800 Pa while that of HGSCs range from 30 to 80 kPa (Azzalini et al. 2021). Because Matrigel is a biomaterial, it can, at least theoretically, show batch-to-batch variability. While this might have been an issue with earlier batches, in our experience modern commercial preparations deliver highly reproducible results. Once suspended in this scaffold, cells grow, differentiate, and undergo at least some degree of morphogenesis; over time (days to weeks), a "mature" organoid develops, reproducing aspects of the tissue from which it derives (Clevers 2016; Neal and Kuo 2016; Neal et al. 2018). Organoids from tumors, sometimes termed "tumoroids," can develop hypoxic or even necrotic cores, recapitulating an important aspect of tumor biology (see above).

Kessler et al. (2015) established the first long-term 3D organoid cultures of normal human FTE. These structures reproduced the native epithelial architecture (folded cysts) of the FT, differentiated into secretory and ciliated cells from single EPCAM+ FTE stem cells, and could be maintained in culture for over 10 months. WNT and NOTCH signaling were found to be essential regulators of stemness and differentiation: WNT/RSPO1 supported expansion and self-renewal of FTE stem cells, whereas NOTCH inhibited ciliogenesis and helped maintain stemness markers. Epidermal growth factor (EGF) and R-spondin 1 (RSPO1) increased sphere number and size; fibroblast growth factor 10 (FGF10) enhanced proliferation; and bone morphogenetic protein (BMP) and TGF-β inhibition was required for long-term expansion. FTE organoids also responded to estradiol and progesterone, reproducing the gene expression changes associated with the menstrual cycle.

The Clevers laboratory subsequently adapted these conditions to reproducibly culture human HGSC organoids (Kopper et al. 2019). They established 56 organoid lines from 32 patients (overall success rate ~65%) with examples of all major OC subtypes, including 17 HGSCs. These cultures maintained the histological, morphological, genomic (CNVs, mutations, and gene expression) and drug sensitivity profiles of the original tumors. They could be genetically manipulated (e.g., by using lentiviral transduction and/or CRISPR-Cas9), deployed for high-throughput drug screening, and used to initiate xenografts in immune-incompetent mice. Similar studies were published shortly thereafter by de Witte et al. (2020) who, in addition to testing standard chemotherapies, used their platform to assess other targeted agents.

In parallel, Zhang et al. (2019) developed conditions for culturing OSE and FTE organoids from normal mice as well as mice induced to delete *Trp53* and express a fragment of large T antigen (T121) that inhibits all "RB pocket proteins" (RB, P107, P130, and P300). They found that OSE and FTE each could give rise to HGSC, although with different growth properties and drug response. They, and several other groups, subsequently used FTE and/or OSE organoids to engineer HGSC with defined genetic defects seen in the human disease. For example, Lõhmussaar et al. (2020) used gene editing on mouse FTE and OSE cells to analyze the importance of the cell-of-origin, as well as genotype, on HGSC properties such as drug sensitivity, tissue differentiation, and tumorigenicity. They confirmed and extended the findings of Zhang et al. that both cell types could give rise to HGSC (as indicated by morphology and molecular markers) when engineered with genetic abnormalities seen in the human disease (e.g., *Trp53; Brca1;Pten* and *Trp53;Brca1;Nf1*). Also, like Zhang et al., they found that FTE-derived tumors typically grew more rapidly in vitro and in mice and were more sensitive to several standard-of-care ovarian cancer drugs. Similar observations were reported later by Galhenage et al. (2023), who used organoids to identify differences in the response of FTE and OSE to replication stress.

Zhang et al. and Iyer et al. took a similar approach to Lõhmussaar et al., using a combination of CRISPR-Cas9-mediated deletion and lentiviral/retroviral overexpression to engineer mouse FTE with several combinations of genetic defects seen in HGSC (Iyer et al. 2021; Zhang et al. 2021). However, these groups used C57Bl6 mice as the source of FTE, which enabled them to monitor organoid-induced tumorigenesis in a syngeneic, immune competent background. Exploiting this system, they observed genotype-dependent differences in sensitivity to chemotherapy, cytokine/chemokine production (secretome), gene expression profiles, TME composition, and response of tumors to combinations of chemotherapy and checkpoint inhibitor agents.

Overall, organoid models of HGSC show great potential for improving our understanding of the disease and developing more effective treatments. However, more research is needed to fully realize the potential of these models and translate their findings into clinical practice. Indeed, as we outline in more detail in the Next-Generation Models section of this work, while organoids are an upgrade compared to traditional 2D cultures, they still do not fully capture the intricacy and diversity of the in vivo microenvironment.

In Vivo Models

In vivo models enable HGSC biology to be studied in the whole organism setting. As for most malignancies, syngeneic models, genetically engineered mouse models (GEMMs) and CDXs/patient-derived xenografts (PDXs) of HGSC have been developed (Fig. 1, bottom panel). Other, less commonly used models also exist, including spontaneous HGSC in hyperovulating chickens (Hawkridge 2014; Paris et al. 2021), and more recently, direct electroporation of mouse FTE with overexpression and gene-editing constructs (Ford and Yamanaka 2022). Studies of in vivo models have provided important insights into the molecular and genetic drivers of HGSC, as well as the role of the TME in the development, progression, and treatment of the disease.

In principle, a major advantage of in vivo models is that they can be used to study the effects of treatments on the whole organism, potentially yielding a better idea of how drugs will perform in patients. Cancer cells interact with many other (normal) cells, both in the TME and in distant organs. Most drugs affect one or more of these normal cell populations in addition to their effects on the cancer cells themselves (drugs targeted against cancer-specific mutations, e.g., the recently developed mutation-specific KRAS inhibitors are an exception, but such mutations are rare in HGSC). It is difficult to predict from in vitro studies alone how drug effects on cancer and normal cells will interact or to model the pharmacokinetic properties of new agents. Despite the potential benefits of in vivo models, mice are not humans, so comparisons will always be imperfect and occasionally misleading. Below, we summarize current in vivo models of HGSC; for more details, readers are advised to consult the primary references.

Syngeneic Models

The most commonly used syngeneic model, ID8, has been around for decades (Roby et al. 2000). This model was generated by serial-passaging of mouse OSE cells until malignant transformation occurred. ID8 cells and their various derivatives generate tumors rapidly upon injection into the mouse ovarian bursa or peritoneum, but in our view, the relevance of this model is highly questionable. OSE, if it is a cell-of-origin for human HGSC, is a much rarer one than

FTE. Equally troubling, ID8 cells are *Trp53* wild-type; as noted above, *TP53* aberration is the molecular sine qua non of HGSC. Researchers have generated ID8 derivatives with *Trp53* deletion and/or bearing alterations of other relevant oncogenes/tumor suppressor genes (Walton et al. 2017). However, malignant cells with additional oncogenic abnormalities introduced are unlikely to have similar properties to tumors initially arising with/from these abnormalities. To put it bluntly, it is difficult to believe that much relevant information about *HGSC* can be deduced from studying tumors arising in the wrong cell-of-origin and lacking the genetic abnormalities seen in the bona fide disease. Nevertheless (and disappointingly, in our view), this model continues to be used, particularly for studies of the HGSC immune response and immune therapies.

Genetically Engineered Models in Mice

Two general types of mouse model have been developed by introducing HGSC-associated genetic defects into FTE or other cell types. Conventional "GEMMs" typically have conditional (lox–stop–lox [LSL]) deletion alleles and/or transgenes driving overexpression of genes amplified in HGSC. Deletion/overexpression is controlled by specific promoters/enhancers that drive Cre recombinase (Cre) expression. Alternatively, as noted above, new syngeneic mouse models have been developed by genetically engineering mouse FTE (or in some cases, OSE) organoids with appropriate disease genes in vitro, followed by implantation into the ovarian bursa. Each type of approach has strengths and weaknesses. GEMMs allow earlier stages of oncogenesis/tumor evolution to be studied in the autochthonous site; engineered cell/injection models cannot provide such information. On the other hand, GEMMs typically suffer from a field effect, wherein all (or most) cells targeted by the Cre driver instantaneously are exposed to deletion of one or more tumor suppressor(s) and/or overexpression of one or more oncogene(s). In contrast, the genetic changes in HGSC (in women) develop sequentially from a(n) initially small number of cells that have undergone these changes. Engineered cell models have the advantage of enabling multiple combinations of genetic defects to be generated rapidly; in contrast, there are relatively few HGSC GEMMs, limiting analyses to a more restricted combination of genetic defects. Notably, conventional GEMMs for studying *CCNE1*-driven disease have not been reported, precluding studies of this fairly common (~20% of HGSC overall) resistant or refractory subgroup.

The first bona fide HGSC GEMM was generated by the Drapkin laboratory using *Pax8 rtTA TetO-Cre* to direct *Trp53* deletion or expression of a *Trp53* gain-of-function mutant (R270H), along with deletion of *Brca1/2* and/or *Pten* (Perets et al. 2013). Lineage tracing confirmed that the *Pax8* promoter/enhancer construct directed expression to FT secretory epithelium, but not OSE, and resulted in several foundational findings. First, it established that FT secretory epithelium could be a cell-of-origin for HGSC. Moreover, HGSC developed via serous tubular intraepithelial carcinoma (STIC) intermediates, as had been proposed based on earlier histological examinations of co-occurring lesions in HGSC patients or in opportunistic salpingectomy patients (Vang et al. 2013; Kahn et al. 2023). Remarkably, salpingectomy was effective at preventing HGSC development in this model, providing preclinical evidence in support of now ongoing clinical trials of salpingectomy in high-risk women (Tang et al. 2025). Interestingly, *Brca1* or *Brca2* heterozygous models gave rise to HGSC, although the latency was longer for *Brca2* heterozygotes compared with homozygotes. Also, combined *Pten/Trp53* deletion resulted in tumors, although with a longer latency than that seen with combinations of all three alleles. All models generated peritoneal and ovarian metastases, and tumors developed CNAs in several chromosomal regions syntenic with human HGSC.

The above studies provided seminal insights into HGSC pathogenesis and pathobiology, but the *Pax8 rtTA TetO-Cre* driver is somewhat cumbersome and can also drive expression in other cell types that limit its ability to model certain gene combinations. For example, Zhang et al. (2019) found that using this driver to express T121 led rapidly to lethal thymomas, most likely because E2F activation is central to this tumor type. Today, the most often used promoter/enhancer driver for HGSC GEMMs is based on *Ovgp-1*, a protein secreted from FT secretory cells. Sherman-Baust et al. (2014) generated mice in which large T antigen was expressed under *Ovgp-1* control. These mice developed p53 signatures and serous tubal intraepithelial carcinomas (STICs), common precursors of ovarian neoplasms in general and HGSC in particular. Subsequent studies by the Cho laboratory used Ovgp1-iCreERT2 to inactivate combinations of tumor suppressor genes (*Brca1*, *Trp53*, *Rb1*, *Nf1*, and *Pten*), resulting in STICs that progress to HGSC or carcinosarcoma with disease features and heterogeneity similar to human HGSC (Zhai et al. 2017; McCool et al. 2020). More recently, an Ovgp1 promoter/enhancer construct driving coexpression of *Trp53R*^{270H} and *Myc* was knocked into the *Trp53* locus in the opposite orientation to the native *Trp53* gene. These mice developed tumors only after a long latency, resembling the typical age of onset of HGSC in women and establishing that *Myc* overexpression alone (in the presence of *Trp53* mutation) is sufficient to initiate HGSC in mice. These tumors also developed multiple aneuploidies, consistent with human disease. However, because the design of the targeting construct renders them global *Trp53* heterozygotes, they also develop various other malignancies, limiting the utility of this model.

Other GEMMs have less relevance to HGSC or even ovarian cancer broadly. *Ovgp1-Cre*-driven deletion of *Pten* and *Apc* leads to endometrioid ovarian carcinomas, consistent with the genetics of that subtype. Kim et al. used an anti-Mullerian hormone receptor (*Amhr*) driver to delete *Pten* and the microRNA regulator *Dicer1* (Kim et al. 2012). Although the authors reported that these mice developed HGSC arising in the FT, the tumors actually initiated in the stromal compartment, not FT secretory cells. These tumors were also *Trp53*-WT, and *DICER1* is not frequently deleted in human HGSC. In our view, while this model might provide insights into effects of DICER1 deficiency on lineage plasticity, it is unlikely to represent events that occur often in human HGSC.

Similarly difficult to interpret are models that use bursal injection of Cre-expressing adenovirus (Ad-Cre) to delete/activate genes associated with ovarian cancer. Tumors arising in such models were initially thought to originate in OSE (Flesken-Nikitin et al. 2003; Xing and Orsulic 2006; Kinross et al. 2012; Szabova et al. 2012). However, lineage-tracing experiments indicate that Ad-Cre can evoke deletion in FTE (Zhang et al. 2019), making it difficult to be sure of the cell-of-origin in such models. Further evidence of the promiscuity of Ad-Cre injection is that codeletion of *Brca1*, *Trp53*, and *Rb1* resulted in rhabdomyosarcomas rather than ovarian cancer (Clark-Knowles et al. 2009). That said, OSE-specific deletion (using *Lgr5-Cre*) of *Trp53* and expression of T121 can cause tumors that resemble HGSC, although these tumors have distinct growth properties and drug response compared with lesions initiating in HGSC (Zhang et al. 2019).

As discussed above, FTE and OSE organoids can also be engineered to exhibit specific combinations of genetic defects and implanted in the autochthonous site (Lõhmussaar et al. 2020; Maniati et al. 2020; Iyer et al. 2021; Zhang et al. 2021). This approach enables rapid assessment of multiple HGSC-associated genetic defects for their ability to evoke tumors, sculpt the TME, and affect the response to conventional, targeted, and/or immune therapies. Overall, GEMMs have been a valuable tool for advancing our understanding of HGSC biology and identifying potential therapeutic targets. Further research using GEMMs, in combination with other model systems and clinical studies, could pave the way for developing more effective treatments for this highly lethal disease.

Patient-Derived Xenografts (PDXs)

PDXs are preclinical models in which tumor cells or tissue fragments from cancer patients are transplanted into immunocompromised (usually NOD/SCID *IL2R*$\gamma^{-/-}$ [NSG], occasionally severe combined immunodeficient mice [SCID] mice) to avoid rejection (Fig. 1, bottom panel). Advantages of these models include the human origin and concomitant relevant, often complex genetics of the tumors that result, and the retention of at least some (but certainly not all) of the heterogeneity/multiclonality of the initiating tumor. PDX models for ovarian cancer were generated as early as 1977, when Davy et al. published a case report on subcutaneous (SQ) engraftment of an ovarian cancer into nude (*nu/nu*) mice (Davy et al. 1977). They used this model to test several chemotherapies and mentioned that they had generated similar grafts from 11 other patients (out of 15). Although they did not specify the subtype of these "ovarian cancers," the fact that they obtained tumors from most samples, along with the relative frequency of HGSC compared to other subtypes, makes it highly likely that at least several (if not most) of these PDXs were HGSC. Massazaa et al. (1989) subsequently established SQ and/or IP PDXs in *nu/nu* mice from four patients and tested their responses to selected chemotherapies. Later, the same group studied PDXs from the same patient at different stages of disease, observing decreased chemosensitivity in transplanted mice concomitant with decreased drug response in the patient (Masazza et al. 1991). They also performed early validation studies of taxol, which at the time still had an NSC number, on select PDXs (Nicoletti et al. 1993). Concomitantly, Fu and Hoffman (1993) established a PDX model by implanting tumor fragments under the ovarian capsule of *nu/nu* mice. For unclear reasons, these early models and techniques were not widely adapted, and CDX models were used far more extensively.

In this century, however, multiple groups have generated PDX models, analyzed the genome and transcriptome of these tumors, and in several cases, correlated drug response of the PDX to that in the patient from whom the sample was obtained (Bankert et al. 2011; Stewart et al. 2011; Topp et al. 2014; Weroha et al. 2014; Dong et al. 2016; George et al. 2017; Winder et al. 2017; Cybulska et al. 2018). Engraftment rates are generally high (~70%–100%), depending in part on the site and method of establishment (isolated tumor cells vs. tumor fragments). HGSC PDXs can be serially transplanted and are relatively stable, yielding a "living biobank" of models. Although multiple tumor subclones can be maintained in a given PDX, barcoding experiments of breast tumor xenografts revealed a significant "bottleneck" following engraftment, leading to subclone loss (Nguyen et al. 2014). The same phenomenon is likely to pertain to HGSC PDXs. Nevertheless, PDXs model the genomic and transcriptomic complexity of HGSC better than CDX models and GEMMs (Weroha et al. 2014; George et al. 2017; Cybulska et al. 2018; Chen et al. 2021). These advantages are offset by the lack of an immune system in recipient mice, a significant deficiency when immune therapies have emerged as ever more important in the clinic. Consequently, various attempts have been made to "humanize" mice to overcome this deficiency and are discussed in the Next-Generation Models section below.

A major use of PDXs has been for preclinical testing of conventional and new therapies. Several studies have shown that the drug sensitivities of PDX or CDX models usually recapitulate that of the parental tumors (Topp et al. 2014; Weroha et al. 2014; George et al. 2017; Liu et al. 2017; Cybulska et al. 2018) making them valuable platforms for drug development. For example, PDX and CDX models have validated the utility of the PARPi niraparib (AlHilli et al. 2016) and olaparib (Kortmann et al. 2011) for HR-defective disease. Kortmann et al. provided an early proof-of-concept for this approach by showing that olaparib markedly inhibited tumor growth in a *BRCA2*-mutated, but not a *BRCA2*-WT HGSC PDX—mirroring the synthetic lethality seen in vitro and in patients. Likewise, AlHilli et al. showed that *BRCA2*-mutated HGSC PDXs responded better to niraparib, but that this effect was only observed for maintenance therapy, with little effect seen in conjunction with carboplatin/paclitaxel chemotherapy. They also pointed to a need for better determination of HRD status, as simple methods (e.g., RAD51 foci) could not predict response. George et al. subsequently established 14 *BRCA*-deficient HGSC PDXs to test HR-targeted therapies. These investigators tested multiple agents, finding that single-agent PARPi, CHK1 inhibitor (CHK1i), and ATR inhibitor each suppressed PDX growth, while combinations enhanced efficacy. Parmar et al. (2019) subsequently found that prexasertib, a CHKi, had monotherapy activity in PARP-resistant PDXs and sensitized them to PARP inhibition. "Luciferized" versions of PDXs have been generated, enabling drug response to be monitored and quantified by bioluminescent imaging (Liu et al. 2017). In addition, PDX models have been used to study mechanisms of resistance and the transcriptomes of resistant cells remaining after chemotherapy (Dobbin et al. 2014).

PDXs can also be used to identify predictive biomarkers of treatment response. For example, the Brugge laboratory used a combined proteomic/computational analysis to identify apoptosis family proteins that predict sensitivity or resistance to phosphoinositide 3-kinase (PI3K)/mammalian target of rapamycin (mTOR) inhibition (Muranen et al. 2012) or mitogen-activated protein kinase kinase (MEK) and B-cell lymphoma 2 (BCL2)/extra large (XL) inhibition (Iavarone et al. 2019). Palmer et al. treated 29 HGSC PDXs with 21 single agents or drug combinations and correlated RNA-seq with tumor response (Palmer et al. 2020). They identified USP51, a deubiquitylase recruited to chromatin after DNA damage that regulates the dynamic assembly/disassembly of TP53BP1 and BRCA1, as a PARP sensitizer. The same analysis revealed that the multidrug efflux pump ABCG2 protects *HGSC* cells from MEK inhibitors.

A major consideration when using PDX and CDX models is where to engraft the tumor. Three major engraftment sites have been used most frequently: SQ, orthotopic (ovarian bursa), and intraperitoneal (IP). Some earlier studies used alternative sites, including the subrenal capsule (Lee et al. 2005) or the mammary fat pad (Stewart et al. 2011), but these have largely been abandoned in more recent work. As discussed previously, the microenvironment of the engraftment site can profoundly affect tumor biology (Shaw et al. 2004; Mitra et al. 2015; Hernandez et al. 2016). For example, Shaw et al. investigated differences between orthotopic and IP engraftment sites. While tumor histology was independent of injection site, they did observe site-specific differences in tumor initiation and growth. Similarly, Mitra et al. injected several classical HGSC lines into *nu*/*nu* mice, either SQ or IP. They found that OVKATE and COV362 only formed tumors SQ, a surprising result considering both lines arose from metastases. A more complete study by Hernandez et al. analyzed the growth rate and gene expression of tumors generated by several classical HGSC lines following SQ, IP, and intrabursal injections into *nu*/*nu* mice. They noted a clear difference in growth kinetics depending on the injection site and cell line tested, with lines that had a more "primary tumor site" gene expression pattern showing preference for IP growth. These authors also showed that expression of specific genes could predict which engraftment site would show higher tumor growth. For example, *CGN* (involved in tight junction formation) was downregulated, while *NR2F2* and *DEAF1* (both transcriptional regulators) were overexpressed, in tumors that grew well SQ. In contrast, *MSRB3* (involved in ROS response) and *MUC1* (encoding the precursor of a mucin) were upregulated in tumors that grew well IP. Curiously, the authors did not provide gene expression data for the intrabursal site but did note major differences in tumor engraftment success as well as growth kinetics depending on cell line. Together, these studies establish the importance of considering the injection site used when evaluating the results of different PDX studies.

Historically, many researchers prefer SQ injection, which technically is the easiest to perform, requires a relatively small number of cells, and gives rise to tumors reliably and quickly. Moreover, SQ tumors often remain localized at the injection site, making it easier to monitor tumor growth and subsequently acquire samples for molecular analysis. Although SQ tumors can be a good method for investigating tumor initiation and response to simple/initial drug regimens, their poor vascularization and "improper" anatomical location are important drawbacks. Orthotopic injections are more biologically relevant, as they place tumor cells in the "correct" environment. However, this approach requires a higher degree of technical aptitude and is more time and resource consuming. The injection site (i.e., the ovary and encapsulating fat pad) can vary in size and disposition between recipient mice due to differences in age, diet, or even oestrus cycle status, and dissemination of tumor cells can be difficult to contain locally. Accurate quantification of PDX growth and dissemination also becomes more complicated, requiring introduction of fluorescent or bioluminescence proteins, such as luciferase. While not particularly problematic in immune-compromised mice, these proteins can be immunogenic, a detail to be considered when using syngeneic models. To study metastatic dissemination, researchers often use IP injections, which can result in tumors that invade the peritoneum, diaphragm, spleen, and/or liver and generate ascites, although sites can vary substantially between animals. IP injections are also easy to master and perform, another advantage of the technique.

PDX models have several intrinsic limitations. While these models are generally stable upon serial passage, stability is not absolute. Dong et al. (2016) propagated nine patient-derived HGSC PDXs through >200 mice (up to four passages). Although tumor histology and most marker expression were retained, PDXs tended to lose hormone receptor gene expression upon passage. Another group also observed differences in gene expression profiles, which they attributed to stromal components, in paired analyses of PDXs and their parent tumors (Liu et al. 2019). This finding is in line with a previous report, which pointed to mouse-specific evolution of human-derived tumors, an important factor to consider when performing serial in vivo experiments (Ben-David et al. 2017).

The main limitation of PDXs, however, is their lack of an immune system. Not surprisingly, Dong et al. (2016) observed altered immune-related gene expression in their serially passaged PDXs, undoubtedly due to the murine host environment. Similarly, transcriptomic profiling demonstrated that HGSC PDXs recapitulate three of the four molecular subtypes in TCGA (differentiated, mesenchymal, and proliferative) but lack the "immunoreactive" signature (Cybulska et al. 2018). While recent years have seen some progress in generating "humanized" mice (i.e., immunodeficient mice which have human immune cells), these models remain far from reproducing the human immune system with high fidelity (for review, see Yin et al. 2020). Notably, only ~70% of cytokines/chemokines/growth factors and their receptors cross-react in mice and humans, so full "humanization" is simply not possible. We briefly discuss humanization efforts for HGSC PDXs below in the Next-Generation Models section of this review.

Overall, PDX models of *HGSC* have proven to be a valuable preclinical tool for studying the biology of ovarian cancer and for testing potential therapies. However, they should be used in conjunction with other preclinical models and clinical trials to validate their findings.

Next-Generation Models

The models discussed above each have several strengths but also serious deficiencies. Next-generation models aim to bridge these gaps by better reproducing the complex cellular heterogeneity and genomic diversity, 3D structure, and TME of HGSC. In this section, we discuss humanized PDXs, tumor slices/explants, organotypic cultures including newer 3D methods such as organoid cocultures, and organ-on-a-chip devices.

Humanized PDXs

Even some early attempts to generate PDX models aimed to conserve elements of the HGSC TME in mice. For example, Bankert et al. (2011) injected "tumor cell aggregates," which included cancer cells and tumor-associated lymphocytes and fibroblasts, into the peritoneum of NSG mice. They noted slowly developing tumors that ultimately metastasized widely (including to the lung) but retained tumor-associated lymphocytes and fibroblasts. The same group later reported that this model could be used to study the response to chemotherapy, tumor vasculature, and the molecular basis of tumor-associated immune suppression (Yokota et al. 2013). It is not clear why other groups have not seen preservation of human cell types beyond cancer cells in their PDX models; perhaps the precise method of preparation of the aggregates is critical.

More recently, attempts were made to either inject autologous or heterologous T cells into PDX-bearing NSG mice and/or to reconstitute elements of human bone marrow (BM) in these mice followed by PDX establishment. Odunsi et al. (2020) reported that ex vivo expanded autologous tumor infiltrating lymphocytes, combined with dual immune checkpoint blockade (ICB) by anti-CTLA4 and anti-PD1, slowed the growth of two PDX models in NSG mice; however, responses were transient (Adekunle et al. 2020). They performed similar studies with expanded autologous T cells from ascites transferred into NSG mice that had been crossed to HLA-A02 transgenic NSG-derived mice that coexpress interleukin 3 (IL3), colony stimulating factor 2 (CSF2), and KIT ligand (KL) under the control of the cytomegalovirus (CMV) promoter (N-HSGM3 mice). In such mice, transferring T cells alone led to a significant antitumor effect, and survival was prolonged upon dual ICB. Nonexpanded ascites T cells were even more efficacious, particularly when combined with ICB, eradicating tumors in one PDX model. Furthermore, 2/3 of these mice resisted rechallenge with parental tumor for >50 days, although progression eventually occurred. Transcriptome profiling implicated alterations in antigen processing and ECM pathways in resistance.

Kleinmanns et al. (2022) transplanted NSG mice and NSG mice expressing IL3, granulocyte macrophage (GM)-CSF, and KL (NSGS mice) with $CD34^+$ cord blood cells. The NSG recipients had more B cells, better erythroid cell production, but lower T cells than the NSGS model, which also showed more granulocytic myeloid-derived suppressor cells. The authors established one orthotopic CDX and two PDX models by bursal injection into successfully engrafted mice. Although no attempt was made to match the MHC of the tumor and the BM-recipient mice, tumor growth was the same in parental or immune reconstituted animals. Treatment with anti-PD1 antibody led to decreased tumor burden but no improvement in survival.

Steinkamp et al. (2023) established three PDX models in NSG mice with defective Kit alleles (NBSGW mice) engrafted with human $CD34^+$ cord blood cells. Interestingly, PDX-bearing mice had a much higher percentage of myeloid cells in their peripheral blood than tumor-free controls; ascites from PDX-bearing mice also had high levels of human-derived myeloid cells. Differential cytokine production correlated with variable infiltration of PDXs by different lymphohematopoietic cell subsets. The authors observed high levels of tumor-derived macrophage colony-stimulating factor (MCSF) and GM-CSF, and the cytokine profiles of ascites from the PDXs resembled those of HGSC patients. Notably, PDXs maintained in NBSGW mice had shorter survival than those in NSG mice, although tumor masses were also smaller. Earlier deaths in NBSGW mice were due to bowel obstructions and/or excessive ascites production.

Taken together, these studies indicate that newer types of humanized mice can more faithfully reproduce the human HGSC TME and might provide improved platforms for testing immune therapies. However, these models remain cumbersome and expensive, limiting the size and number of studies that can be performed on academic laboratory budgets. Future progress will require a consensus on which models are best (and likely, further improvement of these models) and lower prices, funding subsidies, or the availability of centralized repositories (e.g., run by government or private agencies) at reasonable costs.

Slice Cultures/Explants

Tumor slices/explant cultures, in principle, have the advantage of maintaining the cellular composition and architecture of the original tumor, at least for some period. For example, Ricciardelli et al. (2018) developed an explant assay using gelatin sponges that maintained an intact TME for 5 days. They found that chemosensitive/chemoresistant tumors exhibited similar drug sensitivities in explants. More recent studies have reported techniques that substantially extend explant viability, allowing the effects of interventions to be observed. For example, Abreu et al. (2020) maintained explants from 25 ovarian tumors, including 12 HGSCs, in agitation-based cultures (using an orbital shaker) for at least 30 days. During this time, cellular composition, proliferation, apoptosis, biomarker (CA125, WT1, and PAX8), and metabolic activity remained largely constant, although there was initial sloughing of an outer "dead layer" of the explants. Remarkably, the authors also observed consistent levels of multiple immune cell types, including CD4 and CD8 T cells, B cells, and myeloid cells, although these were assessed only by immunostaining rather than more quantitative methods (e.g., flow cytometry). Finally, they were able to deliver two cycles of carboplatin or paclitaxel and see responses, although they did not indicate whether these responses correlated with those of the parental tumor. Subsequent work by the same group used LC-MS to analyze explants from eight HGSC patients and identify potential metabolic biomarkers of high and low and nonresponding slice cultures to carboplatin/paclitaxel therapy (Mendes et al. 2022).

Even more recently, Laforêts et al. (2023) used time-lapse imaging to monitor cell motility in mouse and human HGSC explants treated with various agents. They identified distinct patterns of movement of resident T cells and macrophages, which could be modulated by various treatments (e.g., Toll-like receptor 4 [TLR4] agonists). They also observed that T-cell motility was reduced in explants prepared from chemotherapy-naive and treated mouse HGSC. These results expand the range of phenotypes that can be monitored in slices, which in turn could suggest future mechanistic investigations.

Organotypic Cultures

The use of organotypic cultures for studying ovarian cancer is hardly new: as early as 1985, Niedbala et al. used human mesothelial cells grown on bovine corneal endothelial cell–derived ECM to study the attachment of ovarian cancer cells in ascites, concluding that these cells attached preferentially to ECM (Niedbala et al. 1985). Two years later, they used the same system to study collagen I degradation (Niedbala et al. 1987). Other groups soon joined in. Kanemoto et al. (1991) studied OVCAR-3 adhesion, penetration, and colony formation on a range of ECM extracts, noting that adhesion was affected by laminin or fibronectin mimics. This result was complemented by the studies from the Skubitz laboratory, which reported that anti-β1-integrin antibody blocks ovarian cancer spheroid adhesion to collagen IV and laminin (Casey et al. 2001). Kishikawa et al. (1995) used a primary omental mesothelial monolayer cell culture to classify human ovarian cancer lines as "adhesive" or "invasive," depending on their interactions with the mesothelial monolayer. Interestingly, they showed that clear cell carcinoma lines are adhesive, while the other types, such as poorly differentiated adenocarcinoma, are invasive.

Subsequent studies have increased the complexity of organotypic models, aiming to more closely reproduce the TME. For example, Kenny et al. (2007) incorporated a third cell type, fibroblasts, into their organotypic model. They acquired mesothelial cells and fibroblasts from ovarian cancer surgeries at sites without obvious disease, encapsulated the fibroblasts in ECM, grew the mesothelial cells on top, and assessed the adhesion of a battery of ovarian cancer cell lines. The results indicated that mesothelial cells could serve as a protective barrier against dissemination within the omental space. The same group used this platform in a subsequent study, which showed how initial metastatic spread in the omentum is enabled by matrix metallopeptidase 2 (MMP-2) cleavage of fibronectin and vitronectin (Kenny et al. 2008).

More recently, Malacrida et al. (2021) created "tetra-cultures," which contain primary human mesothelial, fibroblast, and adipocyte cells and HGSC cell lines. The adipocytes were embedded in a type I collagen matrix and deposited at the bottom of a cell culture well. Fibroblasts were seeded on top, followed by omental mesothelial cells. This "triculture" recapitulated elements of the normal omentum and could be maintained for at least 21 days. To simulate omental metastases, AOCS1 and G164 cells were seeded at low density onto the triculture. The resultant "tetraculture" was transcriptionally similar to healthy (without HGSC cells) and diseased (with HGSC) tissue. Based on studies showing that activated platelets are associated with poor prognosis in HGSC (Stone et al. 2012), Malacrida et al. tested the effects of adding human platelets to these cultures. HGSC cells grew faster and were more invasive; RNA-seq revealed upregulation of ECM genes, and confocal imaging showed fibronectin 1 and versican deposits near HGSC colonies. Intriguingly, EMT and ECM genes were induced both in cancer and mesothelial cells, presumably combining to promote invasion. This system can also be used in "order-of-addition" experiments: mesothelial cells were cocultured with platelets, which were then removed before HGSC cells were added. Remarkably, the increased growth/invasive phenotype seen in the complete culture was recapitulated.

Even more recently, Estermann et al. (2023) layered five cell types (immortalized mesothelial, fibroblast, monocyte, and endothelial cells, plus primary, patient-derived adipocytes) into plastic inserts (Fig. 1, middle panel left). Adipocytes were seeded above a basement layer of endothelial cells, on top of which fibroblasts embedded in a collagen matrix were deposited, before mesothelial cells were added. Deposition of alginate-encapsulated macrophage spheroids in the subendothelial space resulted in "milky spots," a common feature of the omentum thought to promote metastatic niches (Clark et al. 2013). When OVCAR8 cells were seeded into this model, they showed limited invasion despite MMP9 upregulation. In contrast, patient-derived tumor cells were invasive, but unfortunately the scope of this largely "proof-of-concept" study was limited to these descriptive observations. Regardless, and despite its limitations (e.g., use of immortalized cells, "wrong" ECM stiffness compared to bona fide *HGSC*, use of alginate spheroids, which limit macrophage dissemination), the ambitiousness of this study is commendable, and it paves way for even more complex models. Indeed, in perhaps the apotheosis of organotypic cultures, Crawford et al. (2024) just reported the creation of human Fallopian tube "assembloids," which recreate the complex 3D organization and function of this organ. Although not an HGSC model per se, this approach has obvious potential utility for future studies of HGSC development.

Organotypic models will likely play an increasingly important role in ovarian cancer research. Future studies should aim to incorporate immune cells into these cultures. In this context, Calvin Kuo's group has created organotypic models for other malignancies that maintain the diversity of the TME for prolonged periods (Neal et al. 2018). Interestingly, in much earlier studies, Ronny Drapkin and coworkers used "organotypic"-inspired culture systems to investigate the cell-of-origin of HGSC (Levanon et al. 2010). Healthy patient samples of FT fimbria were dissociated and placed in air–liquid interface culture on top of a Transwell insert. This model could be maintained for almost a month and effectively reproduced the heterogeneity of FTE, its polarity, secretome, and response to wounding. They also used the model to evaluate differences between the response of secretory and ciliated cells to DNA damage, revealing important differences that may help explain the predisposition of the former to neoplastic transformation.

Additional applications of air–liquid culture methods to study HGSC biology have not been reported. Notably, the Kuo group, together with Mark Davis's laboratory, also developed "artificial lymph nodes" (Wagar et al. 2021). If combined with organotypic cultures containing immune cells, more complex immune processes such as cross priming, which are essential to the antitumor immune response, could become amenable to detailed interrogation.

The increasing use of 3D organoid models is also leading to innovations aimed at more faithfully mimicking in vivo conditions. One area of active research is the development of alternative scaffolds. As discussed above, Matrigel is the most widely available and used commercial hydrogel for organoid culture. As a biomaterial, Matrigel is relatively resistant to modification/perturbation. However, advances in polymer chemistry have given investigators a wealth of synthetic hydrogel alternatives. Researchers can select among different building blocks (e.g., polysaccharides [Xu et al. 2014; Kletzmayr et al. 2020], peptide–proteins [Hedegaard et al.

2020], and polyethylene glycol [PEG] [Zhang et al. 2013; Zhou et al. 2020]), which can be functionalized further using appropriate chemistry to deliver scaffolds with tailored properties (e.g., porosity, stiffness, cleavability, controlled delivery of drugs/growth factors). For more details, we recommend a recent review by Sievers et al. (2023).

Although these innovations are being implemented for organotypic cultures in general, applications to HGSC research have largely been limited to proof-of-concept studies aimed at replacing Matrigel. For example, Brooks et al. (2019) developed an omentum-inspired PEG-maleimide polymer decorated with omentum-specific integrin-binding peptides. They also modulated matrix degradability by integrating a pan-matrix metalloproteinase peptide linker that allows *HGSC* cells to tether to the matrix via tissue-appropriate binding and degrade it to facilitate growth. *HGSC* cells embedded in this matrix more faithfully recapitulate in vivo drug sensitivities, as well as how tumor cells produce their own ECM proteins to promote drug resistance (compared to those in Matrigel). Unfortunately, the study was too limited in scope to fully characterize the mechanistic basis of these phenomena.

Compared to decellularized ECMs, synthetic hydrogels have greater flexibility, but they also require fabrication capabilities beyond those of most academic laboratories. Commercial options exist, but they are expensive and not yet sufficiently widespread to be competitive with Matrigel. Decellularized ECM protein extracts are much easier to use, and indeed, several recent publications have demonstrated the potential of omental extracts to better mimic tumor conditions. For example, Neilson et al. (2023) described "OmGel," a patient-derived omentum hydrogel whose fabrication is similar to Matrigel. Obtained from omentum removed during debulking surgery from patients who had received neoadjuvant therapy, OmGel shows up to 80% similarity in protein composition (by mass spectrometry) between patients. Although OmGel is composed of only 10% matrisome proteins (the rest being other proteins and/or components) compared with 60% in Matrigel, it has a more diverse protein composition, containing 150 matrisome components compared with <80 in the latter. It is not clear whether/how much the neoadjuvant chemotherapy influences the composition of OmGel (or whether it is essential for its properties). However, comporting with the high vascularity of the omentum, blood proteins constitute ~40% of protein content in OmGel compared with 20% in Matrigel. The preparation of OmGel also includes a dialysis step, which results in the loss of growth factors and other small molecules. Perhaps most importantly, OmGel has a similar composition to omentum from metastatic HGSC patients (Pearce et al. 2018), arguing for its biological relevance as a scaffold. Interestingly, established HGSC cell lines cultured on OmGel or Matrigel have a similar phenotype. In contrast, CAFs grow faster and have a more homogeneous, spindly shape on OmGel. Transcriptomic and proteomic analysis revealed that CAFs on OmGel had a more inflammatory phenotype, compared with a more myofibroblast-like phenotype on Matrigel. These results emphasize the complexities to be considered in developing the most biomimetic culture systems.

OmGel was also used in a recent study (still in preprint at the time of writing) to generate "patient-derived immunocompetent cultures" (iPDCs) (Nagaraj et al. 2024). Tumors are subjected to mild digestion and then placed in OmGel; under these conditions, a significant proportion of the stromal cell population, including the immune compartment, remains intact. The study also found that OmGel induced faster growth of patient-derived HGSC cells than basement membrane extract (BME), another commercially available protein extract, which, like Matrigel, derives from the EHS tumor. OmGel cultures also replicated the response of treatment-naive HGSC to various drugs and enabled potential resistance mechanisms to PARPi therapy, including novel *BRCA1* mutations restoring HR proficiency or upregulated cell cycle components, to be revealed. More interestingly, capitalizing on the high-throughput capability of their platform, the authors observed patient-specific effects of ATR inhibitors (ATRi) and the combination of ATRi and ICB on tumor and immune cell viability. This short-lived (maximum 7 days with no possibility to freeze/regenerate), patient-based platform shows great promise for testing treatments, particularly immune-targeting agents, on actual patient samples and investigating underlying mechanisms of response/resistance.

"*Lab-on-a-Chip*" *Models*

"Labs-on-a-chip" (LOCs) are miniaturized devices that integrate multiple laboratory functions onto a single chip, usually a few square centimeters in size. The first LOC was developed in 1979 at Stanford as a gas chromatography system (Terry et al. 1979). But the late 1980s, with the development of microfluidics and, more importantly, microfabrication using soft lithography, marked the true onset of LOC research. Now, almost 40 years later, we are seeing its first applications to ovarian cancer research, where it is used to generate microcompartments that mimic biological compartments such as organs or vasculature.

For example, Saha et al. (2021) reported a microfluidic chip containing a "tumor compartment" and a "vascular compartment," separated by a membrane (Fig. 1, middle right panel). Platelets perfused through the chamber (to mimic the vascular system) could extravasate into the "TME," allowing the authors to assay the platelet effects on EMT, which had been reported in earlier studies (Stone et al. 2012). They found that the platelet protein glycoprotein VI, which recognizes galectin-3, is essential for extravasation into the tumor TME. This interaction was shown to be critical mediator of platelet-induced EMT, and blocking the interaction with antibodies such as revacept, a competitive antagonist of glycoprotein VI, could abrogate these interactions.

The following year, Ibrahim et al. (2022) described "Omentum-on-a-chip," a complex model that could be maintained for up to 14 days. Much like the organotypic omental cultures described above, this chip incorporates immortalized endothelial and adipocyte cells into a bovine fibrinogen matrix, which is then layered with mesothelial cells upon which cancer cells (SKOV3, OV90, or OVCAR3) are seeded. After 3 days, the endothelial and adipocyte cells form a microvasculature that mimics omentum. Lateral microchannels allow nutrient perfusion, while the superior channel, where mesothelial and cancer cells reside, functions like peritoneum. Perhaps not surprisingly, the researchers found that the complexity of vascular branching, as well as the size of the endothelial microvessels, was affected by the presence of the other cell types. All three cell types were needed to approach characteristics of in vivo peritoneal microvascular networks (i.e., branching and connectivity), further underlying how complex models more accurately reproduce real-life conditions. The three cell types were also needed to weaken mesothelial barrier function and permeability and allow tumor cells to effectively invade the mesothelial barrier. Tumor cell invasion also increased microvascular permeability, but only in the presence of conditioned media from tumor cells added to the "peritoneal channel" (i.e., media from a separate dish in which tumor cells had been cultured for over 72 h). This effect was attributed to VEGF secreted by the tumor cells by the authors but was not investigated further in this report. Finally, the authors found that adipocytes were necessary for the cancer cells to develop lipid droplets, an important energy source for metastasis. Although improvements could obviously be made, such as using primary HGSC cells instead of immortalized lines and introducing immune cells, this model is clearly promising in mimicking vascular features of the omentum. More importantly, LOCs like this one offer the clear advantage of perfusing the model, which could give insights into endocrine or lymphohematopoietic cell recruitment to tumor sites. Conceivably, even more complex models, including other cell populations such as an adaptive immune compartment (perhaps not so different from the tonsillar "lymph node" organoids developed by Kuo and Davis described above [Wagar et al. 2021]), could give researchers better systems to interrogate the immune response in HGSC.

Finally, a recent study by Joy et al. (2024) used 3D models of increasing complexity to study CAR-T-cell function (and limitations) in HGSC. The researchers first tested the effects of CAR-T cells on spheroids comprising HGSC cells from omentum grown in low-attachment wells. Under these conditions, CAR-T-cell killing was limited due to defective death receptor signaling. Remarkably, primary fibroblasts added to the spheroid cultures secreted CCL2, which activated the CAR-T cells. Killing was reduced when the spheroids were grown in a collagen matrix, as the fibroblasts then generated a dense ECM that impeded CAR-T-cell penetration. Finally, they developed a microfluidic device to simulate more realistic conditions. A central well containing a spheroid of OVCAR3 cells and fibroblasts was surrounded by endothelial cells in a fibrin gel and left to generate a microvasculature over 7 days. Then, CAR-T cells were perfused through these vessels to mimic dissemination in the omentum. Interestingly, CAR-T cells invaded and killed the cancer cells in this system. The authors noted that even this model was too simplistic, as CCL2 secreted by fibroblasts could also alter macrophage function, which is required for milky spot generation as discussed above. Nevertheless, this single study elegantly shows how systems of increasing sophistication have the capacity to reproduce and study the complex interactions that occur in HGSC patients and provide insight into how to promote CAR-T-cell killing of solid tumor cells, currently a major challenge in the immune therapy field (Posey et al. 2024; Du et al. 2025).

SUMMARY AND PERSPECTIVE

A famous saying attributed to statistician George E.P. Box (1976) holds that "all models are wrong, but some are useful." Hopefully, this review has illustrated how models for HGSC have improved dramatically in the decades after Fogh et al. (1977) developed the first 2D models of this disease. Much about even the most advanced remains "wrong" (or at least imperfect), yet we contend that these models are increasingly more useful. Interestingly, an ongoing single-center trial, OVAREX, is evaluating multiple ex vivo assays, including slice/explants, patient-derived organoids, ascites-derived spheroids, and PDXs, for their ability to identify biomarkers of response to conventional chemotherapy and PARPi and potentially be used to direct treatment in the future (Thorel et al. 2024). The results of this trial are awaited eagerly. Furthermore, as technology advances, we can surely expect the complexity of laboratory models to continue to increase. We might soon be able to avoid animal models entirely as preclinical models increase in sophistication (at least for some applications).

ACKNOWLEDGMENTS

B.G.N. was partially supported by National Institutes of Health (NIH) grant R01 CA257507 during the writing of this review.

REFERENCES

Abreu S, Silva F, Mendes R, Mendes TF, Teixeira M, Santo VE, Boghaert ER, Félix A, Brito C. 2020. Patient-derived ovarian cancer explants: preserved viability and histopathological features in long-term agitation-based cultures. *Sci Rep* **10:** 19462. doi:10.1038/s41598-020-76291-z

Adekunle O, McGray AJR, Anthony M, Yali Z, Jianming W, Adebukola A, Cheryl E, Ruea-Yea H. 2020. Fidelity of human ovarian cancer patient-derived xenografts in a partially humanized mouse model for preclinical testing of immunotherapies. *J Immunother Cancer* **8:** e001237. doi:10.1136/jitc-2020-001237

Ahmed AA, Etemadmoghadam D, Temple J, Lynch AG, Riad M, Sharma R, Stewart C, Fereday S, Caldas C, Defazio A, et al. 2010. Driver mutations in TP53 are ubiquitous in high grade serous carcinoma of the ovary. *J Pathol* **221:** 49–56.

AlHilli MM, Becker MA, Weroha SJ, Flatten KS, Hurley RM, Harrell MI, Oberg AL, Maurer MJ, Hawthorne KM, Hou X, et al. 2016. In vivo anti-tumor activity of the PARP inhibitor niraparib in homologous recombination deficient and proficient ovarian carcinoma. *Gynecol Oncol* **143:** 379–388. doi:10.1016/j.ygyno.2016.08.328

Alley MC, Scudiero DA, Monks A, Hursey ML, Czerwinski MJ, Fine DL, Abbott BJ, Mayo JG, Shoemaker RH, Boyd MR. 1988. Feasibility of drug screening with panels of human tumor cell lines using a microculture tetrazolium assay. *Cancer Res* **48:** 589–601.

Anglesio MS, Wiegand KC, Melnyk N, Chow C, Salamanca C, Prentice LM, Senz J, Yang W, Spillman MA, Cochrane DR, et al. 2013. Type-specific cell line models for type-specific ovarian cancer research. *PLoS One* **8:** e72162. doi:10.1371/journal.pone.0072162

Azzalini E, Abdurakhmanova N, Parisse P, Bartoletti M, Canzonieri V, Stanta G, Casalis L, Bonin S. 2021. Cell-stiffness and morphological architectural patterns in clinical samples of high grade serous ovarian cancers. *Nanomedicine* **37:** 102452. doi:10.1016/j.nano.2021.102452

Bankert RB, Balu-Iyer SV, Odunsi K, Shultz LD, Kelleher RJ Jr, Barnas JL, Simpson-Abelson M, Parsons R, Yokota SJ. 2011. Humanized mouse model of ovarian cancer recapitulates patient solid tumor progression, ascites formation, and metastasis. *PLoS One* **6:** e24420. doi:10.1371/journal.pone.0024420

Bast RC, Feeney M, Lazarus H, Nadler LM, Colvin RB, Knapp RC. 1981. Reactivity of a monoclonal antibody with human ovarian carcinoma. *J Clin Invest* **68:** 1331–1337. doi:10.1172/JCI110380

Bast RC, Klug TL, John ES, Jenison E, Niloff JM, Lazarus H, Berkowitz RS, Leavitt T, Griffiths CT, Parker L, et al. 1983. A radioimmunoassay using a monoclonal antibody to monitor the course of epithelial ovarian cancer. *N Engl J Med* **309:** 883–887. doi:10.1056/NEJM198310133091503

Beaufort CM, Helmijr JCA, Piskorz AM, Hoogstraat M, Ruigrok-Ritstier K, Besselink N, Murtaza M, van IJcken WFJ, Heine AAJ, Smid M, et al. 2014. Ovarian cancer cell line panel (OCCP): clinical importance of in vitro morphological subtypes. *PLoS One* **9:** e103988. doi:10.1371/journal.pone.0103988

Ben-David U, Ha G, Tseng Y-Y, Greenwald NF, Oh C, Shih J, McFarland JM, Wong B, Boehm JS, Beroukhim R, et al. 2017. Patient-derived xenografts undergo mouse-specific tumor evolution. *Nat Genet* **49:** 1567–1575. doi:10.1038/ng.3967

Box GEP. 1976. Science and statistics. *J Am Stat Assoc* **71:** 791–799. doi:10.1080/01621459.1976.10480949

Brooks EA, Gencoglu MF, Corbett DC, Stevens KR, Peyton SR. 2019. An omentum-inspired 3D PEG hydrogel for identifying ECM-drivers of drug resistant ovarian cancer. *APL Bioeng* **3:** 026106. doi:10.1063/1.5091713

Buick RN, Pullano R, Trent JM. 1985. Comparative properties of five human ovarian adenocarcinoma cell lines. *Cancer Res* **45:** 3668–3676.

Casey RC, Burleson KM, Skubitz KM, Pambuccian SE, Oegema TR Jr, Ruff LE, Skubitz AP. 2001. Beta 1-integrins regulate the formation and adhesion of ovarian carcinoma multicellular spheroids. *Am J Pathol* **159:** 2071–2080. doi:10.1016/S0002-9440(10)63058-1

Chen J, Jin Y, Li S, Qiao C, Peng X, Li Y, Gu Y, Wang W, You Y, Yin J, et al. 2021. Patient-derived xenografts are a reliable preclinical model for the personalized treatment of epithelial ovarian cancer. *Front Oncol* **11:** 744256. doi:10.3389/fonc.2021.744256

Cheng Z, Mirza H, Ennis DP, Smith P, Morrill Gavarró L, Sokota C, Giannone G, Goranova T, Bradley T, Piskorz A, et al. 2022. The genomic landscape of early-stage ovarian high-grade serous carcinoma. *Clin Cancer Res* **28:** 2911–2922. doi:10.1158/1078-0432.CCR-21-1643

Cho S, Vashisth M, Abbas A, Majkut S, Vogel K, Xia Y, Ivanovska IL, Irianto J, Tewari M, Zhu K, et al. 2019. Mechanosensing by the lamina protects against nuclear rupture, DNA damage, and cell-cycle arrest. *Dev Cell* **49:** 920–935.e5. doi:10.1016/j.devcel.2019.04.020

Clark R, Krishnan V, Schoof M, Rodriguez I, Theriault B, Chekmareva M, Rinker-Schaeffer C. 2013. Milky spots promote ovarian cancer metastatic colonization of peritoneal adipose in experimental models. *Am J Pathol* **183:** 576–591. doi:10.1016/j.ajpath.2013.04.023

Clark-Knowles KV, Senterman MK, Collins O, Vanderhyden BC. 2009. Conditional inactivation of Brca1, p53 and Rb in mouse ovaries results in the development of leiomyosarcomas. *PLoS One* **4:** e8534. doi:10.1371/journal.pone.0008534

Clevers H. 2016. Modeling development and disease with organoids. *Cell* **165:** 1586–1597. doi:10.1016/j.cell.2016.05.082

Connelly JT, Gautrot JE, Trappmann B, Tan DW-M, Donati G, Huck WTS, Watt FM. 2010. Actin and serum response factor transduce physical cues from the microenvironment to regulate epidermal stem cell fate decisions. *Nat Cell Biol* **12:** 711–718. doi:10.1038/ncb2074

Cooper J, Giancotti FG. 2019. Integrin signaling in cancer: mechanotransduction, stemness, epithelial plasticity, and therapeutic resistance. *Cancer Cell* **35:** 347–367. doi:10.1016/j.ccell.2019.01.007

Crawford AJ, Forjaz A, Bons J, Bhorkar I, Roy T, Schell D, Queiroga V, Ren K, Kramer D, Huang W, et al. 2024. Combined assembloid modeling and 3D whole-organ mapping captures the microanatomy and function of the human fallopian tube. *Sci Adv* **10:** eadp6285. doi:10.1126/sciadv.adp6285

Cybulska P, Stewart JM, Sayad A, Virtanen C, Shaw PA, Clarke B, Stickle N, Bernardini MQ, Neel BG. 2018. A genomically characterized collection of high-grade serous ovarian cancer xenografts for preclinical testing. *Am J Pathol* **188:** 1120–1131. doi:10.1016/j.ajpath.2018.01.019

Dasgupta I, McCollum D. 2019. Control of cellular responses to mechanical cues through YAP/TAZ regulation. *J Biol Chem* **294:** 17693–17706. doi:10.1074/jbc.REV119.007963

Davy M, Mossige J, Johannessen JV. 1977. Heterologous growth of human ovarian cancer. A new in vivo testing system. *Acta Obstet Gynecol Scand* **56:** 55–59. doi:10.3109/00016347709158340

Devor L, Bender. 2021. ES-2 ovarian cancer cells present a genomic profile inconsistent with their reported history. *Obstet Gynecol Res* **4:** 233–238.

de Witte CJ, Espejo Valle-Inclan J, Hami N, Lõhmussaar K, Kopper O, Vreuls CPH, Jonges GN, van Diest P, Nguyen L, Clevers H, et al. 2020. Patient-derived ovarian cancer organoids mimic clinical response and exhibit heterogeneous inter- and intrapatient drug responses. *Cell Rep* **31:** 107762. doi:10.1016/j.celrep.2020.107762

Dobbin ZC, Katre AA, Steg AD, Erickson BK, Shah MM, Alvarez RD, Conner MG, Schneider D, Chen D, Landen CN. 2014. Using heterogeneity of the patient-derived xenograft model to identify the chemoresistant population in ovarian cancer. *Oncotarget* **5:** 8750–8764. doi:10.18632/oncotarget.2373

Domcke S, Sinha R, Levine DA, Sander C, Schultz N. 2013. Evaluating cell lines as tumour models by comparison of genomic profiles. *Nat Commun* **4:** 2126. doi:10.1038/ncomms3126

Dong R, Qiang W, Guo H, Xu X, Kim JJ, Mazar A, Kong B, Wei J-J. 2016. Histologic and molecular analysis of patient derived xenografts of high-grade serous ovarian carcinoma. *J Hematol Oncol* **9:** 92. doi:10.1186/s13045-016-0318-6

Du B, Qin J, Lin B, Zhang J, Li D, Liu M. 2025. CAR-T therapy in solid tumors. *Cancer Cell* **43:** 665–679. doi:10.1016/j.ccell.2025.03.019

Engler AJ, Sen S, Sweeney HL, Discher DE. 2006. Matrix elasticity directs stem cell lineage specification. *Cell* **126:** 677–689. doi:10.1016/j.cell.2006.06.044

Estermann M, Coelho R, Jacob F, Huang Y-L, Liang C-Y, Faia-Torres AB, Septiadi D, Drasler B, Karakocak BB, Dijkhoff IM, et al. 2023. A 3D multi-cellular tissue model of the human omentum to study the formation of ovarian cancer metastasis. *Biomaterials* **294:** 121996. doi:10.1016/j.biomaterials.2023.121996

Fang Y, Eglen RM. 2017. Three-dimensional cell cultures in drug discovery and development. *SLAS Discov* **22:** 456–472. doi:10.1177/1087057117696795

Flesken-Nikitin A, Choi KC, Eng JP, Shmidt EN, Nikitin AY. 2003. Induction of carcinogenesis by concurrent inactivation of p53 and Rb1 in the mouse ovarian surface epithelium. *Cancer Res* **63:** 3459–3463.

Fleury H, Communal L, Carmona E, Portelance L, Arcand SL, Rahimi K, Tonin PN, Provencher D, Mes-Masson AM. 2015. Novel high-grade serous epithelial ovarian cancer cell lines that reflect the molecular diversity of both the sporadic and hereditary disease. *Genes Cancer* **6:** 378–398. doi:10.18632/genesandcancer.76

Flörkemeier I, Antons LK, Weimer JP, Hedemann N, Rogmans C, Krüger S, Scherließ R, Dempfle A, Arnold N, Maass N, et al. 2024. Multicellular ovarian cancer spheroids: novel 3D model to mimic tumour complexity. *Sci Rep* **14:** 23526. doi:10.1038/s41598-024-73680-6

Fogh J, Trempe G. 1975. New human tumor cell lines. In *Human tumor cells in vitro* (ed. Fogh J), pp. 115–159. Springer, Boston.

Fogh J, Fogh JM, Orfeo T. 1977. One hundred and twenty-seven cultured human tumor cell lines producing tumors in nude mice23. *J Natl Cancer Inst* **59:** 221–226. doi:10.1093/jnci/59.1.221

Ford MJ, Yamanaka Y. 2022. Reprogramming mouse oviduct epithelial cells using in vivo electroporation and CRISPR/Cas9-mediated genetic manipulation. In *Stem cell assays: methods and protocols* (ed. Kannan N, Beer P), pp. 367–377. Springer, New York.

Fu X, Hoffman RM. 1993. Human ovarian carcinoma metastatic models constructed in nude mice by orthotopic transplantation of histologically intact patient specimens. *Anticancer Res* **13:** 283–286.

Galhenage P, Zhou Y, Perry E, Loc B, Fietz K, Iyer S, Reinhardt F, Da Silva T, Botchkarev V, Chen J, et al. 2023. Replication stress and defective checkpoints make fallopian tube epithelial cells putative drivers of high-grade serous ovarian cancer. *Cell Rep* **42:** 113144. doi:10.1016/j.celrep.2023.113144

George E, Kim H, Krepler C, Wenz B, Makvandi M, Tanyi JL, Brown E, Zhang R, Brafford P, Jean S, et al. 2017. A patient-derived-xenograft platform to study BRCA-deficient ovarian cancers. *JCI Insight* **2:** e89760. doi:10.1172/jci.insight.89760

Hamilton TC, Young RC, McKoy WM, Grotzinger KR, Green JA, Chu EW, Whang-Peng J, Rogan AM, Green WR, Ozols RF. 1983. Characterization of a human ovarian carcinoma cell line (NIH:OVCAR-3)1 with androgen and estrogen receptors. *Cancer Res* **43:** 5379–5389.

Han SJ, Kwon S, Kim KS. 2021. Challenges of applying multicellular tumor spheroids in preclinical phase. *Cancer Cell Int* **21:** 152. doi:10.1186/s12935-021-01853-8

Hawkridge AM. 2014. The chicken model of spontaneous ovarian cancer. *Proteomics Clin Appl* **8:** 689–699. doi:10.1002/prca.201300135

Hedegaard CL, Redondo-Gómez C, Tan BY, Ng KW, Loessner D, Mata A. 2020. Peptide-protein coassembling matrices as a biomimetic 3D model of ovarian cancer. *Sci Adv* **6:** eabb3298. doi:10.1126/sciadv.abb3298

Hernandez L, Kim MK, Lyle LT, Bunch KP, House CD, Ning F, Noonan AM, Annunziata CM. 2016. Characterization of ovarian cancer cell lines as in vivo models for preclinical studies. *Gynecol Oncol* **142:** 332–340. doi:10.1016/j.ygyno.2016.05.028

Hoadley KA, Yau C, Wolf DM, Cherniack AD, Tamborero D, Ng S, Leiserson MDM, Niu B, McLellan MD, Uzunangelov V, et al. 2014. Multiplatform analysis of 12 cancer types reveals molecular classification within and across tissues of origin. *Cell* **158:** 929–944. doi:10.1016/j.cell.2014.06.049

Iavarone C, Zervantonakis IK, Selfors LM, Palakurthi S, Liu JF, Drapkin R, Matulonis UA, Hallberg D, Velculescu VE, Leverson JD, et al. 2019. Combined MEK and BCL-2/X_L inhibition is effective in high-grade serous ovarian cancer patient-derived xenograft models and BIM levels are predictive of responsiveness. *Mol Cancer Ther* **18:** 642–655. doi:10.1158/1535-7163.MCT-18-0413

Ibrahim LI, Hajal C, Offeddu GS, Gillrie MR, Kamm RD. 2022. Omentum-on-a-chip: a multicellular, vascularized microfluidic model of the human peritoneum for the study of ovarian cancer metastases. *Biomaterials* **288:** 121728. doi:10.1016/j.biomaterials.2022.121728

Ikediobi ON, Davies H, Bignell G, Edkins S, Stevens C, O'Meara S, Santarius T, Avis T, Barthorpe S, Brackenbury L, et al. 2006. Mutation analysis of 24 known cancer genes in the NCI-60 cell line set. *Mol Cancer Ther* **5:** 2606–2612.

Ince TA, Sousa AD, Jones MA, Harrell JC, Agoston ES, Krohn M, Selfors LM, Liu W, Chen K, Yong M, et al. 2015. Characterization of twenty-five ovarian tumour cell lines that phenocopy primary tumours. *Nat Commun* **6:** 7419. doi:10.1038/ncomms8419

Ishihara T, Moore GE, Sandberg AA. 1962. The in vitro chromosome constitution of cells from human tumors. *Cancer Res* **22:** 375–379.

Iyer S, Zhang S, Yucel S, Horn H, Smith SG, Reinhardt F, Hoefsmit E, Assatova B, Casado J, Meinsohn M-C, et al. 2021. Genetically defined syngeneic mouse models of ovarian cancer as tools for the discovery of combination immunotherapy. *Cancer Discov* **11:** 384–407. doi:10.1158/2159-8290.CD-20-0818

Izar B, Tirosh I, Stover EH, Wakiro I, Cuoco MS, Alter I, Rodman C, Leeson R, Su M-J, Shah P, et al. 2020. A single-cell landscape of high-grade serous ovarian cancer. *Nat Med* **26:** 1271–1279. doi:10.1038/s41591-020-0926-0

Janus P, Kuś P, Jaksik R, Vydra N, Toma-Jonik A, Gramatyka M, Kurpas M, Kimmel M, Widłak W. 2024. Transcriptional responses to direct and indirect TGFB1 stimulation in cancerous and noncancerous mammary epithelial cells.

Cell Commun Signal **22:** 522. doi:10.1186/s12964-024-01821-5

Joy JD, Malacrida B, Laforêts F, Kotantaki P, Maniati E, Manchanda R, Annibaldi A, Hopkins S, Garrobo-Calleja I, Gautrot J, et al. 2024. Human 3D ovarian cancer models reveal malignant cell-intrinsic and -extrinsic factors that influence CAR T-cell activity. *Cancer Res* **84:** 2432–2449. doi:10.1158/0008-5472.CAN-23-3007

Kahn RM, Gordhandas S, Godwin K, Stone RL, Worley MJ Jr, Lu KH, Long Roche KC. 2023. Salpingectomy for the primary prevention of ovarian cancer: a systematic review. *JAMA Surg* **158:** 1204–1211. doi:10.1001/jamasurg.2023.4164

Kalli M, Poskus MD, Stylianopoulos T, Zervantonakis IK. 2023. Beyond matrix stiffness: targeting force-induced cancer drug resistance. *Trends Cancer* **9:** 937–954. doi:10.1016/j.trecan.2023.07.006

Kandoth C, McLellan MD, Vandin F, Ye K, Niu B, Lu C, Xie M, Zhang Q, McMichael JF, Wyczalkowski MA, et al. 2013. Mutational landscape and significance across 12 major cancer types. *Nature* **502:** 333–339. doi:10.1038/nature12634

Kanemoto T, Martin GR, Hamilton TC, Fridman R. 1991. Effects of synthetic peptides and protease inhibitors on the interaction of a human ovarian cancer cell line (NIH: OVCAR-3) with a reconstituted basement membrane (Matrigel). *Invasion Metastasis* **11:** 84–92.

Karst AM, Levanon K, Drapkin R. 2011. Modeling high-grade serous ovarian carcinogenesis from the fallopian tube. *Proc Natl Acad Sci* **108:** 7547–7552. doi:10.1073/pnas.1017300108

Kenny HA, Krausz T, Yamada SD, Lengyel E. 2007. Use of a novel 3D culture model to elucidate the role of mesothelial cells, fibroblasts and extra-cellular matrices on adhesion and invasion of ovarian cancer cells to the omentum. *Int J Cancer* **121:** 1463–1472. doi:10.1002/ijc.22874

Kenny HA, Kaur S, Coussens LM, Lengyel E. 2008. The initial steps of ovarian cancer cell metastasis are mediated by MMP-2 cleavage of vitronectin and fibronectin. *J Clin Invest* **118:** 1367–1379. doi:10.1172/JCI33775

Kessler M, Hoffmann K, Brinkmann V, Thieck O, Jackisch S, Toelle B, Berger H, Mollenkopf HJ, Mangler M, Sehouli J, et al. 2015. The Notch and Wnt pathways regulate stemness and differentiation in human fallopian tube organoids. *Nat Commun* **6:** 8989. doi:10.1038/ncomms9989

Kim J, Coffey DM, Creighton CJ, Yu Z, Hawkins SM, Matzuk MM. 2012. High-grade serous ovarian cancer arises from fallopian tube in a mouse model. *Proc Natl Acad Sci* **109:** 3921–3926. doi:10.1073/pnas.1117135109

Kinross KM, Montgomery KG, Kleinschmidt M, Waring P, Ivetac I, Tikoo A, Saad M, Hare L, Roh V, Mantamadiotis T, et al. 2012. An activating Pik3ca mutation coupled with Pten loss is sufficient to initiate ovarian tumorigenesis in mice. *J Clin Invest* **122:** 553–557. doi:10.1172/JCI59309

Kishikawa T, Sakamoto M, Ino Y, Kubushiro K, Nozawa S, Hirohashi S. 1995. Two distinct patterns of peritoneal involvement shown by in vitro and in vivo ovarian cancer dissemination models. *Invasion Metastasis* **15:** 11–21.

Kleinman HK, McGarvey ML, Hassell JR, Star VL, Cannon FB, Laurie GW, Martin GR. 1986. Basement membrane complexes with biological activity. *Biochemistry* **25:** 312–318. doi:10.1021/bi00350a005

Kleinmanns K, Gullaksen S-E, Bredholt G, Davidson B, Torkildsen CF, Grindheim S, Bjørge L, McCormack E. 2022. Humanized ovarian cancer patient-derived xenografts for improved preclinical evaluation of immunotherapies. *Cancers (Basel)* **14:** 3092. doi:10.3390/cancers14133092

Kletzmayr A, Clement Frey F, Zimmermann M, Eberli D, Millan C. 2020. An automatable hydrogel culture platform for evaluating efficacy of antibody-based therapeutics in overcoming chemoresistance. *Biotechnol J* **15:** 1900439. doi:10.1002/biot.201900439

Konstantinopoulos PA, Ceccaldi R, Shapiro GI, D'Andrea AD. 2015. Homologous recombination deficiency: exploiting the fundamental vulnerability of ovarian cancer. *Cancer Discov* **5:** 1137–1154. doi:10.1158/2159-8290.CD-15-0714

Kopper O, de Witte CJ, Lõhmussaar K, Valle-Inclan JE, Hami N, Kester L, Balgobind AV, Korving J, Proost N, Begthel H, et al. 2019. An organoid platform for ovarian cancer captures intra- and interpatient heterogeneity. *Nat Med* **25:** 838–849. doi:10.1038/s41591-019-0422-6

Korch C, Spillman MA, Jackson TA, Jacobsen BM, Murphy SK, Lessey BA, Jordan VC, Bradford AP. 2012. DNA profiling analysis of endometrial and ovarian cell lines reveals misidentification, redundancy and contamination. *Gynecol Oncol* **127:** 241–248. doi:10.1016/j.ygyno.2012.06.017

Kortmann U, McAlpine JN, Xue H, Guan J, Ha G, Tully S, Shafait S, Lau A, Cranston AN, O'Connor MJ, et al. 2011. Tumor growth inhibition by Olaparib in *BRCA2* germline-mutated patient-derived ovarian cancer tissue xenografts. *Clin Cancer Res* **17:** 783–791. doi:10.1158/1078-0432.CCR-10-1382

Ku JL, Park JG. 2005. Biology of SNU cell lines. *Cancer Res Treat* **37:** 1–19.

Kurman RJ. 2013. Origin and molecular pathogenesis of ovarian high-grade serous carcinoma. *Ann Oncol* **24:** x16–x21. doi:10.1093/annonc/mdt463

Laforêts F, Kotantaki P, Malacrida B, Elorbany S, Manchanda R, Donnadieu E, Balkwill F. 2023. Semi-supervised analysis of myeloid and T cell behavior in ex vivo ovarian tumor slices reveals changes in cell motility after treatments. *iScience* **26:** 106514. doi:10.1016/j.isci.2023.106514

Langland GT, Yannone SM, Langland RA, Nakao A, Guan Y, Long SB, Vonguyen L, Chen DJ, Gray JW, Chen F. 2010. Radiosensitivity profiles from a panel of ovarian cancer cell lines exhibiting genetic alterations in p53 and disparate DNA-dependent protein kinase activities. *Oncol Rep* **23:** 1021–1026.

Lau DH, Lewis AD, Ehsan MN, Sikic BI. 1991. Multifactorial mechanisms associated with broad cross-resistance of ovarian carcinoma cells selected by cyanomorpholino doxorubicin. *Cancer Res* **51:** 5181–5187.

Lee C-H, Xue H, Sutcliffe M, Gout PW, Huntsman DG, Miller DM, Gilks CB, Wang YZ. 2005. Establishment of subrenal capsule xenografts of primary human ovarian tumors in SCID mice: potential models. *Gynecol Oncol* **96:** 48–55. doi:10.1016/j.ygyno.2004.09.025

Levanon K, Ng V, Piao HY, Zhang Y, Chang MC, Roh MH, Kindelberger DW, Hirsch MS, Crum CP, Marto JA, et al. 2010. Primary ex vivo cultures of human fallopian tube epithelium as a model for serous ovarian carcinogenesis. *Oncogene* **29:** 1103–1113. doi:10.1038/onc.2009.402

Li ML, Aggeler J, Farson DA, Hatier C, Hassell J, Bissell MJ. 1987. Influence of a reconstituted basement membrane and its components on casein gene expression and secretion in mouse mammary epithelial cells. *Proc Natl Acad Sci* **84:** 136–140. doi:10.1073/pnas.84.1.136

Li S, Sampson C, Liu C, Piao HL, Liu HX. 2023. Integrin signaling in cancer: bidirectional mechanisms and therapeutic opportunities. *Cell Commun Signal* **21:** 266. doi:10.1186/s12964-023-01264-4

Liao J, Qian F, Tchabo N, Mhawech-Fauceglia P, Beck A, Qian Z, Wang X, Huss WJ, Lele SB, Morrison CD, et al. 2014. Ovarian cancer spheroid cells with stem cell-like properties contribute to tumor generation, metastasis and chemotherapy resistance through hypoxia-resistant metabolism. *PLoS One* **9:** e84941.

Liu JF, Palakurthi S, Zeng Q, Zhou S, Ivanova E, Huang W, Zervantonakis IK, Selfors LM, Shen Y, Pritchard CC, et al. 2017. Establishment of patient-derived tumor xenograft models of epithelial ovarian cancer for preclinical evaluation of novel therapeutics. *Clin Cancer Res* **23:** 1263–1273. doi:10.1158/1078-0432.CCR-16-1237

Liu Y, Chanana P, Davila JI, Hou X, Zanfagnin V, McGehee CD, Goode EL, Polley EC, Haluska P, Weroha SJ, et al. 2019. Gene expression differences between matched pairs of ovarian cancer patient tumors and patient-derived xenografts. *Sci Rep* **9:** 6314. doi:10.1038/s41598-019-42680-2

Lõhmussaar K, Kopper O, Korving J, Begthel H, Vreuls CPH, van Es JH, Clevers H. 2020. Assessing the origin of high-grade serous ovarian cancer using CRISPR-modification of mouse organoids. *Nat Commun* **11:** 2660. doi:10.1038/s41467-020-16432-0

Louie KG, Behrens BC, Kinsella TJ, Hamilton TC, Grotzinger KR, McKoy WM, Winker MA, Ozols RF. 1985. Radiation survival parameters of antineoplastic drug-sensitive and -resistant human ovarian cancer cell lines and their modification by buthionine sulfoximine. *Cancer Res* **45:** 2110–2115.

Mai Z, Lin Y, Lin P, Zhao X, Cui L. 2024. Modulating extracellular matrix stiffness: a strategic approach to boost cancer immunotherapy. *Cell Death Dis* **15:** 307. doi:10.1038/s41419-024-06697-4

Malacrida B, Nichols S, Maniati E, Jones R, Delanie-Smith R, Roozitalab R, Tyler EJ, Thomas M, Boot G, Mackerodt J, et al. 2021. A human multi-cellular model shows how platelets drive production of diseased extracellular matrix and tissue invasion. *iScience* **24:** 102676. doi:10.1016/j.isci.2021.102676

Maniati E, Berlato C, Gopinathan G, Heath O, Kotantaki P, Lakhani A, McDermott J, Pegrum C, Delaine-Smith RM, Pearce OMT, et al. 2020. Mouse ovarian cancer models recapitulate the human tumor microenvironment and patient response to treatment. *Cell Rep* **30:** 525–540.e7. doi:10.1016/j.celrep.2019.12.034

Masazza G, Lucchini V, Tomasoni A, Peccatori F, Lampasona V, Giudici G, Mangioni C, Biondi A, Giavazzi R. 1991. Malignant behavior and resistance to cisplatin of human ovarian carcinoma xenografts established from the same patient at different stages of the disease. *Cancer Res* **51:** 6358–6362.

Massazza G, Tomasoni A, Lucchini V, Allavena P, Erba E, Colombo N, Mantovani A, D'Incalci M, Mangioni C, Giavazzi R. 1989. Intraperitoneal and subcutaneous xenografts of human ovarian carcinoma in nude mice and their potential in experimental therapy. *Int J Cancer* **44:** 494–500. doi:10.1002/ijc.2910440320

McCool KW, Freeman ZT, Zhai Y, Wu R, Hu K, Liu C-J, Tomlins SA, Fearon ER, Magnuson B, Kuick R, et al. 2020. Murine oviductal high-grade serous carcinomas mirror the genomic alterations, gene expression profiles, and immune microenvironment of their human counterparts. *Cancer Res* **80:** 877–889. doi:10.1158/0008-5472.CAN-19-2558

Mendes R, Graça G, Silva F, Guerreiro ACL, Gomes-Alves P, Serpa J, Boghaert ER, Alves PM, Félix A, Brito C, et al. 2022. Exploring metabolic signatures of ex vivo tumor tissue cultures for prediction of chemosensitivity in ovarian cancer. *Cancers (Basel)* **14:** 4460. doi:10.3390/cancers14184460

Mitra AK, Davis DA, Tomar S, Roy L, Gurler H, Xie J, Lantvit DD, Cardenas H, Fang F, Liu Y, et al. 2015. In vivo tumor growth of high-grade serous ovarian cancer cell lines. *Gynecol Oncol* **138:** 372–377. doi:10.1016/j.ygyno.2015.05.040

Moses HL, Roberts AB, Derynck R. 2016. The discovery and early days of TGF-β: a historical perspective. *Cold Spring Harb Perspect Biol* **8:** a021865. doi:10.1101/cshperspect.a021865

Motoyama T. 1981. Biological characterization including sensitivity to mitomycin C of cultured human ovarian cancers (transl.). *Nihon Sanka Fujinka Gakkai Zasshi* **33:** 1197–1204.

Muir A, Vander Heiden MG. 2018. The nutrient environment affects therapy. *Science* **360:** 962–963. doi:10.1126/science.aar5986

Muranen T, Selfors LM, Worster DT, Iwanicki MP, Song L, Morales FC, Gao S, Mills GB, Brugge JS. 2012. Inhibition of PI3K/mTOR leads to adaptive resistance in matrix-attached cancer cells. *Cancer Cell* **21:** 227–239. doi:10.1016/j.ccr.2011.12.024

Murarka M, Vesley-Gross ZI, Essler JL, Smith PG, Hooda J, Drapkin R, Otto CM. 2019. Testing ovarian cancer cell lines to train dogs to detect ovarian cancer from blood plasma: a pilot study. *J Vet Behav* **32:** 42–48.

Nagaraj AS, Salko M, Sirskikar A, Erkan EP, Pietilä EA, Niemiec I, Bao J, Marchi G, Szabó A, Nowlan K, et al. 2024. Patient-derived functional immuno-oncology platform identifies responders to ATR inhibitor and immunotherapy combinations in ovarian cancer. bioRxiv doi:10.1101/2024.02.15.579904

Natarajan S, Foreman KM, Soriano MI, Rossen NS, Shehade H, Fregoso DR, Eggold JT, Krishnan V, Dorigo O, Krieg AJ, et al. 2019. Collagen remodeling in the hypoxic tumor-mesothelial niche promotes ovarian cancer metastasis. *Cancer Res* **79:** 2271–2284. doi:10.1158/0008-5472.CAN-18-2616

Neal JT, Kuo CJ. 2016. Organoids as models for neoplastic transformation. *Annu Rev Pathol* **11:** 199–220. doi:10.1146/annurev-pathol-012615-044249

Neal JT, Li X, Zhu J, Giangarra V, Grzeskowiak CL, Ju J, Liu IH, Chiou S-H, Salahudeen AA, Smith AR, et al. 2018. Organoid modeling of the tumor immune microenvironment. *Cell* **175:** 1972–1988.e16. doi:10.1016/j.cell.2018.11.021

Neilson LJ, Cartwright D, Risteli M, Jokinen EM, McGarry L, Sandvik T, Nikolatou K, Hodge K, Atkinson S, Vias M, et al. 2023. Omentum-derived matrix enables the study of metastatic ovarian cancer and stromal cell functions in a physiologically relevant environment. *Matrix Biol Plus* **19–20:** 100136. doi:10.1016/j.mbplus.2023.100136

Nelson L, Tighe A, Golder A, Littler S, Bakker B, Moralli D, Murtuza Baker S, Donaldson IJ, Spierings DCJ, Wardenaar R, et al. 2020. A living biobank of ovarian cancer ex vivo models reveals profound mitotic heterogeneity. *Nat Commun* **11:** 822. doi:10.1038/s41467-020-14551-2

Nguyen LV, Cox CL, Eirew P, Knapp DJHF, Pellacani D, Kannan N, Carles A, Moksa M, Balani S, Shah S, et al. 2014. DNA barcoding reveals diverse growth kinetics of human breast tumour subclones in serially passaged xenografts. *Nat Commun* **5:** 5871. doi:10.1038/ncomms6871

Nicoletti MI, Lucchini V, Massazza G, Abbott BJ, D'Incalci M, Giavazzi R. 1993. Antitumor activity of taxol (NSC-125973) in human ovarian carcinomas growing in the peritoneal cavity of nude mice. *Ann Oncol* **4:** 151–155. doi:10.1093/oxfordjournals.annonc.a058419

Niedbala MJ, Crickard K, Bernacki RJ. 1985. Interactions of human ovarian tumor cells with human mesothelial cells grown on extracellular matrix: an in vitro model system for studying tumor cell adhesion and invasion. *Exp Cell Res* **160:** 499–513. doi:10.1016/0014-4827(85)90197-1

Niedbala MJ, Crickard K, Bernacki RJ. 1987. In vitro degradation of extracellular matrix by human ovarian carcinoma cells. *Clin Exp Metastasis* **5:** 181–197. doi:10.1007/BF00058063

Odunsi A, McGray AJR, Anthony M, Yali Z, Jianming W, Adebukola A, Cheryl E, Ruea-Yea H. 2020. Fidelity of human ovarian cancer patient-derived xenografts in a partially humanized mouse model for preclinical testing of immunotherapies. *J ImmunoTher Cancer* **8:** e001237.

Ohta I, Gorai I, Miyamoto Y, Yang J, Zheng JH, Kawata N, Hirahara F, Shirotake S. 2001. Cyclophosphamide and 5-fluorouracil act synergistically in ovarian clear cell adenocarcinoma cells. *Cancer Lett* **162:** 39–48.

Orkin RW, Gehron P, McGoodwin EB, Martin GR, Valentine T, Swarm R. 1977. A murine tumor producing a matrix of basement membrane. *J Exp Med* **145:** 204–220. doi:10.1084/jem.145.1.204

Palmer AC, Plana D, Gao H, Korn JM, Yang G, Green J, Zhang X, Velazquez R, McLaughlin ME, Ruddy DA, et al. 2020. A proof of concept for biomarker-guided targeted therapy against ovarian cancer based on patient-derived tumor xenografts. *Cancer Res* **80:** 4278–4287. doi:10.1158/0008-5472.CAN-19-3850

Papp E, Hallberg D, Konecny GE, Bruhm DC, Adleff V, Noë M, Kagiampakis I, Palsgrove D, Conklin D, Kinose Y, et al. 2018. Integrated genomic, epigenomic, and expression analyses of ovarian cancer cell lines. *Cell Rep* **25:** 2617–2633. doi:10.1016/j.celrep.2018.10.096

Paris EA, Bahr JM, Bitterman P, Basu S, Abramowicz JS, Barua A. 2021. Incidence of malignant transformation in the oviductal fimbria in laying hens, a preclinical model of spontaneous ovarian cancer. *PLoS One* **16:** e0255007. doi:10.1371/journal.pone.0255007

Parmar K, Kochupurakkal BS, Lazaro JB, Wang ZC, Palakurthi S, Kirschmeier PT, Yang C, Sambel LA, Färkkilä A, Reznichenko E, et al. 2019. The CHK1 inhibitor prexasertib exhibits monotherapy activity in high-grade serous ovarian cancer models and sensitizes to PARP inhibition. *Clin Cancer Res* **25:** 6127–6140. doi:10.1158/1078-0432.CCR-19-0448

Pearce OMT, Delaine-Smith RM, Maniati E, Nichols S, Wang J, Böhm S, Rajeeve V, Ullah D, Chakravarty P, Jones RR, et al. 2018. Deconstruction of a metastatic tumor microenvironment reveals a common matrix response in human cancers. *Cancer Discov* **8:** 304–319. doi:10.1158/2159-8290.CD-17-0284

Perets R, Wyant GA, Muto KW, Bijron JG, Poole BB, Chin KT, Chen JYH, Ohman AW, Stepule CD, Kwak S, et al. 2013. Transformation of the fallopian tube secretory epithelium leads to high-grade serous ovarian cancer in Brca;Tp53;Pten models. *Cancer Cell* **24:** 751–765. doi:10.1016/j.ccr.2013.10.013

Pietilä EA, Gonzalez-Molina J, Moyano-Galceran L, Jamalzadeh S, Zhang K, Lehtinen L, Turunen SP, Martins TA, Gultekin O, Lamminen T, et al. 2021. Co-evolution of matrisome and adaptive adhesion dynamics drives ovarian cancer chemoresistance. *Nat Commun* **12:** 3904. doi:10.1038/s41467-021-24009-8

Posey AD Jr, Young RM, June CH. 2024. Future perspectives on engineered T cells for cancer. *Trends Cancer* **10:** 687–695. doi:10.1016/j.trecan.2024.05.007

Provencher DM, Lounis H, Champoux L, Tétrault M, Manderson EN, Wang JC, Eydoux P, Savoie R, Tonin PN, Mes-Masson AM. 2000. Characterization of four novel epithelial ovarian cancer cell lines. *In Vitro Cell Dev Biol Anim* **36:** 357–361.

Quevedo R, Smirnov P, Tkachuk D, Ho C, El-Hachem N, Safikhani Z, Pugh TJ, Haibe-Kains B. 2020. Assessment of genetic drift in large pharmacogenomic studies. *Cell Syst* **11:** 393–401.e2. doi:10.1016/j.cels.2020.08.012

Ricciardelli C, Lokman NA, Sabit I, Gunasegaran K, Bonner WM, Pyragius CE, Macpherson AM, Oehler MK. 2018. Novel ex vivo ovarian cancer tissue explant assay for prediction of chemosensitivity and response to novel therapeutics. *Cancer Lett* **421:** 51–58. doi:10.1016/j.canlet.2018.02.006

Roby KF, Taylor CC, Sweetwood JP, Cheng Y, Pace JL, Tawfik O, Persons DL, Smith PG, Terranova PF. 2000. Development of a syngeneic mouse model for events related to ovarian cancer. *Carcinogenesis* **21:** 585–591. doi:10.1093/carcin/21.4.585

Saha B, Mathur T, Tronolone JJ, Chokshi M, Lokhande GK, Selahi A, Gaharwar AK, Afshar-Kharghan V, Sood AK, Bao G, et al. 2021. Human tumor microenvironment chip evaluates the consequences of platelet extravasation and combinatorial antitumor-antiplatelet therapy in ovarian cancer. *Sci Adv* **7:** eabg5283. doi:10.1126/sciadv.abg5283

Schilder RJ, Hall L, Monks A, Handel LM, Fornace AJ Jr, Ozols RF, Fojo AT, Hamilton TC. 1990. Metallothionein gene expression and resistance to cisplatin in human ovarian cancer. *Int J Cancer* **45:** 416–422.

Shaw TJ, Senterman MK, Dawson K, Crane CA, Vanderhyden BC. 2004. Characterization of intraperitoneal, orthotopic, and metastatic xenograft models of human ovarian cancer. *Mol Ther* **10:** 1032–1042. doi:10.1016/j.ymthe.2004.08.013

Sherman-Baust CA, Kuhn E, Valle BL, Shih I-M, Kurman RJ, Wang T-L, Amano T, Ko MSH, Miyoshi I, Araki Y, et al. 2014. A genetically engineered ovarian cancer mouse model based on fallopian tube transformation mimics human high-grade serous carcinoma development. *J Pathol* **233:** 228–237. doi:10.1002/path.4353

Shield K, Ackland ML, Ahmed N, Rice GE. 2009. Multicellular spheroids in ovarian cancer metastases: biology and pathology. *Gynecol Oncol* **113:** 143–148. doi:10.1016/j.ygyno.2008.11.032

Sievers J, Mahajan V, Welzel PB, Werner C, Taubenberger A. 2023. Precision hydrogels for the study of cancer cell mechanobiology. *Adv Healthcare Mater* **12:** 2202514. doi:10.1002/adhm.202202514

Steinkamp MP, Lagutina I, Brayer KJ, Schultz F, Burke D, Pankratz VS, Adams SF, Hudson LG, Ness SA, Wandinger-Ness A. 2023. Humanized patient-derived xenograft models of disseminated ovarian cancer recapitulate key aspects of the tumor immune environment within the peritoneal cavity. *Cancer Res Commun* **3:** 309–324. doi:10.1158/2767-9764.CRC-22-0300

Stewart JM, Shaw PA, Gedye C, Bernardini MQ, Neel BG, Ailles LE. 2011. Phenotypic heterogeneity and instability of human ovarian tumor-initiating cells. *Proc Natl Acad Sci* **108:** 6468–6473. doi:10.1073/pnas.1005529108

Stone RL, Nick AM, McNeish IA, Balkwill F, Han HD, Bottsford-Miller J, Rupaimoole R, Armaiz-Pena GN, Pecot CV, Coward J, et al. 2012. Paraneoplastic thrombocytosis in ovarian cancer. *N Engl J Med* **366:** 610–618. doi:10.1056/NEJMoa1110352

Sutherland RM, McCredie JA, Inch WR. 1971. Growth of multicell spheroids in tissue culture as a model of nodular carcinomas. *J Natl Cancer Inst* **46:** 113–120.

Szabova L, Yin C, Bupp S, Guerin TM, Schlomer JJ, Householder DB, Baran ML, Yi M, Song Y, Sun W, et al. 2012. Perturbation of Rb, p53, and Brca1 or Brca2 cooperate in inducing metastatic serous epithelial ovarian cancer. *Cancer Res* **72:** 4141–4153. doi:10.1158/0008-5472.CAN-11-3834

Tadić V, Zhang W, Brozovic A. 2024. The high-grade serous ovarian cancer metastasis and chemoresistance in 3D models. *Biochim Biophys Acta Rev Cancer* **1879:** 189052. doi:10.1016/j.bbcan.2023.189052

Tang Y, Sun H, Fu P, Zhou T, Liu R. 2025. Prophylactic salpingectomy as a preventative strategy for ovarian cancer in the general population: a systematic review and meta-analysis. *J Gynecol Oncol* **36:** e8. doi:10.3802/jgo.2025.36.e8

Terry SC, Jerman JH, Angell JB. 1979. A gas chromatographic air analyzer fabricated on a silicon wafer. *IEEE Trans Electron Devices* **26:** 1880–1886. doi:10.1109/T-ED.1979.19791

The Cancer Genome Atlas Research Network; Bell D, Berchuck A, Birrer M, Chien J, Cramer DW, Dao F, Dhir R, DiSaia P, Gabra H, et al. 2011. Integrated genomic analyses of ovarian carcinoma. *Nature* **474:** 609–615. doi:10.1038/nature10166

Thorel L, Divoux J, Lequesne J, Babin G, Morice P-M, Florent R, Desmartin G, Lecouflet L, Marde Alagama C, Leconte A, et al. 2024. The OVAREX study: establishment of ex vivo ovarian cancer models to validate innovative therapies and to identify predictive biomarkers. *BMC Cancer* **24:** 701. doi:10.1186/s12885-024-12429-w

Tomas E, Shepherd TG. 2023. Insights into high-grade serous carcinoma pathobiology using three-dimensional culture model systems. *J Ovarian Res* **16:** 70. doi:10.1186/s13048-023-01145-x

Topp MD, Hartley L, Cook M, Heong V, Boehm E, McShane L, Pyman J, McNally O, Ananda S, Harrell M, et al. 2014. Molecular correlates of platinum response in human high-grade serous ovarian cancer patient-derived xenografts. *Mol Oncol* **8:** 656–668. doi:10.1016/j.molonc.2014.01.008

van den Berg-Bakker CAM, Hagemeijer A, Franken-Postma EM, Smit VTHBM, Kuppen PJK, Claasen HHVR, Cornelisse CJ, Schrier PI. 1993. Establishment and characterization of 7 ovarian carcinoma cell lines and one granulosa tumor cell line: growth features and cytogenetics. *Int J Cancer* **53:** 613–620.

Vang R, Shih I-M, Kurman RJ. 2013. Fallopian tube precursors of ovarian low- and high-grade serous neoplasms. *Histopathology* **62:** 44–58. doi:10.1111/his.12046

Vázquez-García I, Uhlitz F, Ceglia N, Lim JLP, Wu M, Mohibullah N, Niyazov J, Ruiz AEB, Boehm KM, Bojilova V, et al. 2022. Ovarian cancer mutational processes drive site-specific immune evasion. *Nature* **612:** 778–786. doi:10.1038/s41586-022-05496-1

Wagar LE, Salahudeen A, Constantz CM, Wendel BS, Lyons MM, Mallajosyula V, Jatt LP, Adamska JZ, Blum LK, Gupta N, et al. 2021. Modeling human adaptive immune responses with tonsil organoids. *Nat Med* **27:** 125–135. doi:10.1038/s41591-020-01145-0

Walton JB, Farquharson M, Mason S, Port J, Kruspig B, Dowson S, Stevenson D, Murphy D, Matzuk M, Kim J, et al. 2017. CRISPR/Cas9-derived models of ovarian high grade serous carcinoma targeting Brca1, Pten and Nf1, and correlation with platinum sensitivity. *Sci Rep* **7:** 16827. doi:10.1038/s41598-017-17119-1

Weroha SJ, Becker MA, Enderica-Gonzalez S, Harrington SC, Oberg AL, Maurer MJ, Perkins SE, AlHilli M, Butler KA, McKinstry S, et al. 2014. Tumorgrafts as in vivo surrogates for women with ovarian cancer. *Clin Cancer Res* **20:** 1288–1297. doi:10.1158/1078-0432.CCR-13-2611

Westin EH, Gallo RC, Arya SK, Eva A, Souza LM, Baluda MA, Aaronson SA, Wong-Staal F. 1982. Differential expression of the amv gene in human hematopoietic cells. *Proc Natl Acad Sci* **79:** 2194–2198.

Winder A, Unno K, Yu Y, Lurain J, Kim JJ. 2017. The allosteric AKT inhibitor, MK2206, decreases tumor growth and invasion in patient derived xenografts of endometrial cancer. *Cancer Biol Ther* **18:** 958–964. doi:10.1080/15384047.2017.1281496

Wright WC, Daniels WP, Fogh J. 1981. Distinction of seventy-one cultured human tumor cell lines by polymorphic enzyme analysis. *JNCI: J Natl Cancer Inst* **66:** 239–247.

Xing D, Orsulic S. 2006. A mouse model for the molecular characterization of brca1-associated ovarian carcinoma. *Cancer Res* **66:** 8949–8953. doi:10.1158/0008-5472.CAN-06-1495

Xu J, Lamouille S, Derynck R. 2009. TGF-β-induced epithelial to mesenchymal transition. *Cell Res* **19:** 156–172. doi:10.1038/cr.2009.5

Xu G, Yin F, Wu H, Hu X, Zheng L, Zhao J. 2014. In vitro ovarian cancer model based on three-dimensional agarose hydrogel. *J Tissue Eng* **5:** 2041731413520438. doi:10.1177/2041731413520438

Yanagibashi T, Gorai I, Nakazawa T, Miyagi E, Hirahara F, Kitamura H, Minaguchi H. 1997. Complexity of expression of the intermediate filaments of six new human ovarian carcinoma cell lines: new expression of cytokeratin 20. *Brit J Cancer* **76:** 829–835.

Yee C, Dickson KA, Muntasir MN, Ma Y, Marsh DJ. 2022. Three-dimensional modelling of ovarian cancer: from cell lines to organoids for discovery and personalized medicine. *Front Bioeng Biotechnol* **10:** 836984. doi:10.3389/fbioe.2022.836984

Yin L, Wang XJ, Chen DX, Liu XN, Wang XJ. 2020. Humanized mouse model: a review on preclinical applications for cancer immunotherapy. *Am J Cancer Res* **10:** 4568–4584.

Yokota SJ, Facciponte JG, Kelleher RJ, Shultz LD, Loyall JL, Parsons RR, Odunsi K, Frelinger JG, Lord EM, Gerber SA, et al. 2013. Changes in ovarian tumor cell number, tumor vasculature, and T cell function monitored in vivo using a novel xenograft model. *Cancer Immun* **13:** 11.

Yoshiya N. 1986. Establishment of a cell line from human ovarian cancer (undifferentiated carcinoma of FIGO classification) and analysis of its cell-biological characteristics and sensitivity to anticancer drugs. *Nihon Sanka Fujinka Gakkai Zasshi* **38:** 1747–1753.

Yuan Y, Kim WH, Han HS, Lee JH, Park HS, Chung JK, Kang SB, Park JG. 1997. Establishment and characterization of human ovarian carcinoma cell lines. *Gynecol Oncol* **66:** 378–387.

Zhai Y, Wu R, Kuick R, Sessine MS, Schulman S, Green M, Fearon ER, Cho KR. 2017. High-grade serous carcinomas arise in the mouse oviduct via defects linked to the human disease. *J Pathol* **243:** 16–25. doi:10.1002/path.4927

Zhang T, Chen J, Zhang Q, Dou J, Gu N. 2013. Poly(ethylene glycol)-cross linked poly(methyl vinyl ether-co-maleic acid) hydrogels for three-dimensional human ovarian cancer cell culture. *Colloids Surf A Physicochem Eng Asp* **422:** 81–89. doi:10.1016/j.colsurfa.2013.01.030

Zhang S, Dolgalev I, Zhang T, Ran H, Levine DA, Neel BG. 2019. Both fallopian tube and ovarian surface epithelium are cells-of-origin for high-grade serous ovarian carcinoma. *Nat Commun* **10:** 5367. doi:10.1038/s41467-019-13116-2

Zhang S, Iyer S, Ran H, Dolgalev I, Gu S, Wei W, Foster CJR, Loomis CA, Olvera N, Dao F, et al. 2021. Genetically defined, syngeneic organoid platform for developing combination therapies for ovarian cancer. *Cancer Discov* **11:** 362–383. doi:10.1158/2159-8290.CD-20-0455

Zhou N, Ma X, Bernaerts KV, Ren P, Hu W, Zhang T. 2020. Expansion of ovarian cancer stem-like cells in poly(ethylene glycol)-cross-linked poly(methyl vinyl ether-*alt*-maleic acid) and alginate double-network hydrogels. *ACS Biomater Sci Eng* **6:** 3310–3326. doi:10.1021/acsbiomaterials.9b01967

Prevention of Epithelial Ovarian Cancer

Thomas A. Sellers,[1] Lauren C. Peres,[2] Cassandra A. Hathaway,[2] and Shelley S. Tworoger[2]

[1]Division of Oncological Sciences, Knight Cancer Institute, Oregon Health & Science University, Portland, Oregon 97239, USA

[2]Department of Cancer Epidemiology, Moffitt Cancer Center & Research Institute, Tampa, Florida 33612, USA

Correspondence: Shelley.Tworoger@moffitt.org

Given the challenges with achieving effective and durable treatment for epithelial ovarian cancer, primary prevention is highly desirable. Fortunately, decades of research have provided evidence for several strategies that can be deployed to optimize risk reduction. These include surgery, chemoprevention, and lifestyle factor modifications. These broad categories vary in terms of the magnitude of risk reduction possible, the possible short-term and long-term side effects, the degree of difficulty, and acceptability. Thus, the concept of a risk-based model to personalize preventive interventions is advocated to guide discussion between care providers and women at risk. For women with inherited major gene mutations that greatly increase risk of ovarian cancer, surgical approaches have favorable risk to benefit ratios. Chemoprevention and lifestyle factor modifications portend a lower degree of risk reduction but confer lower risk of undesirable side effects. Since complete prevention is not currently possible, better methods for early detection remain a high priority.

As reviewed elsewhere in the literature, epithelial ovarian cancer (EOC) is a leading cause of death among women in the United States and around the world. The incidence rates are not in the top 10 female cancers, but the absence of specific signs or symptoms or an effective screening test means that most women are diagnosed at advanced stages. Although there are drugs that demonstrate efficacy against ovarian cancer, mainly high-grade serous tumors, the results are typically insufficient to effect a cure, and the disease relapses. Thus, primary prevention remains a laudable goal to reduce incidence and mortality from ovarian cancer. This work will review the options known to reduce risk, as well as areas of active investigation that harbor the potential to provide additional strategies but for which sufficient evidence among humans is lacking.

Cancer prevention efforts can be applied in the context of preventing the cancer from occurring, detecting tumors at an earlier and more treatable stage, or preventing relapse among cancer patients. In this review, we will focus on primary prevention, for which the target population is individuals at risk for, but without a history of, ovarian cancer. Prevention strategies can be considered in two broad categories. The public health approach attempts to shift the distribution of risk factors in the population. This translates to broad efforts to minimize exposure to factors that increase risk and enhance adoption of healthy, risk-reducing behaviors. Because of the broad scale of intervention, these

Cite this article as *Cold Spring Harb Perspect Med* doi: 10.1101/cshperspect.a038216

often focus on lifestyle. The expected benefit at the individual level is typically modest, but the risk of the intervention is generally low.

For women with a strong genetic predisposition to ovarian cancer, population-based strategies are insufficient, requiring a personalized prevention approach that considers tailored interventions. These interventions often have higher potential side effects but may be more acceptable in the face of greater personal risk. Genetic predisposition can reflect single-gene mutations that segregate in a Mendelian manner or the effects of multiple genetic variants, typically in noncoding regions of the genome, that each confers modest effects on risk but whose combined effects can be quantified by a polygenic risk score (Jones et al. 2017). Thus, as prevention interventions are reviewed, we will consider the public health versus high-risk approach. Further, ovarian cancer is a heterogeneous disease with various cells of origin and genetic abnormalities. For example, high-grade serous ovarian cancer, which accounts for ~70% of EOC, is characterized by *TP53* abnormalities, whereas clear cell tumors typically have *ARID1A* mutations. Therefore, we will note differences in prevention interventions by histological subtype when applicable.

SURGERY

The most effective approaches for reducing the risk of ovarian cancer are surgical procedures that remove tissues that can give rise to these tumors. The cells of origin for ovarian tumors are described in detail in the literature (see Austria and Dubeau 2023; Sasamoto and Elias 2023), but are thought to include endometriotic tissue, the distal end of the fallopian tube, ovarian surface epithelium, and potentially gastrointestinal cells. Here we review four types of surgical procedures and their effectiveness: bilateral salpingo-oophorectomy (BSO), hysterectomy, blockage or removal of the fallopian tubes, and endometriosis excision. Given the nature of the procedures and the importance of patient preference, these interventions are not generally amenable to randomized controlled trials. Thus, the majority of evidence is derived from observational (epidemiologic) studies.

Bilateral Salpingo-Oophorectomy (BSO) and Hysterectomy

Hysterectomy entails the surgical removal of the uterus, but this procedure is often combined with removal of one or both ovaries and fallopian tubes (called a BSO), the cervix, and other surrounding structures. They are commonly performed in the United States (Novetsky et al. 2011) for a range of benign conditions, and the number of procedures performed every year are growing exponentially (Karia et al. 2021). Hysterectomy without oophorectomy does not appear to reduce ovarian cancer risk overall, although exploratory analyses indicate potential benefit among women with endometriosis or fibroids or for the endometrioid/clear cell carcinoma histotype (Dixon-Suen et al. 2019; Huo et al. 2019). Conversely, when hysterectomy includes a BSO, risk reduction is greater than 90% (Falconer et al. 2015). A unilateral salpingo-oophorectomy (USO) is associated with a 30%–35% lower risk of ovarian cancer, suggesting a dose-response for the procedure (Rice et al. 2013, 2014). Women with a genetic predisposition to ovarian cancer (e.g., *BRCA1* or *BRCA2* mutations, Lynch syndrome) benefit significantly from risk-reducing surgery. In two meta-analyses of *BRCA1* or *BRCA2* mutation carriers, risk of ovarian or fallopian tube cancer was reduced by 50% (Rebbeck et al. 2009), and overall survival was longer after BSO compared with no surgery (hazard ratio [HR] = 0.32) (Eleje et al. 2018). Most, but not all, studies suggest that there is a cost savings for risk-reducing BSO in women with *BRCA* mutations compared to surveillance (Schrauder et al. 2019; Hurry et al. 2020; Bommer et al. 2022). In a large population-based study, the absolute risk reduction of ovarian cancer comparing women with hysterectomy or hysterectomy plus BSO was 0.38%, with a need to treat 260 women to prevent one case (Cusimano et al. 2022). A summary of ovarian cancer risk reduction for BSO compared to no surgery or hysterectomy only is shown in Table 1.

Women undergoing hysterectomy before menopause have negative consequences of early menopause, including increased risk of coronary heart disease (Evans et al. 2016; do Valle

Table 1. Ovarian cancer risk reduction after bilateral salpingo-oophorectomy (BSO) compared to hysterectomy alone

Genetic risk	Study reference	*N* Subjects	Relative risk (RR) of ovarian cancer comparing women with vs. without BSO (95% confidence interval [CI])	Risk reduction
High (*BRCA1* or *BRCA2* positive)	Rutter et al. 2003	249	0.29 (0.12–0.73)	71%
	Finch et al. 2006	1828	0.20 (0.07–0.58)	80%
	Finkelman et al. 2012	3787	0.08 (0.04–0.16)	92%
	Eleje et al. 2018	8087	0.17 (0.04–0.75)	83%
	Crosbie et al. 2021	891	0.03 (0.01–0.10)	97%
Average or low	Rutter et al. 2003	598	0.05 (0.01–0.22)	95%
	Parker et al. 2009[a]	29,390	0.04 (0.01–0.09)	96%
	Jacoby et al. 2011[a]	25,448	0.07 (0.02–0.22)	93%
	Falconer et al. 2015	37,348	0.06 (0.03–0.12)	94%
	Cusimano et al. 2021[a]	195,282	0.23 (0.14–0.38)	77%
Unknown	Evans et al. 2009	803	0.08 (0.01–0.57)	92%

[a]Only among women with hysterectomy.

et al. 2021). Further, a 44% increased risk of cardiovascular mortality was observed in women with hysterectomy and BSO before menopause compared with women without surgery. All-cause mortality for premenopausal women receiving BSO was also increased (Evans et al. 2016), especially among those who were not treated with estrogen-replacement therapy (Rocca et al. 2006). For women with surgery either before or after menopause, hysterectomy plus BSO was associated with increased mortality compared with a hysterectomy without BSO. This is largely due to increased mortality from coronary heart disease, which has been linked to reductions in endogenous estrogens in experimental studies (Parker et al. 2009). Another negative consequence of BSO, particularly in premenopausal women, is increased fracture rates due to lower bone density (Melton et al. 2003), especially the earlier in life menopause occurs (Gallagher 2007). One study modeled risk estimates for ovarian cancer and other causes of death (through age 80) in a hypothetical cohort of 10,000 women aged 50–54 choosing hysterectomy with BSO (vs. ovarian conservation). While 47 fewer women would have died from ovarian cancer, nearly 1000 more women would have died from coronary heart disease or hip fractures, due to their higher prevalence (Parker et al. 2007). Other complications of hysterectomy plus BSO include increased depressive symptoms (Hickey et al. 2016, 2021; Wilson et al. 2018; Kotsopoulos et al. 2020), reduced sexual function (Islam et al. 2021; Kershaw et al. 2021), increased risk of cognitive impairment, dementia, and Parkinson's disease (Rocca et al. 2007, 2012; Phung et al. 2010; Evans et al. 2016), and pelvic organ prolapse and urinary dysfunction (Cooper et al. 2011). Several studies suggest that premature estrogen deficiency plays a key role in many of these associations, and estrogen therapy may offset some of the negative side effects (Rivera et al. 2009; Phung et al. 2010; Rocca et al. 2012).

Procedures to Block or Remove the Fallopian Tubes

Tubal procedures are most commonly used in the setting of permanent contraception, but also for medical need (e.g., tubal infection, ectopic pregnancy) (Dilley et al. 2017). While these surgeries have decreased over time (Chan and Westhoff 2010), tubal sterilizations are still one of the most commonly performed gynecologic surgeries (Cullen et al. 2009). Methods to occlude or obstruct the tube are thought to reduce ovarian cancer risk via blockage of retrograde menstruation and endometriosis into the peritoneal cavity. Overall, tubal ligations are associated with a 30% lower risk of ovarian cancer, but this evidence suggests it is stronger for the endometrioid and clear cell histotypes (Rice et al. 2012; Wentzensen et al. 2016).

With increasing awareness of the fallopian tube as a cell of origin, particularly for high-grade serous cancer (Kurman and Shih 2010; Soong et al. 2018a,b,c, 2019), recommendations by the Society of Gynecologic Oncology state that women with a genetic predisposition to ovarian cancer who forego or delay risk-reducing BSO should be counseled to consider bilateral salpingectomy (BS) when childbearing is complete, followed by oophorectomy in the future. For women without a genetic predisposition to ovarian cancer, risk-reducing BS should be discussed and considered at the time of abdominal or pelvic surgery, hysterectomy, or in lieu of tubal ligation (www.sgo.org/clinical-practice/guidelines/sgo-clinical-practice-statement-salpingectomy-for-ovarian-cancer-prevention). Several studies examined the association of salpingectomy, indicated for a specific tubal problem, with ovarian cancer risk. Overall, the lower risk of ovarian cancer with BS was stronger than for tubal ligation, with a suggestively stronger association for BS versus unilateral salpingectomy (Morelli et al. 2013; Yoon et al. 2016; Castellano et al. 2017; Anggraeni et al. 2018; Fortner et al. 2020; Darelius et al. 2021; Falconer et al. 2021). However, one study found that the risk-reducing effects of a BS was only seen for high-grade serous carcinomas (HGSCs) but not for other histotypes, consistent with the fallopian tube origin of HGSC (Darelius et al. 2021). Further, the indications for salpingectomy (e.g., ectopic pregnancy) may have led to bias in risk estimates (Poole et al. 2015). A meta-analysis of 11 studies found inconclusive evidence of ovarian cancer risk reduction after BS (Darelius et al. 2017). Despite recent widespread implementation, it will be many years before we have risk estimates for opportunistic BS (Dilley et al. 2017).

Appropriate preoperative counseling regarding future reproductive choices is critical for BS and tubal ligation (Committee on Gynecologic Practice 2015). Addition of either procedure at time of hysterectomy slightly increases operative times and minimally increases blood loss, but does not increase surgical complications such as infections, increased hospital stay, or changes in ovarian function (Morelli et al. 2013; McAlpine et al. 2014; Behnamfar and Jabbari 2017; Hanley et al. 2017; Tehranian et al. 2017; Ding et al. 2018; Subramaniam et al. 2018; Zerden et al. 2018; van Lieshout et al. 2019). One Canadian study found that women who underwent opportunistic BS (with or without hysterectomy), compared to hysterectomy alone, were about 20% more likely to fill a prescription for an analgesic in the 2 wk after discharge from the hospital; however, no other differences in complications were observed (Hanley et al. 2018).

Tubal ligation appears to be associated with few long-term complications. Hypothesized concerns include reduced ovarian reserve or early menopause and Doppler blood flow changes (Chan et al. 2003; Gelbaya et al. 2006), neither of which have been confirmed (Bulent Tiras et al. 2001), although there may be an increased rate of polycystic ovary features (Revel et al. 2004) as well as higher premenstrual symptoms, including noncyclic pelvic pain (Dias et al. 2014). Similar concerns may arise for BS. While few studies have examined long-term outcomes following opportunistic BS, several small studies have not observed adverse effects (Strandell et al. 2001; Sezik et al. 2007; Yi et al. 2012; Morelli et al. 2013; Yuan et al. 2019). A small randomized trial looked at differences in hormone concentrations for women undergoing a hysterectomy with BS or hysterectomy alone and found no differences between groups (Van Lieshout et al. 2018). Ongoing randomized trials are currently examining surgical complications, effects on ovarian function, and risk of EOC for opportunistic BS (Idahl et al. 2019). Observational cohorts of women undergoing permanent contraception or hysterectomy should also be formed to additionally study long-term outcomes.

Endometriosis Excision

Endometriosis is strongly associated with risk of endometrioid and clear cell ovarian cancer (Pearce et al. 2012) and is hypothesized to be a precursor lesion for these histotypes (Ruderman and Pavone 2017). However, it is unclear whether surgical treatment for endometriosis lowers risk (Mandai et al. 2009; Kim et al. 2014; Wilbur et al. 2017). One Swedish nested case-control study observed a reduction in ovarian cancer risk among women with endometriosis after a unilateral oophorectomy (odds ratio [OR] = 0.19, 95% confidence interval [CI] = 0.05–0.46) or after radical extirpation of all visible endometriosis (OR = 0.30, 95% CI = 0.12–0.74) (Melin et al. 2013). Treatment for endometriosis is complex, with surgical interventions generally limited to women with pelvic pain and/or infertility because of increased complications and recurrent lesions or scarring that can lead to worse pain (Guo 2015; Kho et al. 2018). Definitive treatment for endometriosis includes removal of ovaries; however, as discussed above, this has many other negative side effects and is not indicated except in extreme situations. Overall, research should focus on nonsurgical approaches (e.g., hormones) to lower ovarian cancer risk in women with endometriosis (Vercellini et al. 2018).

Recommendations

Women with a strong family history of breast or ovarian cancer are recommended to receive genetic testing, and those with certain genetic mutations (e.g., in *BRCA1* or *BRCA2*) should consider risk-reducing salpingo-oophorectomy at age 45 to 50 or earlier based on the specific genetic mutation or family history of earlier onset ovarian cancer (Daly et al. 2017). Few studies have examined risk-reducing BSO for women with Lynch syndrome, although a study of over 6000 women suggested limited benefit with respect to ovarian cancer risk and mortality for this population (Dominguez-Valentin et al. 2021). For women without a risk-conferring mutation, BSO cannot be recommended. A critical need is the development of well-calibrated and discriminatory predictive models to identify which women are at highest risk, for whom surgical interventions may have a positive benefit: risk ratio. The continuation of offering opportunistic BS at time of permanent contraception or hysterectomy is warranted, but future research must better elucidate short- and long-term consequences of this procedure.

CHEMOPREVENTION

The National Cancer Institute defines chemoprevention as "The use of drugs, vitamins, or other agents to try to reduce the risk of, or delay the development or recurrence of, cancer." Here, we focus on primary prevention. With one exception, we do not include reports on target identification, mechanisms of action, or preclinical models of agents that have not been tested in humans. Interested readers are directed to a review of this topic (Kathawala et al. 2018).

Oral Contraceptives

The epidemiological evidence that use of oral contraceptives is inversely associated with the risk of ovarian cancer is highly consistent (Reid et al. 2017), and risk decreases by 20% for each 5 yr of use. Importantly, reduced risk persists for decades after use has ceased, although it does wane with time (Collaborative Group on Epidemiological Studies of Ovarian Cancer et al. 2008). Most studies evaluated early, high-dose formulations of oral contraceptives, and some evidence from analyses of more recent birth cohorts suggests that newer, low-dose formulations might not substantially decrease risk until at least 10 yr of use (Bethea et al. 2017; Koushik et al. 2017; Shafrir et al. 2017). The decreased risk is evident across all histotypes of ovarian cancer, although the effect is lower for mucinous cancers (Risch et al. 1996; Riman et al. 2002; Tung et al. 2003; Parazzini et al. 2004; Collaborative Group on Epidemiological Studies of Ovarian Cancer et al. 2008; Yang et al. 2011; Wentzensen et al. 2016; Hemmingsen et al. 2021). It has been estimated that oral contraceptive use corresponds to the prevention of approximately 30,000 cases of ovarian cancer per year and has already prevented an estimated 200,000 cases and 100,000 deaths over the last 50 yr (Collaborative Group on Epidemiological Studies of Ovarian Cancer et al. 2008). Progestin-only contraceptives have been less studied, due to their low prevalence of use, but available data suggest they also may lower risk (Liang et al. 1983; Cancer and Steroid Hormone Study of the Centers for Disease Control and the National

Institute of Child Health and Human Development 1987; Rosenberg et al. 1994).

The use of oral contraceptives among women who carry a mutation in *BRCA1* or *BRCA2* has attracted much interest. Studies have shown clear reductions in ovarian cancer risk in *BRCA1/2* patients on oral contraceptives (Huber et al. 2020; Schrijver et al. 2021) but increases in the risk of breast cancer, particularly for women with *BRCA1* mutations (Cibula et al. 2011; Huber et al. 2020; Karlsson et al. 2021). In recent years, there has been a shift in the United States to using intrauterine devices (IUDs) rather than oral contraceptives (Howard et al. 2017; Webb et al. 2017; King et al. 2021). A meta-analysis of nine case-control and two cohort studies concluded that use of IUDs was associated with a 32% lower risk (Wheeler et al. 2019) of ovarian cancer, although most of these studies were conducted before hormonal IUDs were commonly used, necessitating further research.

Aspirin

The possible benefit of nonsteroidal anti-inflammatory agents to lower risk of ovarian cancer has been examined in several epidemiologic studies, and pooled analyses suggest a 10% risk reduction with daily use of aspirin (Trabert et al. 2014a). Further, the Nurses' Health Studies observed that women who reported recent, regular use of low-dose aspirin (100 mg or less) had a 23% lower risk of developing ovarian cancer when compared with women who did not regularly take aspirin (Barnard et al. 2018). These associations do not differ by ovarian cancer histotypes. There does not appear to be benefits of non-aspirin NSAIDs, and a possible increased risk among those with 10 or more years of use (Barnard et al. 2018; Trabert et al. 2019) merits further study. However, the consistency of risk reduction and the recommendation for daily low-dose aspirin use for cardiovascular disease risk reduction in certain populations provides support for adoption (US Preventive Services Task Force 2022). Although low-dose aspirin is considered safe, there is an evolving understanding of risk-benefit ratios across certain populations (e.g., by age) as some groups are more susceptible to side effects, like gastrointestinal bleeding (US Preventive Services Task Force 2022).

Vaccines

Although not yet studied in humans, two reports described a strategy that has been tested in mice and has shown encouraging evidence of efficacy for prevention (Mazumder et al. 2017, 2020). This novel strategy is based on the hypothesis that targeting ovarian-specific self-proteins that are no longer active in generating an autoimmune response beyond a certain age but are expressed at high levels in cancer may serve as vaccine targets for immunoprevention. Expression of the extracellular domain of anti-Müllerian hormone receptor II (AMHR2-ED) is confined exclusively to nonmalignant human ovarian tissues, decreases at menopause, and found at high levels in ~90% of human EOC. Vaccination of mice with AMHR2-ED inhibited tumor growth and enhanced overall survival (Mazumder et al. 2017, 2020). Although early, the promising results support the potential of preemptive immunity against EOC in women at high genetic risk.

LIFESTYLE FACTORS

Modifying exposure to certain lifestyle factors, including diet, obesity, physical activity, smoking, alcohol, pelvic inflammatory disease (PID) and infectious agents, and body or talcum powders, provides an additional public health approach for the primary prevention of ovarian cancer. The epidemiologic evidence linking these factors to ovarian cancer is mostly weak-to-moderate. Therefore, altering exposure to these factors would result in only a modest risk reduction, yet the risk of side effects or adverse consequences is minimal compared to the other prevention approaches discussed above. Moreover, modifying exposure to these lifestyle factors could have additional health benefits beyond ovarian cancer prevention. Below, we detail the current evidence on modifiable lifestyle factors and their association with risk of ovarian cancer, focusing primarily on findings from large consortia or systematic reviews and meta-analyses that have compiled effect estimates across studies.

Diet and Nutrition

Despite numerous studies of diet in ovarian carcinogenesis, the relationship with specific foods and nutrients is not firmly established. There is some evidence that a higher intake of vegetables is associated with lower ovarian cancer risk (Kushi et al. 1999; Larsson et al. 2004; Pan et al. 2004), but a large European cohort (Schulz et al. 2005) and a pooled analysis of 12 prospective studies (Koushik et al. 2005) did not reach similar conclusions. Other studies suggested that cruciferous vegetable intake (Pan et al. 2004; Hu et al. 2015; McManus et al. 2018) and flavonoid intake, particularly from tea (Cassidy et al. 2014; Hua et al. 2016; Zhan et al. 2017), may also lower risk, although generally no associations have been observed for coffee consumption (Tworoger et al. 2008; Berretta et al. 2018; Salari-Moghaddam et al. 2019; Shafiei et al. 2019). The literature on dietary fat intake, including different types of dietary fat, has been inconclusive. A meta-analysis (Qiu et al. 2016) reported an increased risk of ovarian cancer for higher intakes of total fat as well as *trans*-fat; however, these associations were primarily present in case-control but not prospective cohort studies. This association was recently investigated in two cohort studies not included in the prior meta-analysis (Rice et al. 2020; Yammine et al. 2020). In the Nurses' Health Studies, no clear association between dietary fat and ovarian cancer risk was observed (Rice et al. 2020); however, data from the European Prospective Investigation into Cancer and Nutrition cohort showed that industrial *trans*-fatty acids and fatty acids from deep-frying fats were associated with an increased risk of ovarian cancer (Yammine et al. 2020). An analysis of the Women's Health Initiative dietary modification trial found that compared to a usual diet, the adoption of a low-fat diet for more than 4.1 yr was associated with a 40% decrease in ovarian cancer risk among postmenopausal women (Prentice et al. 2007). Dietary fiber was inversely associated with ovarian cancer risk in a meta-analysis (Xu et al. 2018). Dairy foods and lactose may increase risk (Larsson et al. 2006; Qin et al. 2016), although an analysis of 12 prospective studies did not find an association for specific dairy foods or calcium (Genkinger et al. 2006). There is also no indication that red meat consumption is associated with ovarian cancer risk, although the findings for processed meat, poultry, and fish are mixed (Kolahdooz et al. 2010; Wallin et al. 2011).

In addition to single foods and nutrients, some studies have explored dietary patterns or metrics of dietary quality with ovarian cancer risk. Three dietary quality indices, the Healthy Eating Index (HEI)-2005, the Alternate HEI, and the Alternate Mediterranean Diet Score, were not associated with ovarian cancer risk in a large, prospective cohort, the Nurses' Health Study (Xie et al. 2014); likewise, no association was observed for the HEI-2005 in a population-based case-control study in New Jersey (Chandran et al. 2011). As these studies were composed of predominantly white women, their findings may not be generalizable to other racial/ethnic groups. In a population-based case-control study of African-American women, higher Alternate HEI-2010 scores, but not HEI-2005 or HEI-2010 scores, were associated with a decreased risk of ovarian cancer (OR for the highest vs. lowest quartile = 0.66, 95% CI = 0.45, 0.98) (Qin et al. 2017). Another dietary pattern that has been examined in ovarian cancer is the dietary inflammatory index, a measure of the inflammatory potential of the diet as calculated either through a literature- (Shivappa et al. 2014) or empirically derived (Tabung et al. 2016) approach. In four case-control studies (Shivappa et al. 2016, 2018; Peres et al. 2017; Nagle et al. 2019), a more proinflammatory diet prior to diagnosis modestly increased risk of ovarian cancer, particularly among postmenopausal women; however, no association was observed in the prospective Nurses' Health Study (Tabung et al. 2017). There were no differences by histotype in any of these studies.

Obesity

Obesity, defined as a body mass index (BMI) ≥ 30 kg/m^2, is associated with a modest increased risk of ovarian cancer overall (Olsen et al. 2007;

Aune et al. 2015; Liu et al. 2015). Data from 34 prospective and population-based case-control studies suggested that obese women had a 13% increased risk of ovarian cancer (relative risk [RR] = 1.13, 95% CI = 1.06, 1.20) (Collaborative Group on Epidemiological Studies of Ovarian Cancer 2012). Other anthropometric measurements, such as waist circumference or waist-to-hip ratio, have not shown consistent associations with risk (Aune et al. 2015; Baumeister et al. 2021). A Mendelian randomization study did not find strong evidence of an association between genetically predicted waist-to-hip ratio and risk of ovarian cancer (Gao et al. 2016).

While conferring a modest increased risk of ovarian cancer overall, obesity appears to primarily influence risk of the less common epithelial histotypes (e.g., endometrioid, clear cell, mucinous, and low-grade serous carcinoma). In the Ovarian Cancer Association Consortium (OCAC), a 5 kg/m^2 increase in BMI was associated with an increased risk of endometrioid, mucinous, and low-grade serous carcinoma, but no association was found for HGSC (Olsen et al. 2013). Also, Mendelian randomization studies found that higher genetically predicted BMI was associated with increased risk of non-HGSC but not HGSC (Dixon et al. 2016; Freuer et al. 2021). The Ovarian Cancer Cohort Consortium (Wentzensen et al. 2016) also noted a suggestive, but not statistically significant, positive association with endometrioid, mucinous, and clear cell, but not serous tumors. Moreover, studies have shown that BMI is either weakly or not associated with subgroups of women that are more likely to have HGSC than non-HGSC tumors, such as *BRCA1* or *BRCA2* mutation carriers (McGee et al. 2012) and postmenopausal women (Olsen et al. 2013; Liu et al. 2015).

BMI in early life and weight changes over the life span have also been investigated to elucidate the most critical window of susceptibility for this exposure on ovarian cancer risk. Studies have shown that a higher BMI in childhood (Aarestrup et al. 2019), adolescence, and early adulthood (Engeland et al. 2003; Aune et al. 2015) confers an increased risk of ovarian cancer. A study using data from the Nurses' Health Studies showed that early life adiposity (BMI at age 18) and BMI changes between ages 10 and 18 were more strongly associated with ovarian cancer risk than changes in BMI in adulthood (Huang et al. 2019). A 2015 meta-analysis observed no association for weight gain in adulthood (Aune et al. 2015), while another meta-analysis of prospective observational studies noted a positive association for adult weight gain only among postmenopausal women who did not use or had low use of hormone therapy (Keum et al. 2015). Conversely, other studies have shown an increased risk for adult weight gain (Schouten et al. 2003; Minlikeeva et al. 2018; Christakoudi et al. 2021) including in African-American (Schildkraut et al. 2016) and Chinese women (Ma et al. 2013).

Although obesity appears to only modestly influence risk of the less common EOC histotypes, maintaining a healthy weight and preventing excess weight gain at any time throughout the life span is recommended. Additional work is needed to clarify the most critical time periods that would portend the greatest benefit of modifying weight for ovarian cancer risk reduction.

Physical Activity

Engaging in physical activity has numerous health benefits including weight management, cardiovascular health, bone strength, reductions in inflammation, and improved quality of life. The role of physical activity on ovarian cancer is uncertain as findings have been inconclusive. A meta-analysis found that women with the highest versus lowest levels of recreational physical activity had a ∼20% lower risk of ovarian cancer (Olsen et al. 2007). Studies published on recreational physical activity since this meta-analysis have been mostly null (Carnide et al. 2009; Lahmann et al. 2009; Leitzmann et al. 2009; Rossing et al. 2010; Moorman et al. 2011; Xiao et al. 2013; Hildebrand et al. 2015; Abbott et al. 2016; Huang et al. 2016; Grundy et al. 2020). Interestingly, in the Nurses' Health Studies, premenopausal physical activity demonstrated a U-shaped relationship with later risk, with very sedentary women having a higher risk, particularly of nonserous histotypes, and those with moderate activity having a higher risk, particularly of serous disease; the latter may be due to increased ovulation with moderate activity (Huang et al. 2016). In the same cohort of women, no association with ovarian cancer risk was observed for resistance training, an aspect of physical activity associated with reduced inflammation (Phillips et al. 2012; Tomeleri et al. 2018), nor early life physical activity (Buras et al. 2021; Wang et al. 2021a). In addition, the role of physical inactivity or sedentary behavior has been investigated. Data from nine studies in the OCAC suggests that physical inactivity increases the risk of ovarian cancer by 34% (Cannioto et al. 2016). Other studies have demonstrated an increased risk for sedentary behavior or prolonged sitting (Zhang et al. 2004; Patel et al. 2006; Hildebrand et al. 2015), although the NIH-AARP Diet and Health Study did not observe an association (Xiao et al. 2013). A systematic review and meta-analysis of seven studies reported a 29% increased risk of ovarian cancer for women with prolonged sitting time, comparing the highest to the lowest tertile of sedentary behavior (Biller et al. 2021). Given the modest evidence for the impact of physical activity on ovarian cancer risk reduction and the wealth of health benefits outside of cancer prevention, incorporating physical activity and exercise into daily life is recommended for general health.

Smoking

Traditionally, ovarian cancer has not been thought of as smoking-associated due to the consistent lack of an association with ovarian cancer risk overall. However, investigations by histotype revealed that cigarette smoking increases the risk for mucinous ovarian carcinoma, but not the other epithelial histotypes (Collaborative Group on Epidemiological Studies of Ovarian Cancer et al. 2012; Faber et al. 2013; Wentzensen et al. 2016; Licaj et al. 2017). There is also an indication that smoking may confer a weak protective effect for clear cell and endometrioid carcinomas (Collaborative Group on Epidemiological Studies of Ovarian Cancer et al. 2012; Faber et al. 2013; Wentzensen et al. 2016). A recent investigation of early life exposure to tobacco smoke and ovarian cancer risk in the Nurses' Health Studies showed that parental smoking at home during childhood and adolescence was associated with a modestly increased risk of ovarian cancer (HR = 1.15, 95% CI = 1.04, 1.27) (Wang et al. 2021b). Avoiding cigarette smoking, or quitting if a current smoker, offers a variety of health benefits, including prevention of mucinous ovarian carcinoma.

Alcohol

The literature on the influence of alcohol consumption on ovarian cancer risk is mixed. However, a pooled analysis in the OCAC (Kelemen et al. 2013) and a meta-analysis of studies until 2012 (Rota et al. 2012) did not find an association between alcohol and ovarian cancer risk, except for a possible modest inverse association with endometrioid carcinoma (Rota et al. 2012). There is also little evidence supporting an association for specific types of alcohol (e.g., wine, beer, liquor) or the duration or frequency of exposure. Thus, modifying alcohol use may not be an effective strategy to reduce the risk of ovarian cancer.

Pelvic Inflammatory Disease and Associated Infectious Agents

PID is inflammation of the female upper reproductive tract that is induced by infectious agents, most notably chlamydia and gonorrhea (Brunham et al. 2015). A meta-analysis of six cohort studies and seven case-control studies reported a 24% increased risk of ovarian cancer for women with PID (RR = 1.24, 95% CI = 1.06, 1.44) (Zhou et al. 2017). Prior studies investigating antibodies to the bacterium that cause PID have shown an association between seropositivity for *Chlamydia trachomatis* and ovarian cancer risk (Ness et al. 2003), although other studies have reported null results (Ness et al. 2008; Idahl et al. 2011). Recent studies (Fortner et al. 2019; Trabert et al. 2019) reported an increased risk of ovarian cancer for women with a prior or current *C. trachomatis* infection, but not *Mycoplasma genitalium*, herpes simplex virus type 2, or human papillomavirus infection. In the European Prospective Investigation into Cancer and Nutrition cohort, an increased risk of serous and mucinous ovarian cancers was observed for *C. trachomatis* infection, while herpes simplex virus type 2 was associated with an increased risk of endometrioid ovarian cancer (Idahl et al. 2020). Taking precautions against acquiring sexually transmitted infections that have the potential to cause PID is recommended with respect to future ovarian cancer risk.

Body/Talcum Powders

Application of talcum or body powders to perineal areas has been associated with an increased ovarian cancer risk in several case-control studies (Cramer et al. 1999; Gates et al. 2008; Merritt et al. 2008; Rosenblatt et al. 2011; Terry et al. 2013), although cohort studies generally do not support this relationship (Gates et al. 2008; Houghton et al. 2014; Gonzalez et al. 2016). In a pooled analysis of four large U.S. cohort studies, there was a positive but not statistically significant association of self-reported powder use applied to genital areas and risk of ovarian cancer (HR = 1.08, 95% CI = 0.99, 1.17), which was stronger for women in an intact reproductive system (i.e., no hysterectomy or tubal ligation; HR = 1.13, 95% CI = 1.01, 1.26) (O'Brien et al. 2020). A recent meta-analysis reported that the summary relative risk for genital talc use and ovarian cancer risk for case-control studies was 1.26 (95% CI = 1.17, 1.35) (Berge et al. 2018). Minorities are more likely to report body or talc powder use in comparison to white women (Peres et al. 2018), yet few studies have investigated this association among minority populations. In a contemporary population-based case-control study of African-American women, a positive association between body powders applied to genital areas and ovarian cancer risk was observed (Schildkraut et al. 2016). However, this association was found only in women interviewed after 2014, when media coverage of the talc-ovarian cancer lawsuits became prevalent. This study highlights concerns of recall and reporting bias in case-control studies and leads to additional questions on whether this association can be quantified without bias in the aftermath of heightened media coverage. More recently, data from the Ovarian Cancer in Women of African Ancestry, which included the aforementioned case-control study of African-American women and four other studies, showed no differences in the association between genital powder use and ovarian cancer risk by race (African-American women, OR = 1.22, 95% CI = 0.97, 1.53; White women, OR = 1.36, 95% CI = 1.19, 1.57) (Davis et al. 2021). Moreover, none of these studies show a clear dose-response relationship between genital powder use and ovarian cancer risk, and the mechanistic link between talcum or body powders and ovarian cancer remains unclear; further research is needed to understand this potential relationship.

Given the inconsistent findings across epidemiologic studies and the paucity of research on the biologic mechanism as to how talcum or body powders contribute to carcinogenesis, it is still unclear whether altering exposure will have a measurable impact on risk reduction. However, as there are few modifiable risk factors for ovarian cancer, avoiding the use of body or talcum powders may provide another primary prevention approach for ovarian cancer.

EMERGING RISK FACTORS

High Inflammatory State

There is increasing evidence supporting inflammation as a mechanism of ovarian cancer development. For example, very high, but not moderate, levels of C-reactive protein (CRP), a nonspecific marker of inflammation, has been consistently associated with increased ovarian cancer risk, as reported in a meta-analysis and pooled analysis of prospective studies (Peres et al. 2019; Wang et al. 2020). Moreover, prior work has linked several other inflammatory cytokines with increased ovarian cancer risk (Clendenen et al. 2011; Trabert et al. 2014b; Peres et al. 2021) and tumorigenesis (Schauer et al. 2013; Chandler et al. 2015; Korneev et al. 2017). These associations were still observed when blood was collected more than 15 yr before ovarian cancer occurred. However, a meta-analysis of the IL-6, tumor necrosis factor (TNF)-α, and soluble TNF-α receptor 2 did not observe consistent associations (Zeng et al. 2016; Wang et al. 2020). Future studies are needed to fully understand the role inflammation plays on ovarian cancer development.

Chronic Stress/Distress

Recently, evidence has shown that chronic stress and associated distress may play a role in ovarian cancer risk. An initial registry study showed a 2.4-fold higher standardized incidence rate for ovarian cancer in those with a diagnosis of posttraumatic stress disorder (PTSD). This was subsequently found, in two prospective longitudinal cohorts, that risk of ovarian cancer was two times higher for women with high PTSD symptoms than for women without a history of PTSD (Roberts et al. 2019). Further, depression was associated with a 30% higher ovarian cancer risk (Huang et al. 2015). Other psychosocial factors associated with distress, including being socially isolated versus integrated as well as widowhood (compared to being married or in a long-term relationship) were also related to increased ovarian cancer risk (Trudel-Fitzgerald et al. 2019). However, more work is needed to understand these findings as not all studies on stressors and other types of distress (e.g., anxiety) have been associated with ovarian cancer risk (Poole et al. 2016; Trudel-Fitzgerald et al. 2017).

SUMMARY AND CONCLUSION

In this review, we present prevention strategies across a spectrum of interventions ranging from surgery to chemoprevention to alteration of risk factor profiles. According to the American College of Obstetricians and Gynecologists (ACOG), BSO should be recommended for women with inherited mutations in *BRCA1* (between the ages of 35 and 40) and *BRCA2* (between the ages of 40 and 45) (Committee on Practice Bulletins–Gynecology, Committee on Genetics, Society of Gynecologic Oncology 2017). Since polygenic risk prediction is currently insufficient to be used in clinical practice even when considered with known risk factors (Clyde et al. 2016), it is critical to identify both new genetic variants and novel risk factors (e.g., gut microbiome, systemic immune surveillance) to improve the clinical utility to become sufficiently refined to recommend surgical interventions for certain populations of women. The public health approach of less aggressive interventions is recommended when risk is elevated to low penetrance genetic factors. Figure 1 shows this concept. A summary of recom-

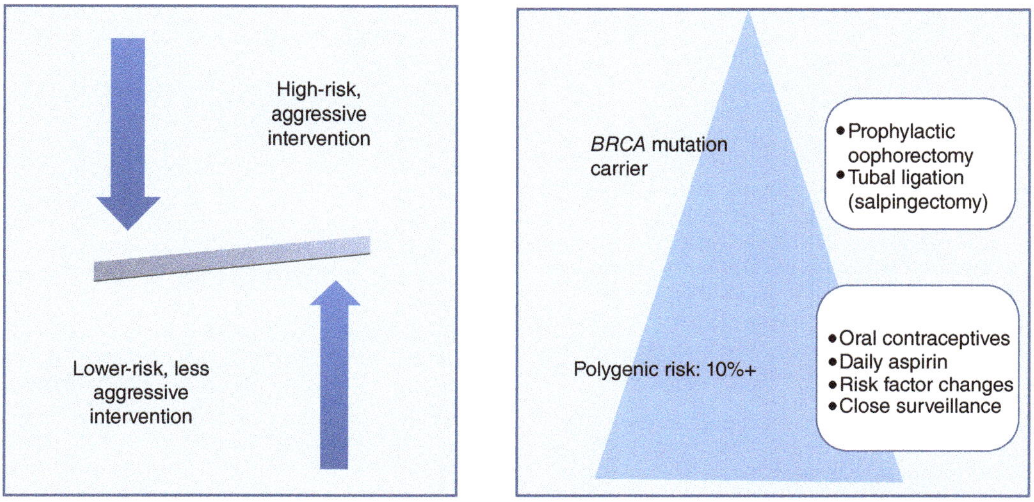

Figure 1. Risk-based prevention applied to epithelial ovarian cancer.

Table 2. Summary of prevention strategies ordered from greatest to lowest risk reduction

Recommendation	Pros	Cons
Bilateral salpingo-oophorectomy	Greatest level of risk reduction	Recommended for mutation carriers only Symptoms of sudden menopause Increased risk for nonmalignant disease
Oral contraceptives	Easily deployed and well-accepted Moderate risk reduction and long-lasting	Risk of side effects Insufficient for women at greatest risk
Low-dose aspirin	Easily deployed and low-cost intervention	Risk of side effects Modest risk reduction
Weight management	Portends additional health benefits beyond ovarian cancer risk reduction Low risk of adverse consequences or negative side effects	Modest risk reduction Risk reduction primarily for less common, non-high-grade serous carcinoma (HGSC) tumors
Avoiding sexually transmitted infections that cause pelvic inflammatory disease (PID)	Low risk of adverse consequences or negative side effects	Modest risk reduction Additional work needed to identify infectious agents with largest impact on risk
Avoiding cigarette smoking	Well-accepted Portends additional health benefits beyond ovarian cancer risk reduction	Modest risk reduction only for mucinous tumors

mendations based on the current evidence is presented in Table 2.

REFERENCES

*Reference is also in this subject collection.

Aarestrup J, Trabert B, Ulrich LG, Wentzensen N, Sørensen TIA, Baker JL. 2019. Childhood overweight, tallness, and growth increase risks of ovarian cancer. *Cancer Epidemiol Biomarkers Prev* **28:** 183–188. doi:10.1158/1055-9965.EPI-18-0024

Abbott SE, Bandera EV, Qin B, Peres LC, Moorman PG, Barnholtz-Sloan J, Schwartz AG, Funkhouser E, Peters ES, Cote ML, et al. 2016. Recreational physical activity and ovarian cancer risk in African American women. *Cancer Med* **5:** 1319–1327. doi:10.1002/cam4.677

Anggraeni TD, Al Fattah AN, Surya R. 2018. Prophylactic salpingectomy and ovarian cancer: an evidence-based analysis. *South Asian J Cancer* **7:** 42–45. doi:10.4103/sajc.sajc_187_17

Aune D, Navarro Rosenblatt DA, Chan DS, Abar L, Vingeliene S, Vieira AR, Greenwood DC, Norat T. 2015. Anthropometric factors and ovarian cancer risk: a systematic review and nonlinear dose-response meta-analysis of prospective studies. *Int J Cancer* **136:** 1888–1898. doi:10.1002/ijc.29207

*Austria T, Dubeau L. 2023. Embryological insights into the origin of epithelial cancers of the female reproductive tract. *Cold Spring Harb Perspect Med* doi:10.1101/cshperspect.a040642

Barnard ME, Poole EM, Curhan GC, Eliassen AH, Rosner BA, Terry KL, Tworoger SS. 2018. Association of analgesic use with risk of ovarian cancer in the nurses' health studies. *JAMA Oncol* **4:** 1675–1682. doi:10.1001/jamaoncol.2018.4149

Baumeister SE, Schlecht I, Trabert B, Nolde M, Meisinger C, Leitzmann MF. 2021. Anthropometric risk factors for ovarian cancer in the NIH-AARP diet and health study. *Cancer Causes Control* **32:** 231–239. doi:10.1007/s10552-020-01377-y

Behnamfar F, Jabbari H. 2017. Evaluation of ovarian function after hysterectomy with or without salpingectomy: a feasible study. *J Res Med Sci* **22:** 68. doi:10.4103/jrms.JRMS_81_17

Berge W, Mundt K, Luu H, Boffetta P. 2018. Genital use of talc and risk of ovarian cancer: a meta-analysis. *Eur J Cancer Prev* **27:** 248–257. doi:10.1097/CEJ.0000000000000340

Berretta M, Micek A, Lafranconi A, Rossetti S, Di Francia R, De Paoli P, Rossi P, Facchini G. 2018. Coffee consumption is not associated with ovarian cancer risk: a dose-response meta-analysis of prospective cohort studies. *Oncotarget* **9:** 20807–20815. doi:10.18632/oncotarget.24829

Bethea TN, Palmer JR, Adams-Campbell LL, Rosenberg L. 2017. A prospective study of reproductive factors and exogenous hormone use in relation to ovarian cancer risk among black women. *Cancer Causes Control* **28:** 385–391. doi:10.1007/s10552-016-0840-4

Biller VS, Leitzmann MF, Sedlmeier AM, Berger FF, Ortmann O, Jochem C. 2021. Sedentary behaviour in relation to ovarian cancer risk: a systematic review and meta-analysis. *Eur J Epidemiol* **36:** 769–780. doi:10.1007/s10654-020-00712-6

Bommer C, Lupatsch J, Bürki N, Schwenkglenks M. 2022. Cost-utility analysis of risk-reducing strategies to prevent breast and ovarian cancer in BRCA-mutation carriers in Switzerland. *Eur J Health Econ* **23:** 807–821. doi:10.1007/s10198-021-01396-9

Brunham RC, Gottlieb SL, Paavonen J. 2015. Pelvic inflammatory disease. *N Engl J Med* **372:** 2039–2048. doi:10.1056/NEJMra1411426

Bulent Tiras M, Noyan V, Ozdemir H, Guner H, Yildiz A, Yildirim M. 2001. The changes in ovarian hormone levels and ovarian artery blood flow rate after laparoscopic tubal sterilization. *Eur J Obstet Gynecol Reprod Biol* **99:** 219–221. doi:10.1016/S0301-2115(01)00410-9

Buras AL, Hathaway CA, Wang T, Townsend MK, Tworoger SS. 2021. The association of resistance training with risk of ovarian cancer. *Cancer Med* **10:** 2489–2495. doi:10.1002/cam4.3804

Cancer and Steroid Hormone Study of the Centers for Disease Control and the National Institute of Child Health and Human Development. 1987. The reduction in risk of ovarian cancer associated with oral-contraceptive use. *N Engl J Med* **316:** 650–655. doi:10.1056/NEJM198703123161102

Cannioto R, LaMonte MJ, Risch HA, Hong CC, Sucheston-Campbell LE, Eng KH, Brian Szender J, Chang-Claude J, Schmalfeldt B, Klapdor R, et al. 2016. Chronic recreational physical inactivity and epithelial ovarian cancer risk: evidence from the Ovarian Cancer Association Consortium. *Cancer Epidemiol Biomarkers Prev* **25:** 1114–1124. doi:10.1158/1055-9965.EPI-15-1330

Carnide N, Kreiger N, Cotterchio M. 2009. Association between frequency and intensity of recreational physical activity and epithelial ovarian cancer risk by age period. *Eur J Cancer Prev* **18:** 322–330.

Cassidy A, Huang T, Rice MS, Rimm EB, Tworoger SS. 2014. Intake of dietary flavonoids and risk of epithelial ovarian cancer. *Am J Clin Nutr* **100:** 1344–1351. doi:10.3945/ajcn.114.088708

Castellano T, Zerden M, Marsh L, Boggess K. 2017. Risks and benefits of salpingectomy at the time of sterilization. *Obstet Gynecol Surv* **72:** 663–668. doi:10.1097/OGX.0000000000000503

Chan LM, Westhoff CL. 2010. Tubal sterilization trends in the United States. *Fertil Steril* **94:** 1–6. doi:10.1016/j.fertnstert.2010.03.029

Chan CC, Ng EH, Li CF, Ho PC. 2003. Impaired ovarian blood flow and reduced antral follicle count following laparoscopic salpingectomy for ectopic pregnancy. *Hum Reprod* **18:** 2175–2180. doi:10.1093/humrep/deg411

Chandler RL, Damrauer JS, Raab JR, Schisler JC, Wilkerson MD, Didion JP, Starmer J, Serber D, Yee D, Xiong J, et al. 2015. Coexistent ARID1A-PIK3CA mutations promote ovarian clear-cell tumorigenesis through pro-tumorigenic inflammatory cytokine signalling. *Nat Commun* **6:** 6118. doi:10.1038/ncomms7118

Chandran U, Bandera EV, Williams-King MG, Paddock LE, Rodriguez-Rodriguez L, Lu SE, Faulkner S, Pulick K, Olson SH. 2011. Healthy eating index and ovarian cancer risk. *Cancer Causes Control* **22:** 563–571. doi:10.1007/s10552-011-9728-5

Christakoudi S, Pagoni P, Ferrari P, Cross AJ, Tzoulaki I, Muller DC, Weiderpass E, Freisling H, Murphy N, Dossus L, et al. 2021. Weight change in middle adulthood and risk of cancer in the European Prospective Investigation into Cancer and Nutrition (EPIC) cohort. *Int J Cancer* **148:** 1637–1651. doi:10.1002/ijc.33339

Cibula D, Zikan M, Dusek L, Majek O. 2011. Oral contraceptives and risk of ovarian and breast cancers in BRCA mutation carriers: a meta-analysis. *Expert Rev Anticancer Ther* **11:** 1197–1207. doi:10.1586/era.11.38

Clendenen TV, Lundin E, Zeleniuch-Jacquotte A, Koenig KL, Berrino F, Lukanova A, Lokshin AE, Idahl A, Ohlson N, Hallmans G, et al. 2011. Circulating inflammation markers and risk of epithelial ovarian cancer. *Cancer Epidemiol Biomarkers Prev* **20:** 799–810. doi:10.1158/1055-9965.EPI-10-1180

Clyde MA, Palmieri Weber R, Iversen ES, Poole EM, Doherty JA, Goodman MT, Ness RB, Risch HA, Rossing MA, Terry KL, et al. 2016. Risk prediction for epithelial ovarian cancer in 11 United States-based case-control studies: incorporation of epidemiologic risk factors and 17 confirmed genetic loci. *Am J Epidemiol* **184:** 579–589. doi:10.1093/aje/kww091

Collaborative Group on Epidemiological Studies of Ovarian Cancer. 2012. Ovarian cancer and body size: individual participant meta-analysis including 25,157 women with ovarian cancer from 47 epidemiological studies. *PLoS Med* **9:** e1001200. doi:10.1371/journal.pmed.1001200

Collaborative Group on Epidemiological Studies of Ovarian Cancer; Beral V, Doll R, Hermon C, Peto R, Reeves G. 2008. Ovarian cancer and oral contraceptives: collaborative reanalysis of data from 45 epidemiological studies including 23,257 women with ovarian cancer and 87,303 controls. *Lancet* **371:** 303–314. doi:10.1016/S0140-6736(08)60167-1

Collaborative Group on Epidemiological Studies of Ovarian Cancer; Beral V, Gaitskell K, Hermon C, Moser K, Reeves G, Peto R. 2012. Ovarian cancer and smoking: individual participant meta-analysis including 28,114 women with ovarian cancer from 51 epidemiological studies. *Lancet Oncol* **13:** 946–956. doi:10.1016/S1470-2045(12)70322-4

Committee on Gynecologic Practice. 2015. Committee opinion no. 620: salpingectomy for ovarian cancer prevention. *Obstet Gynecol* **125:** 279–281. doi:10.1097/01.AOG.0000459871.88564.09

Committee on Practice Bulletins–Gynecology, Committee on Genetics, Society of Gynecologic Oncology. 2017. Practice bulletin no 182: hereditary breast and ovarian cancer syndrome. *Obstet Gynecol* **130:** e110–e126. doi:10.1097/AOG.0000000000002296

Cooper K, Lee A, Chien P, Raja E, Timmaraju V, Bhattacharya S. 2011. Outcomes following hysterectomy or endometrial ablation for heavy menstrual bleeding: retrospective analysis of hospital episode statistics in Scotland.

BJOG **118:** 1171–1179. doi:10.1111/j.1471-0528.2011.03011.x

Cramer DW, Liberman RF, Titus-Ernstoff L, Welch WR, Greenberg ER, Baron JA, Harlow BL. 1999. Genital talc exposure and risk of ovarian cancer. *Int J Cancer* **81:** 351–356. doi:10.1002/(SICI)1097-0215(19990505)81:3<351::AID-IJC7>3.0.CO;2-M

Crosbie EJ, Flaum N, Harkness EF, Clayton RD, Holland C, Martin-Hirsch P, Wood N, Keating P, Woodward ER, Lalloo F, et al. 2021. Specialist oncological surgery for removal of the ovaries and fallopian tubes in BRCA1 and BRCA2 pathogenic variant carriers may reduce primary peritoneal cancer risk to very low levels. *Int J Cancer* **148:** 1155–1163. doi:10.1002/ijc.33378

Cullen KA, Hall MJ, Golosinskiy A. 2009. Ambulatory surgery in the United States, 2006. *Natl Health Stat Report* **11:** 1–25.

Cusimano MC, Ferguson SE, Moineddin R, Chiu M, Aktar S, Liu N, Baxter NN. 2022. Ovarian cancer incidence and death in average-risk women undergoing bilateral salpingo-oophorectomy at benign hysterectomy. *Am J Obstet Gynecol* **226:** 220.e1–220.e26. doi:10.1016/j.ajog.2021.09.020

Daly MB, Pilarski R, Berry M, Buys SS, Farmer M, Friedman S, Garber JE, Kauff ND, Khan S, Klein C, et al. 2017. NCCN guidelines insights: genetic/familial high-risk assessment: breast and ovarian, version 2.2017. *J Natl Compr Canc Netw* **15:** 9–20. doi:10.6004/jnccn.2017.0003

Darelius A, Lycke M, Kindblom JM, Kristjansdottir B, Sundfeldt K, Strandell A. 2017. Efficacy of salpingectomy at hysterectomy to reduce the risk of epithelial ovarian cancer: a systematic review. *BJOG* **124:** 880–889. doi:10.1111/1471-0528.14601

Darelius A, Kristjansdottir B, Dahm-Kahler P, Strandell A. 2021. Risk of epithelial ovarian cancer type I and II after hysterectomy, salpingectomy and tubal ligation—a nationwide case-control study. *Int J Cancer* **149:** 1544–1552. doi:10.1002/ijc.33714

Davis CP, Bandera EV, Bethea TN, Camacho F, Joslin CE, Wu AH, Beeghly-Fadiel A, Moorman PG, Myers ER, Ochs-Balcom HM, et al. 2021. Genital powder use and risk of epithelial ovarian cancer in the ovarian cancer in women of African Ancestry Consortium. *Cancer Epidemiol Biomarkers Prev* **30:** 1660–1668. doi:10.1158/1055-9965.EPI-21-0162

Dias DS, Dias R, Nahás-Neto J, Nahás EA, Leite NJ, Bueloni-Dias FN, Modotti WP. 2014. Clinical and psychological repercussions of videolaparoscopic tubal ligation: observational, single cohort, retrospective study. *Sao Paulo Med J* **132:** 321–331. doi:10.1590/1516-3180-2014-1326687

Dilley SE, Straughn JM Jr, Leath CA III. 2017. The evolution of and evidence for opportunistic salpingectomy. *Obstet Gynecol* **130:** 814–824. doi:10.1097/AOG.0000000000002243

Ding DC, Huang C, Chu TY, Wei YC, Chen PC, Hong MK. 2018. Trends of opportunistic salpingectomy. *JSLS* **22:** e2018.00004. doi:10.4293/JSLS.2018.00004

Dixon SC, Nagle CM, Thrift AP, Pharoah PD, Pearce CL, Zheng W, Painter JN; AOCS Group & Australian Cancer Study (Ovarian Cancer); Chenevix-Trench G, Fasching PA, et al. 2016. Adult body mass index and risk of ovarian cancer by subtype: mendelian randomization study. *Int J Epidemiol* **45:** 884–895. doi:10.1093/ije/dyw158

Dixon-Suen SC, Webb PM, Wilson LF, Tuesley K, Stewart LM, Jordan SJ. 2019. The association between hysterectomy and ovarian cancer risk: a population-based record-linkage study. *J Natl Cancer Inst* **111:** 1097–1103. doi:10.1093/jnci/djz015

Dominguez-Valentin M, Crosbie EJ, Engel C, Aretz S, Macrae F, Winship I, Capella G, Thomas H, Nakken S, Hovig E, et al. 2021. Risk-reducing hysterectomy and bilateral salpingo-oophorectomy in female heterozygotes of pathogenic mismatch repair variants: a prospective lynch syndrome database report. *Genet Med* **23:** 705–712. doi:10.1038/s41436-020-01029-1

do Valle HA, Kaur P, Kwon JS, Cheifetz R, Dawson L, Hanley GE. 2021. Risk of cardiovascular disease among women carrying BRCA mutations after risk-reducing bilateral salpingo-oophorectomy: a population-based study. *Gynecol Oncol* **162:** 707–714. doi:10.1016/j.ygyno.2021.06.022

Eleje GU, Eke AC, Ezebialu IU, Ikechebelu JI, Ugwu EO, Okonkwo OO. 2018. Risk-reducing bilateral salpingo-oophorectomy in women with BRCA1 or BRCA2 mutations. *Cochrane Database Syst Rev* **8:** CD012464.

Engeland A, Tretli S, Bjorge T. 2003. Height, body mass index, and ovarian cancer: a follow-up of 1.1 million Norwegian women. *J Natl Cancer Inst* **95:** 1244–1248. doi:10.1093/jnci/djg010

Evans DG, Clayton R, Donnai P, Shenton A, Lalloo F. 2009. Risk-reducing surgery for ovarian cancer: outcomes in 300 surgeries suggest a low peritoneal primary risk. *Eur J Hum Genet* **17:** 1381–1385. doi:10.1038/ejhg.2009.60

Evans EC, Matteson KA, Orejuela FJ, Alperin M, Balk EM, El-Nashar S, Gleason JL, Grimes C, Jeppson P, Mathews C, et al. 2016. Salpingo-oophorectomy at the time of benign hysterectomy: a systematic review. *Obstet Gynecol* **128:** 476–485. doi:10.1097/AOG.0000000000001592

Faber MT, Kjær SK, Dehlendorff C, Chang-Claude J, Andersen KK, Høgdall E, Webb PM, Jordan SJ; Australian Cancer Study (Ovarian Cancer); Australian Ovarian Cancer Study Group, et al. 2013. Cigarette smoking and risk of ovarian cancer: a pooled analysis of 21 case-control studies. *Cancer Causes Control* **24:** 989–1004. doi:10.1007/s10552-013-0174-4

Falconer H, Yin L, Gronberg H, Altman D. 2015. Ovarian cancer risk after salpingectomy: a nationwide population-based study. *J Natl Cancer Inst* **107:** dju410. doi:10.1093/jnci/dju410

Falconer H, Yin L, Salehi S, Altman D. 2021. Association between pelvic inflammatory disease and subsequent salpingectomy on the risk for ovarian cancer. *Eur J Cancer* **145:** 38–43. doi:10.1016/j.ejca.2020.11.046

Finch A, Beiner M, Lubinski J, Lynch HT, Moller P, Rosen B, Murphy J, Ghadirian P, Friedman E, Foulkes WD, et al. 2006. Salpingo-oophorectomy and the risk of ovarian, fallopian tube, and peritoneal cancers in women with a BRCA1 or BRCA2 mutation. *JAMA* **296:** 185–192. doi:10.1001/jama.296.2.185

Finkelman BS, Rubinstein WS, Friedman S, Friebel TM, Dubitsky S, Schonberger NS, Shoretz R, Singer CF, Blum JL, Tung N, et al. 2012. Breast and ovarian cancer risk and risk reduction in Jewish BRCA1/2 mutation carriers. *J Clin Oncol* **30:** 1321–1328. doi:10.1200/JCO.2011.37.8133

Fortner RT, Terry KL, Bender N, Brenner N, Hufnagel K, Butt J, Waterboer T, Tworoger SS. 2019. Sexually transmitted infections and risk of epithelial ovarian cancer: results from the Nurses' Health Studies. *Br J Cancer* **120:** 855–860. doi:10.1038/s41416-019-0422-9

Fortner RT, Rice MS, Knutsen SF, Orlich MJ, Visvanathan K, Patel AV, Gaudet MM, Tjønneland A, Kvaskoff M, Kaaks R, et al. 2020. Ovarian cancer risk factor associations by primary anatomic site: the Ovarian Cancer Cohort Consortium. *Cancer Epidemiol Biomarkers Prev* **29:** 2010–2018. doi:10.1158/1055-9965.EPI-20-0354

Freuer D, Linseisen J, O'Mara TA, Leitzmann M, Baurecht H, Baumeister SE, Meisinger C. 2021. Body fat distribution and risk of breast, endometrial, and ovarian cancer: a two-sample Mendelian randomization study. *Cancers (Basel)* **13:** 5053. doi:10.3390/cancers13205053

Gallagher JC. 2007. Effect of early menopause on bone mineral density and fractures. *Menopause* **14:** 567–571. doi:10.1097/gme.0b013e31804c793d

Gao C, Patel CJ, Michailidou K, Peters U, Gong J, Schildkraut J, Schumacher FR, Zheng W, Boffetta P, Stucker I, et al. 2016. Mendelian randomization study of adiposity-related traits and risk of breast, ovarian, prostate, lung and colorectal cancer. *Int J Epidemiol* **45:** 896–908. doi:10.1093/ije/dyw129

Gates MA, Tworoger SS, Terry KL, Titus-Ernstoff L, Rosner B, De Vivo I, Cramer DW, Hankinson SE. 2008. Talc use, variants of the GSTM1, GSTT1, and NAT2 genes, and risk of epithelial ovarian cancer. *Cancer Epidemiol Biomarkers Prev* **17:** 2436–2444. doi:10.1158/1055-9965.EPI-08-0399

Gelbaya TA, Nardo LG, Fitzgerald CT, Horne G, Brison DR, Lieberman BA. 2006. Ovarian response to gonadotropins after laparoscopic salpingectomy or the division of fallopian tubes for hydrosalpinges. *Fertil Steril* **85:** 1464–1468. doi:10.1016/j.fertnstert.2005.10.036

Genkinger JM, Hunter DJ, Spiegelman D, Anderson KE, Arslan A, Beeson WL, Buring JE, Fraser GE, Freudenheim JL, Goldbohm RA, et al. 2006. Dairy products and ovarian cancer: a pooled analysis of 12 cohort studies. *Cancer Epidemiol Biomarkers Prev* **15:** 364–372. doi:10.1158/1055-9965.EPI-05-0484

Gonzalez NL, O'Brien KM, D'Aloisio AA, Sandler DP, Weinberg CR. 2016. Douching, talc use, and risk of ovarian cancer. *Epidemiology* **27:** 797–802. doi:10.1097/EDE.0000000000000528

Grundy A, Ho V, Abrahamowicz M, Parent ME, Siemiatycki J, Arseneau J, Gilbert L, Gotlieb WH, Provencher DM, Koushik A. 2020. Lifetime recreational moderate-to-vigorous physical activity and ovarian cancer risk: a case-control study. *Int J Cancer* **146:** 1800–1809.

Guo SW. 2015. Endometriosis and ovarian cancer: potential benefits and harms of screening and risk-reducing surgery. *Fertil Steril* **104:** 813–830. doi:10.1016/j.fertnstert.2015.08.006

Hanley GE, McAlpine JN, Pearce CL, Miller D. 2017. The performance and safety of bilateral salpingectomy for ovarian cancer prevention in the United States. *Am J Obstet Gynecol* **216:** 270.e1–270.e9. doi:10.1016/j.ajog.2016.10.035

Hanley GE, Kwon JS, Finlayson SJ, Huntsman DG, Miller D, McAlpine JN. 2018. Extending the safety evidence for opportunistic salpingectomy in prevention of ovarian cancer: a cohort study from British Columbia, Canada. *Am J Obstet Gynecol* **219:** 172.e1–172.e8. doi:10.1016/j.ajog.2018.05.019

Hemmingsen CH, Kjaer SK, Bennetsen AKK, Dehlendorff C, Baandrup L. 2021. The association of reproductive factors with risk of non-epithelial ovarian cancer and comparison with serous ovarian cancer. *Gynecol Oncol* **162:** 469–474. doi:10.1016/j.ygyno.2021.05.008

Hickey M, Schoenaker DA, Joffe H, Mishra GD. 2016. Depressive symptoms across the menopause transition: findings from a large population-based cohort study. *Menopause* **23:** 1287–1293. doi:10.1097/GME.0000000000000712

Hickey M, Moss KM, Brand A, Wrede CD, Domchek SM, Meiser B, Mishra GD, Joffe H. 2021. What happens after menopause? (WHAM): a prospective controlled study of depression and anxiety up to 12 months after premenopausal risk-reducing bilateral salpingo-oophorectomy. *Gynecol Oncol* **161:** 527–534. doi:10.1016/j.ygyno.2021.02.001

Hildebrand JS, Gapstur SM, Gaudet MM, Campbell PT, Patel AV. 2015. Moderate-to-vigorous physical activity and leisure-time sitting in relation to ovarian cancer risk in a large prospective US cohort. *Cancer Causes Control* **26:** 1691–1697. doi:10.1007/s10552-015-0656-7

Houghton SC, Reeves KW, Hankinson SE, Crawford L, Lane D, Wactawski-Wende J, Thomson CA, Ockene JK, Sturgeon SR. 2014. Perineal powder use and risk of ovarian cancer. *J Natl Cancer Inst* **106:** dju208. doi:10.1093/jnci/dju208

Howard B, Grubb E, Lage MJ, Tang B. 2017. Trends in use of and complications from intrauterine contraceptive devices and tubal ligation or occlusion. *Reprod Health* **14:** 70. doi:10.1186/s12978-017-0334-1

Hu J, Hu Y, Hu Y, Zheng S. 2015. Intake of cruciferous vegetables is associated with reduced risk of ovarian cancer: a meta-analysis. *Asia Pac J Clin Nutr* **24:** 101–109.

Hua X, Yu L, You R, Yang Y, Liao J, Chen D, Yu L. 2016. Association among dietary flavonoids, flavonoid subclasses and ovarian cancer risk: a meta-analysis. *PLoS ONE* **11:** e0151134. doi:10.1371/journal.pone.0151134

Huang T, Poole EM, Okereke OI, Kubzansky LD, Eliassen AH, Sood AK, Wang M, Tworoger SS. 2015. Depression and risk of epithelial ovarian cancer: results from two large prospective cohort studies. *Gynecol Oncol* **139:** 481–486. doi:10.1016/j.ygyno.2015.10.004

Huang T, Eliassen AH, Hankinson SE, Okereke OI, Kubzansky LD, Wang M, Poole EM, Chavarro JE, Tworoger SS. 2016. A prospective study of leisure-time physical activity and risk of incident epithelial ovarian cancer: impact by menopausal status. *Int J Cancer* **138:** 843–852. doi:10.1002/ijc.29834

Huang T, Tworoger SS, Willett WC, Stampfer MJ, Rosner BA. 2019. Associations of early life and adulthood adiposity with risk of epithelial ovarian cancer. *Ann Oncol* **30:** 303–309. doi:10.1093/annonc/mdy546

Huber D, Seitz S, Kast K, Emons G, Ortmann O. 2020. Use of oral contraceptives in BRCA mutation carriers and risk for ovarian and breast cancer: a systematic review. *Arch*

Gynecol Obstet **301:** 875–884. doi:10.1007/s00404-020-05458-w

Huo X, Yao L, Han X, Li W, Liu J, Zhou L, Gou Y, Yang K, Liu H. 2019. Hysterectomy and risk of ovarian cancer: a systematic review and meta-analysis. *Arch Gynecol Obstet* **299:** 599–607. doi:10.1007/s00404-018-5020-1

Hurry M, Eccleston A, Dyer M, Hoskins P. 2020. Canadian cost-effectiveness model of BRCA-driven surgical prevention of breast/ovarian cancers compared to treatment if cancer develops. *Int J Technol Assess Health Care* **36:** 104–112. doi:10.1017/S0266462319003519

Idahl A, Lundin E, Jurstrand M, Kumlin U, Elgh F, Ohlson N, Ottander U. 2011. *Chlamydia trachomatis* and *Mycoplasma genitalium* plasma antibodies in relation to epithelial ovarian tumors. *Infect Dis Obstet Gynecol* **2011:** 824627. doi:10.1155/2011/824627

Idahl A, Darelius A, Sundfeldt K, Pålsson M, Strandell A. 2019. Hysterectomy and opportunistic salpingectomy (HOPPSA): study protocol for a register-based randomized controlled trial. *Trials* **20:** 10. doi:10.1186/s13063-018-3083-8

Idahl A, Le Cornet C, González Maldonado S, Waterboer T, Bender N, Tjønneland A, Hansen L, Boutron-Ruault MC, Fournier A, Kvaskoff M, et al. 2020. Serologic markers of *Chlamydia trachomatis* and other sexually transmitted infections and subsequent ovarian cancer risk: results from the EPIC cohort. *Int J Cancer* **147:** 2042–2052. doi:10.1002/ijc.32999

Islam RM, Davis SR, Bell RJ, Tejada-Berges T, Wrede CD, Domchek SM, Meiser B, Kirk J, Krejany EO, Hickey M. 2021. A prospective controlled study of sexual function and sexually related personal distress up to 12 months after premenopausal risk-reducing bilateral salpingo-oophorectomy. *Menopause* **28:** 748–755. doi:10.1097/GME.0000000000001766

Jacoby VL, Grady D, Wactawski-Wende J, Manson JE, Allison MA, Kuppermann M, Sarto GE, Robbins J, Phillips L, Martin LW, et al. 2011. Oophorectomy vs ovarian conservation with hysterectomy: cardiovascular disease, hip fracture, and cancer in the Women's Health Initiative Observational Study. *Arch Intern Med* **171:** 760–768. doi:10.1001/archinternmed.2011.121

Jones MR, Kamara D, Karlan BY, Pharoah PDP, Gayther SA. 2017. Genetic epidemiology of ovarian cancer and prospects for polygenic risk prediction. *Gynecol Oncol* **147:** 705–713. doi:10.1016/j.ygyno.2017.10.001

Karia PS, Joshu CE, Visvanathan K. 2021. Uptake and predictors of opportunistic salpingectomy for ovarian cancer risk reduction in the United States. *Cancer Prev Res (Phila)* **14:** 1101–1110. doi:10.1158/1940-6207.CAPR-21-0121

Karlsson T, Johansson T, Höglund J, Ek WE, Johansson A. 2021. Time-dependent effects of oral contraceptive use on breast, ovarian, and endometrial cancers. *Cancer Res* **81:** 1153–1162. doi:10.1158/0008-5472.CAN-20-2476

Kathawala RJ, Kudelka A, Rigas B. 2018. Correction: the chemoprevention of ovarian cancer: the need and the options. *Curr Pharmacol Rep* **4:** 414. doi:10.1007/s40495-018-0159-9

Kelemen LE, Bandera EV, Terry KL, Rossing MA, Brinton LA, Doherty JA, Ness RB, Kjær SK, Chang-Claude J, Köbel M, et al. 2013. Recent alcohol consumption and risk of incident ovarian carcinoma: a pooled analysis of 5,342 cases and 10,358 controls from the Ovarian Cancer Association Consortium. *BMC Cancer* **13:** 28. doi:10.1186/1471-2407-13-28

Kershaw V, Hickey I, Wyld L, Jha S. 2021. The impact of risk reducing bilateral salpingo-oophorectomy on sexual function in BRCA1/2 mutation carriers and women with Lynch syndrome: a systematic review and meta-analysis. *Eur J Obstet Gynecol Reprod Biol* **265:** 7–17. doi:10.1016/j.ejogrb.2021.08.001

Keum N, Greenwood DC, Lee DH, Kim R, Aune D, Ju W, Hu FB, Giovannucci EL. 2015. Adult weight gain and adiposity-related cancers: a dose-response meta-analysis of prospective observational studies. *J Natl Cancer Inst* **107:** djv088. doi:10.1093/jnci/djv088

Kho RM, Andres MP, Borrelli GM, Neto JS, Zanluchi A, Abrão MS. 2018. Surgical treatment of different types of endometriosis: comparison of major society guidelines and preferred clinical algorithms. *Best Pract Res Clin Obstet Gynaecol* **51:** 102–110. doi:10.1016/j.bpobgyn.2018.01.020

Kim HS, Kim TH, Chung HH, Song YS. 2014. Risk and prognosis of ovarian cancer in women with endometriosis: a meta-analysis. *Br J Cancer* **110:** 1878–1890. doi:10.1038/bjc.2014.29

King LA, Michels KA, Graubard BI, Trabert B. 2021. Trends in oral contraceptive and intrauterine device use among reproductive-aged women in the US from 1999 to 2017. *Cancer Causes Control* **32:** 587–595. doi:10.1007/s10552-021-01410-8

Kolahdooz F, van der Pols JC, Bain CJ, Marks GC, Hughes MC, Whiteman DC, Webb PM; Australian Cancer Study (Ovarian Cancer) and the Australian Ovarian Cancer Study Group. 2010. Meat, fish, and ovarian cancer risk: results from 2 Australian case-control studies, a systematic review, and meta-analysis. *Am J Clin Nutr* **91:** 1752–1763. doi:10.3945/ajcn.2009.28415

Korneev KV, Atretkhany KN, Drutskaya MS, Grivennikov SI, Kuprash DV, Nedospasov SA. 2017. TLR-signaling and proinflammatory cytokines as drivers of tumorigenesis. *Cytokine* **89:** 127–135. doi:10.1016/j.cyto.2016.01.021

Kotsopoulos J, Gronwald J, Lubinski J, McCuaig J, Lynch HT, Neuhausen SL, Foulkes WD, Weitzel JN, Senter L, Tung N, et al. 2020. Does preventive oophorectomy increase the risk of depression in BRCA mutation carriers? *Menopause* **27:** 156–161. doi:10.1097/GME.0000000000001437

Koushik A, Hunter DJ, Spiegelman D, Anderson KE, Arslan AA, Beeson WL, van den Brandt PA, Buring JE, Cerhan JR, Colditz GA, et al. 2005. Fruits and vegetables and ovarian cancer risk in a pooled analysis of 12 cohort studies. *Cancer Epidemiol Biomarkers Prev* **14:** 2160–2167. doi:10.1158/1055-9965.EPI-05-0218

Koushik A, Grundy A, Abrahamowicz M, Arseneau J, Gilbert L, Gotlieb WH, Lacaille J, Mes-Masson AM, Parent ME, Provencher DM, et al. 2017. Hormonal and reproductive factors and the risk of ovarian cancer. *Cancer Causes Control* **28:** 393–403. doi:10.1007/s10552-016-0848-9

Kurman RJ, Shih I-M. 2010. The origin and pathogenesis of epithelial ovarian cancer: a proposed unifying theory.

Am J Surg Pathol **34:** 433–443. doi:10.1097/PAS.0b013e3181cf3d79

Kushi LH, Mink PJ, Folsom AR, Anderson KE, Zheng W, Lazovich D, Sellers TA. 1999. Prospective study of diet and ovarian cancer. *Am J Epidemiol* **149:** 21–31. doi:10.1093/oxfordjournals.aje.a009723

Lahmann PH, Friedenreich C, Schulz M, Cust AE, Lukanova A, Kaaks R, Tjønneland A, Johnsen NF, Overvad K, Fournier A, et al. 2009. Physical activity and ovarian cancer risk: the European prospective investigation into cancer and nutrition. *Cancer Epidemiol Biomarkers Prev* **18:** 351–354. doi:10.1158/1055-9965.EPI-08-0958

Larsson SC, Holmberg L, Wolk A. 2004. Fruit and vegetable consumption in relation to ovarian cancer incidence: the Swedish mammography cohort. *Br J Cancer* **90:** 2167–2170. doi:10.1038/sj.bjc.6601872

Larsson SC, Orsini N, Wolk A. 2006. Milk, milk products and lactose intake and ovarian cancer risk: a meta-analysis of epidemiological studies. *Int J Cancer* **118:** 431–441. doi:10.1002/ijc.21305

Leitzmann MF, Koebnick C, Moore SC, Danforth KN, Brinton LA, Hollenbeck AR, Schatzkin A, Lacey JV. 2009. Prospective study of physical activity and the risk of ovarian cancer. *Cancer Causes Control* **20:** 765–773. doi:10.1007/s10552-008-9291-x

Liang AP, Levenson AG, Layde PM, Shelton JD, Hatcher RA, Potts M, Michelson MJ. 1983. Risk of breast, uterine corpus, and ovarian cancer in women receiving medroxyprogesterone injections. *JAMA* **249:** 2909–2912. doi:10.1001/jama.1983.03330450039022

Licaj I, Jacobsen BK, Selmer RM, Maskarinec G, Weiderpass E, Gram IT. 2017. Smoking and risk of ovarian cancer by histological subtypes: an analysis among 300,000 Norwegian women. *Br J Cancer* **116:** 270–276. doi:10.1038/bjc.2016.418

Liu Z, Zhang TT, Zhao JJ, Qi SF, Du P, Liu DW, Tian QB. 2015. The association between overweight, obesity and ovarian cancer: a meta-analysis. *Jpn J Clin Oncol* **45:** 1107–1115.

Ma X, Beeghly-Fadiel A, Shu XO, Li H, Yang G, Gao YT, Zheng W. 2013. Anthropometric measures and epithelial ovarian cancer risk among Chinese women: results from the Shanghai Women's Health Study. *Br J Cancer* **109:** 751–755. doi:10.1038/bjc.2013.384

Mandai M, Yamaguchi K, Matsumura N, Baba T, Konishi I. 2009. Ovarian cancer in endometriosis: molecular biology, pathology, and clinical management. *Int J Clin Oncol* **14:** 383–391. doi:10.1007/s10147-009-0935-y

Mazumder S, Johnson JM, Swank V, Dvorina N, Martelli E, Ko J, Tuohy VK. 2017. Primary immunoprevention of epithelial ovarian carcinoma by vaccination against the extracellular domain of anti-Müllerian hormone receptor II. *Cancer Prev Res (Phila)* **10:** 612–624. doi:10.1158/1940-6207.CAPR-17-0154

Mazumder S, Swank V, Komar AA, Johnson JM, Tuohy VK. 2020. Immunotherapy of ovarian cancer with a monoclonal antibody specific for the extracellular domain of anti-Müllerian hormone receptor II. *Oncotarget* **11:** 1894–1910. doi:10.18632/oncotarget.27585

McAlpine JN, Hanley GE, Woo MM, Tone AA, Rozenberg N, Swenerton KD, Gilks CB, Finlayson SJ, Huntsman DG, Miller DM, et al. 2014. Opportunistic salpingectomy: uptake, risks, and complications of a regional initiative for ovarian cancer prevention. *Am J Obstet Gynecol* **210:** 471.e1–471.e11. doi:10.1016/j.ajog.2014.01.003

McGee J, Kotsopoulos J, Lubinski J, Lynch HT, Rosen B, Tung N, Kim-Sing C, Karlan B, Foulkes WD, Ainsworth P, et al. 2012. Anthropometric measures and risk of ovarian cancer among BRCA1 and BRCA2 mutation carriers. *Obesity (Silver Spring)* **20:** 1288–1292. doi:10.1038/oby.2011.394

McManus H, Moysich KB, Tang L, Joseph J, McCann SE. 2018. Usual cruciferous vegetable consumption and ovarian cancer: a case-control study. *Nutr Cancer* **70:** 678–683. doi:10.1080/01635581.2018.1464346

Melin AS, Lundholm C, Malki N, Swahn ML, Sparèn P, Bergqvist A. 2013. Hormonal and surgical treatments for endometriosis and risk of epithelial ovarian cancer. *Acta Obstet Gynecol Scand* **92:** 546–554. doi:10.1111/aogs.12123

Melton LJ III, Khosla S, Malkasian GD, Achenbach SJ, Oberg AL, Riggs BL. 2003. Fracture risk after bilateral oophorectomy in elderly women. *J Bone Miner Res* **18:** 900–905. doi:10.1359/jbmr.2003.18.5.900

Merritt MA, Green AC, Nagle CM, Webb PM; Australian Cancer Study (Ovarian Cancer) and Australian Ovarian Cancer Study Group. 2008. Talcum powder, chronic pelvic inflammation and NSAIDs in relation to risk of epithelial ovarian cancer. *Int J Cancer* **122:** 170–176. doi:10.1002/ijc.23017

Minlikeeva AN, Moysich KB, Mayor PC, Etter JL, Cannioto RA, Ness RB, Starbuck K, Edwards RP, Segal BH, Lele S, et al. 2018. Anthropometric characteristics and ovarian cancer risk and survival. *Cancer Causes Control* **29:** 201–212. doi:10.1007/s10552-017-0997-5

Moorman PG, Jones LW, Akushevich L, Schildkraut JM. 2011. Recreational physical activity and ovarian cancer risk and survival. *Ann Epidemiol* **21:** 178–187. doi:10.1016/j.annepidem.2010.10.014

Morelli M, Venturella R, Mocciaro R, Di Cello A, Rania E, Lico D, D'Alessandro P, Zullo F. 2013. Prophylactic salpingectomy in premenopausal low-risk women for ovarian cancer: primum non nocere. *Gynecol Oncol* **129:** 448–451. doi:10.1016/j.ygyno.2013.03.023

Nagle CM, Ibiebele T, Shivappa N, Hébert JR, DeFazio A, Webb PM, Australian Ovarian Cancer Study. 2019. The association between the inflammatory potential of diet and risk of developing, and survival following, a diagnosis of ovarian cancer. *Eur J Nutr* **58:** 1747–1756. doi:10.1007/s00394-018-1779-x

Ness RB, Goodman MT, Shen C, Brunham RC. 2003. Serologic evidence of past infection with *Chlamydia trachomatis*, in relation to ovarian cancer. *J Infect Dis* **187:** 1147–1152. doi:10.1086/368380

Ness RB, Shen C, Bass D, Jackson C, Moysich K, Edwards R, Brunham RC. 2008. *Chlamydia trachomatis* serology in women with and without ovarian cancer. *Infect Dis Obstet Gynecol* **2008:** 219672.

Novetsky AP, Boyd LR, Curtin JP. 2011. Trends in bilateral oophorectomy at the time of hysterectomy for benign disease. *Obstet Gynecol* **118:** 1280–1286. doi:10.1097/AOG.0b013e318236fe61

O'Brien KM, Tworoger SS, Harris HR, Anderson GL, Weinberg CR, Trabert B, Kaunitz AM, D'Aloisio AA, Sandler

DP, Wentzensen N. 2020. Association of powder use in the genital area with risk of ovarian cancer. *JAMA* **323:** 49–59. doi:10.1001/jama.2019.20079

Olsen CM, Green AC, Whiteman DC, Sadeghi S, Kolahdooz F, Webb PM. 2007. Obesity and the risk of epithelial ovarian cancer: a systematic review and meta-analysis. *Eur J Cancer* **43:** 690–709. doi:10.1016/j.ejca.2006.11.010

Olsen CM, Nagle CM, Whiteman DC, Ness R, Pearce CL, Pike MC, Rossing MA, Terry KL, Wu AH; Australian Cancer Study (Ovarian Cancer), et al. 2013. Obesity and risk of ovarian cancer subtypes: evidence from the Ovarian Cancer Association Consortium. *Endocr Relat Cancer* **20:** 251–262. doi:10.1530/ERC-12-0395

Pan SY, Ugnat AM, Mao Y, Wen SW, Johnson KC, Canadian Cancer Registries Epidemiology Research Group. 2004. A case-control study of diet and the risk of ovarian cancer. *Cancer Epidemiol Biomarkers Prev* **13:** 1521–1527. doi:10.1158/1055-9965.1521.13.9

Parazzini F, Chiaffarino F, Negri E, Surace M, Benzi G, Franceschi S, Fedele L, La Vecchia C. 2004. Risk factors for different histological types of ovarian cancer. *Int J Gynecol Cancer* **14:** 431–436. doi:10.1111/j.1048-891x.2004.14302.x

Parker WH, Broder MS, Liu Z, Shoupe D, Farquhar C, Berek JS. 2007. Ovarian conservation at the time of hysterectomy for benign disease. *Clin Obstet Gynecol* **50:** 354–361. doi:10.1097/GRF.0b013e31804a838d

Parker WH, Broder MS, Chang E, Feskanich D, Farquhar C, Liu Z, Shoupe D, Berek JS, Hankinson S, Manson JE. 2009. Ovarian conservation at the time of hysterectomy and long-term health outcomes in the nurses' health study. *Obstet Gynecol* **113:** 1027–1037. doi:10.1097/AOG.0b013e3181a11c64

Patel AV, Rodriguez C, Pavluck AL, Thun MJ, Calle EE. 2006. Recreational physical activity and sedentary behavior in relation to ovarian cancer risk in a large cohort of US women. *Am J Epidemiol* **163:** 709–716. doi:10.1093/aje/kwj098

Pearce CL, Templeman C, Rossing MA, Lee A, Near AM, Webb PM, Nagle CM, Doherty JA, Cushing-Haugen KL, Wicklund KG, et al. 2012. Association between endometriosis and risk of histological subtypes of ovarian cancer: a pooled analysis of case-control studies. *Lancet Oncol* **13:** 385–394. doi:10.1016/S1470-2045(11)70404-1

Peres LC, Bandera EV, Qin B, Guertin KA, Shivappa N, Hebert JR, Abbott SE, Alberg AJ, Barnholtz-Sloan J, Bondy M, et al. 2017. Dietary inflammatory index and risk of epithelial ovarian cancer in African American women. *Int J Cancer* **140:** 535–543. doi:10.1002/ijc.30467

Peres LC, Risch H, Terry KL, Webb PM, Goodman MT, Wu AH, Alberg AJ, Bandera EV, Barnholtz-Sloan J, Bondy ML, et al. 2018. Racial/ethnic differences in the epidemiology of ovarian cancer: a pooled analysis of 12 case-control studies. *Int J Epidemiol* **47:** 460–472. doi:10.1093/ije/dyx252

Peres LC, Mallen AR, Townsend MK, Poole EM, Trabert B, Allen NE, Arslan AA, Dossus L, Fortner RT, Gram IT, et al. 2019. High levels of C-reactive protein are associated with an increased risk of ovarian cancer: results from the Ovarian Cancer Cohort Consortium. *Cancer Res* **79:** 5442–5451. doi:10.1158/0008-5472.CAN-19-1554

Peres LC, Townsend MK, Birmann BM, Conejo-Garcia JR, Kim Y, Kubzansky LD, Magpantay LI, Martinez-Maza O, Tworoger SS. 2021. Circulating biomarkers of inflammation and ovarian cancer risk in the Nurses' Health Studies. *Cancer Epidemiol Biomarkers Prev* **30:** 710–718. doi:10.1158/1055-9965.EPI-20-1390

Phillips MD, Patrizi RM, Cheek DJ, Wooten JS, Barbee JJ, Mitchell JB. 2012. Resistance training reduces subclinical inflammation in obese, postmenopausal women. *Med Sci Sports Exerc* **44:** 2099–2110. doi:10.1249/MSS.0b013e3182644984

Phung TK, Waltoft BL, Laursen TM, Settnes A, Kessing LV, Mortensen PB, Waldemar G. 2010. Hysterectomy, oophorectomy and risk of dementia: a nationwide historical cohort study. *Dement Geriatr Cogn Disord* **30:** 43–50. doi:10.1159/000314681

Poole EM, Rice MS, Crum CP, Tworoger SS. 2015. Salpingectomy as a potential ovarian cancer risk-reducing procedure. *J Natl Cancer Inst* **107:** dju490. doi:10.1093/jnci/dju490

Poole EM, Kubzansky LD, Sood AK, Okereke OI, Tworoger SS. 2016. A prospective study of phobic anxiety, risk of ovarian cancer, and survival among patients. *Cancer Causes Control* **27:** 661–668. doi:10.1007/s10552-016-0739-0

Prentice RL, Thomson CA, Caan B, Hubbell FA, Anderson GL, Beresford SA, Pettinger M, Lane DS, Lessin L, Yasmeen S, et al. 2007. Low-fat dietary pattern and cancer incidence in the women's health initiative dietary modification randomized controlled trial. *J Natl Cancer Inst* **99:** 1534–1543. doi:10.1093/jnci/djm159

Qin B, Moorman PG, Alberg AJ, Barnholtz-Sloan JS, Bondy M, Cote ML, Funkhouser E, Peters ES, Schwartz AG, Terry P, et al. 2016. Dairy, calcium, vitamin D and ovarian cancer risk in African-American women. *Br J Cancer* **115:** 1122–1130. doi:10.1038/bjc.2016.289

Qin B, Moorman PG, Kelemen LE, Alberg AJ, Barnholtz-Sloan JS, Bondy M, Cote ML, Funkhouser E, Peters ES, Schwartz AG, et al. 2017. Dietary quality and ovarian cancer risk in African-American Women. *Am J Epidemiol* **185:** 1281–1289. doi:10.1093/aje/kwx022

Qiu W, Lu H, Qi Y, Wang X. 2016. Dietary fat intake and ovarian cancer risk: a meta-analysis of epidemiological studies. *Oncotarget* **7:** 37390–37406. doi:10.18632/oncotarget.8940

Rebbeck TR, Kauff ND, Domchek SM. 2009. Meta-analysis of risk reduction estimates associated with risk-reducing salpingo-oophorectomy in BRCA1 or BRCA2 mutation carriers. *J Natl Cancer Inst* **101:** 80–87. doi:10.1093/jnci/djn442

Reid BM, Miller BS, Dorn LD, Desjardins C, Donzella B, Gunnar M. 2017. Early growth faltering in post-institutionalized youth and later anthropometric and pubertal development. *Pediatr Res* **82:** 278–284. doi:10.1038/pr.2017.35

Revel A, Abramov Y, Yagel S, Nadjari M. 2004. Utero-ovarian morphology and blood flow after tubal ligation by the Pomeroy technique. *Contraception* **69:** 151–156. doi:10.1016/j.contraception.2003.09.016

Rice MS, Murphy MA, Tworoger SS. 2012. Tubal ligation, hysterectomy and ovarian cancer: a meta-analysis. *J Ovarian Res* **5:** 13. doi:10.1186/1757-2215-5-13

Rice MS, Murphy MA, Vitonis AF, Cramer DW, Titus LJ, Tworoger SS, Terry KL. 2013. Tubal ligation, hysterectomy and epithelial ovarian cancer in the New England case-control study. *Int J Cancer* **133:** 2415–2421. doi:10.1002/ijc.28249

Rice MS, Hankinson SE, Tworoger SS. 2014. Tubal ligation, hysterectomy, unilateral oophorectomy, and risk of ovarian cancer in the Nurses' Health Studies. *Fertil Steril* **102:** 192–198.e3. doi:10.1016/j.fertnstert.2014.03.041

Rice MS, Poole EM, Willett WC, Tworoger SS. 2020. Adult dietary fat intake and ovarian cancer risk. *Int J Cancer* **146:** 2756–2772. doi:10.1002/ijc.32635

Riman T, Dickman PW, Nilsson S, Correia N, Nordlinder H, Magnusson CM, Persson IR. 2002. Risk factors for invasive epithelial ovarian cancer: results from a Swedish case-control study. *Am J Epidemiol* **156:** 363–373. doi:10.1093/aje/kwf048

Risch HA, Marrett LD, Jain M, Howe GR. 1996. Differences in risk factors for epithelial ovarian cancer by histologic type: results of a case-control study. *Am J Epidemiol* **144:** 363–372. doi:10.1093/oxfordjournals.aje.a008937

Rivera CM, Grossardt BR, Rhodes DJ, Brown RD Jr, Roger VL, Melton LJ III, Rocca WA. 2009. Increased cardiovascular mortality after early bilateral oophorectomy. *Menopause* **16:** 15–23. doi:10.1097/gme.0b013e31818888f7

Roberts AL, Huang T, Koenen KC, Kim Y, Kubzansky LD, Tworoger SS. 2019. Posttraumatic stress disorder is associated with increased risk of ovarian cancer: a prospective and retrospective longitudinal cohort study. *Cancer Res* **79:** 5113–5120. doi:10.1158/0008-5472.CAN-19-1222

Rocca WA, Grossardt BR, de Andrade M, Malkasian GD, Melton LJ III. 2006. Survival patterns after oophorectomy in premenopausal women: a population-based cohort study. *Lancet Oncol* **7:** 821–828. doi:10.1016/S1470-2045(06)70869-5

Rocca WA, Bower JH, Maraganore DM, Ahlskog JE, Grossardt BR, de Andrade M, Melton LJ III. 2007. Increased risk of cognitive impairment or dementia in women who underwent oophorectomy before menopause. *Neurology* **69:** 1074–1083. doi:10.1212/01.wnl.0000276984.19542.e6

Rocca WA, Grossardt BR, Shuster LT, Stewart EA. 2012. Hysterectomy, oophorectomy, estrogen, and the risk of dementia. *Neurodegener Dis* **10:** 175–178. doi:10.1159/000334764

Rosenberg L, Palmer JR, Zauber AG, Warshauer ME, Lewis JL Jr, Strom BL, Harlap S, Shapiro S. 1994. A case-control study of oral contraceptive use and invasive epithelial ovarian cancer. *Am J Epidemiol* **139:** 654–661. doi:10.1093/oxfordjournals.aje.a117055

Rosenblatt KA, Weiss NS, Cushing-Haugen KL, Wicklund KG, Rossing MA. 2011. Genital powder exposure and the risk of epithelial ovarian cancer. *Cancer Causes Control* **22:** 737–742. doi:10.1007/s10552-011-9746-3

Rossing MA, Cushing-Haugen KL, Wicklund KG, Doherty JA, Weiss NS. 2010. Recreational physical activity and risk of epithelial ovarian cancer. *Cancer Causes Control* **21:** 485–491.

Rota M, Pasquali E, Scotti L, Pelucchi C, Tramacere I, Islami F, Negri E, Boffetta P, Bellocco R, Corrao G, et al. 2012. Alcohol drinking and epithelial ovarian cancer risk. A systematic review and meta-analysis. *Gynecol Oncol* **125:** 758–763. doi:10.1016/j.ygyno.2012.03.031

Ruderman R, Pavone ME. 2017. Ovarian cancer in endometriosis: an update on the clinical and molecular aspects. *Minerva Ginecol* **69:** 286–294.

Rutter JL, Wacholder S, Chetrit A, Lubin F, Menczer J, Ebbers S, Tucker MA, Struewing JP, Hartge P. 2003. Gynecologic surgeries and risk of ovarian cancer in women with BRCA1 and BRCA2 Ashkenazi founder mutations: an Israeli population-based case-control study. *J Natl Cancer Inst* **95:** 1072–1078. doi:10.1093/jnci/95.14.1072

Salari-Moghaddam A, Milajerdi A, Surkan PJ, Larijani B, Esmaillzadeh A. 2019. Caffeine, type of coffee, and risk of ovarian cancer: a dose-response meta-analysis of prospective studies. *J Clin Endocrinol Metab* **104:** 5349–5359. doi:10.1210/jc.2019-00637

* Sasamoto N, Elias KM. 2023. Early detection of ovarian cancer. *Cold Spring Harb Perspect Med* doi:10.1101/cshperspect.a041337

Schauer IG, Zhang J, Xing Z, Guo X, Mercado-Uribe I, Sood AK, Huang P, Liu J. 2013. Interleukin-1β promotes ovarian tumorigenesis through a p53/NF-κB-mediated inflammatory response in stromal fibroblasts. *Neoplasia* **15:** 409–420. doi:10.1593/neo.121228

Schildkraut JM, Abbott SE, Alberg AJ, Bandera EV, Barnholtz-Sloan JS, Bondy ML, Cote ML, Funkhouser E, Peres LC, Peters ES, et al. 2016. Association between body powder use and ovarian cancer: the African American Cancer Epidemiology Study (AACES). *Cancer Epidemiol Biomarkers Prev* **25:** 1411–1417. doi:10.1158/1055-9965.EPI-15-1281

Schouten LJ, Goldbohm RA, van den Brandt PA. 2003. Height, weight, weight change, and ovarian cancer risk in the Netherlands cohort study on diet and cancer. *Am J Epidemiol* **157:** 424–433. doi:10.1093/aje/kwf224

Schrauder MG, Brunel-Geuder L, Häberle L, Wunderle M, Hoyer J, Csorba R, Reis A, Schulz-Wendtland R, Beckmann MW, Lux MP. 2019. Cost effectiveness of bilateral risk-reducing mastectomy and salpingo-oophorectomy. *Eur J Med Res* **24:** 32. doi:10.1186/s40001-019-0391-8

Schrijver LH, Antoniou AC, Olsson H, Mooij TM, Roos-Blom MJ, Azarang L, Adlard J, Ahmed M, Barrowdale D, Davidson R, et al. 2021. Oral contraceptive use and ovarian cancer risk for BRCA1/2 mutation carriers: an international cohort study. *Am J Obstet Gynecol* **225:** 51.e1–51.e17. doi:10.1016/j.ajog.2021.01.014

Schulz M, Lahmann PH, Boeing H, Hoffmann K, Allen N, Key TJ, Bingham S, Wirfält E, Berglund G, Lundin E, et al. 2005. Fruit and vegetable consumption and risk of epithelial ovarian cancer: the European prospective investigation into cancer and nutrition. *Cancer Epidemiol Biomarkers Prev* **14:** 2531–2535. doi:10.1158/1055-9965.EPI-05-0159

Sezik M, Ozkaya O, Demir F, Sezik HT, Kaya H. 2007. Total salpingectomy during abdominal hysterectomy: effects on ovarian reserve and ovarian stromal blood flow. *J Obstet Gynaecol Res* **33:** 863–869. doi:10.1111/j.1447-0756.2007.00669.x

Shafiei F, Salari-Moghaddam A, Milajerdi A, Larijani B, Esmaillzadeh A. 2019. Coffee and caffeine intake and risk of ovarian cancer: a systematic review and meta-analysis. *Int J Gynecol Cancer* **29:** 579–584. doi:10.1136/ijgc-2018-000102

Shafrir AL, Schock H, Poole EM, Terry KL, Tamimi RM, Hankinson SE, Rosner BA, Tworoger SS. 2017. A prospective cohort study of oral contraceptive use and ovarian cancer among women in the United States born from 1947 to 1964. *Cancer Causes Control* **28:** 371–383. doi:10.1007/s10552-017-0876-0

Shivappa N, Steck SE, Hurley TG, Hussey JR, Hébert JR. 2014. Designing and developing a literature-derived, population-based dietary inflammatory index. *Public Health Nutr* **17:** 1689–1696. doi:10.1017/S1368980013002115

Shivappa N, Hébert JR, Rosato V, Rossi M, Montella M, Serraino D, La Vecchia C. 2016. Dietary inflammatory index and ovarian cancer risk in a large Italian case-control study. *Cancer Causes Control* **27:** 897–906. doi:10.1007/s10552-016-0767-9

Shivappa N, Hébert JR, Paddock LE, Rodriguez-Rodriguez L, Olson SH, Bandera EV. 2018. Dietary inflammatory index and ovarian cancer risk in a New Jersey case-control study. *Nutrition* **46:** 78–82. doi:10.1016/j.nut.2017.08.011

Soong TR, Dinulescu DM, Xian W, Crum CP. 2018a. Frontiers in the pathology and pathogenesis of ovarian cancer: cancer precursors and "precursor escape." *Hematol Oncol Clin North Am* **32:** 915–928. doi:10.1016/j.hoc.2018.07.013

Soong TR, Howitt BE, Miron A, Horowitz NS, Campbell F, Feltmate CM, Muto MG, Berkowitz RS, Nucci MR, Xian W, et al. 2018b. Evidence for lineage continuity between early serous proliferations (ESPs) in the fallopian tube and disseminated high-grade serous carcinomas. *J Pathol* **246:** 344–351. doi:10.1002/path.5145

Soong TR, Kolin DL, Teschan NJ, Crum CP. 2018c. Back to the future? the fallopian tube, precursor escape and a dualistic model of high-grade serous carcinogenesis. *Cancers (Basel)* **10:** 468. doi:10.3390/cancers10120468

Soong TR, Howitt BE, Horowitz N, Nucci MR, Crum CP. 2019. The fallopian tube, "precursor escape" and narrowing the knowledge gap to the origins of high-grade serous carcinoma. *Gynecol Oncol* **152:** 426–433. doi:10.1016/j.ygyno.2018.11.033

Strandell A, Lindhard A, Waldenstrom U, Thorburn J. 2001. Prophylactic salpingectomy does not impair the ovarian response in IVF treatment. *Hum Reprod* **16:** 1135–1139. doi:10.1093/humrep/16.6.1135

Subramaniam A, Blanchard CT, Erickson BK, Szychowski J, Leath CA, Biggio JR, Huh WK. 2018. Feasibility of complete salpingectomy compared with standard postpartum tubal ligation at cesarean delivery: a randomized controlled trial. *Obstet Gynecol* **132:** 20–27. doi:10.1097/AOG.0000000000002646

Tabung FK, Smith-Warner SA, Chavarro JE, Wu K, Fuchs CS, Hu FB, Chan AT, Willett WC, Giovannucci EL. 2016. Development and validation of an empirical dietary inflammatory index. *J Nutr* **146:** 1560–1570. doi:10.3945/jn.115.228718

Tabung FK, Huang T, Giovannucci EL, Smith-Warner SA, Tworoger SS, Poole EM. 2017. The inflammatory potential of diet and ovarian cancer risk: results from two prospective cohort studies. *Br J Cancer* **117:** 907–911. doi:10.1038/bjc.2017.246

Tehranian A, Zangbar RH, Aghajani F, Sepidarkish M, Rafiei S, Esfidani T. 2017. Effects of salpingectomy during abdominal hysterectomy on ovarian reserve: a randomized controlled trial. *Gynecol Surg* **14:** 17. doi:10.1186/s10397-017-1019-z

Terry KL, Karageorgi S, Shvetsov YB, Merritt MA, Lurie G, Thompson PJ, Carney ME, Weber RP, Akushevich L, Lo-Ciganic WH, et al. 2013. Genital powder use and risk of ovarian cancer: a pooled analysis of 8,525 cases and 9,859 controls. *Cancer Prev Res (Phila)* **6:** 811–821. doi:10.1158/1940-6207.CAPR-13-0037

Tomeleri CM, Souza MF, Burini RC, Cavaglieri CR, Ribeiro AS, Antunes M, Nunes JP, Venturini D, Barbosa DS, Sardinha LB, et al. 2018. Resistance training reduces metabolic syndrome and inflammatory markers in older women: a randomized controlled trial. *J Diabetes* **10:** 328–337. doi:10.1111/1753-0407.12614

Trabert B, Ness RB, Lo-Ciganic WH, Murphy MA, Goode EL, Poole EM, Brinton LA, Webb PM, Nagle CM, Jordan SJ, et al. 2014a. Aspirin, nonaspirin nonsteroidal anti-inflammatory drug, and acetaminophen use and risk of invasive epithelial ovarian cancer: a pooled analysis in the Ovarian Cancer Association Consortium. *J Natl Cancer Inst* **106:** djt431. doi:10.1093/jnci/djt431

Trabert B, Pinto L, Hartge P, Kemp T, Black A, Sherman ME, Brinton LA, Pfeiffer RM, Shiels MS, Chaturvedi AK, et al. 2014b. Pre-diagnostic serum levels of inflammation markers and risk of ovarian cancer in the prostate, lung, colorectal and ovarian cancer (PLCO) screening trial. *Gynecol Oncol* **135:** 297–304. doi:10.1016/j.ygyno.2014.08.025

Trabert B, Waterboer T, Idahl A, Brenner N, Brinton LA, Butt J, Coburn SB, Hartge P, Hufnagel K, Inturrisi F, et al. 2019. Antibodies against *Chlamydia trachomatis* and ovarian cancer risk in two independent populations. *J Natl Cancer Inst* **111:** 129–136. doi:10.1093/jnci/djy084

Trudel-Fitzgerald C, Poole EM, Idahl A, Lundin E, Sood AK, Kawachi I, Kubzansky LD, Tworoger SS. 2017. The association of work characteristics with ovarian cancer risk and mortality. *Psychosom Med* **79:** 1059–1067. doi:10.1097/PSY.0000000000000464

Trudel-Fitzgerald C, Poole EM, Sood AK, Okereke OI, Kawachi I, Kubzansky LD, Tworoger SS. 2019. Social integration, marital status, and ovarian cancer risk: a 20-year prospective cohort study. *Psychosom Med* **81:** 833–840. doi:10.1097/PSY.0000000000000747

Tung KH, Goodman MT, Wu AH, McDuffie K, Wilkens LR, Kolonel LN, Nomura AM, Terada KY, Carney ME, Sobin LH. 2003. Reproductive factors and epithelial ovarian cancer risk by histologic type: a multiethnic case-control study. *Am J Epidemiol* **158:** 629–638. doi:10.1093/aje/kwg177

Tworoger SS, Gertig DM, Gates MA, Hecht JL, Hankinson SE. 2008. Caffeine, alcohol, smoking, and the risk of incident epithelial ovarian cancer. *Cancer* **112:** 1169–1177. doi:10.1002/cncr.23275

US Preventive Services Task Force. 2022. Aspirin use to prevent cardiovascular disease: US Preventive Services Task Force Recommendation Statement. *JAMA* **327:** 1577–1584. doi:10.1001/jama.2022.4983

Van Lieshout LAM, Pijlman B, Vos MC, de Groot MJM, Houterman S, Coppus S, Harmsen MG, Vandenput I, Piek JMJ. 2018. Opportunistic salpingectomy in women undergoing hysterectomy: results from the HYSTUB randomised controlled trial. *Maturitas* **107:** 1–6. doi:10.1016/j.maturitas.2017.09.012

van Lieshout LAM, Steenbeek MP, De Hullu JA, Vos MC, Houterman S, Wilkinson J, Piek JM. 2019. Hysterectomy with opportunistic salpingectomy versus hysterectomy alone. *Cochrane Database Syst Rev* **8:** CD012858.

Vercellini P, Viganò P, Buggio L, Makieva S, Scarfone G, Cribiù FM, Parazzini F, Somigliana E. 2018. Perimenopausal management of ovarian endometriosis and associated cancer risk: when is medical or surgical treatment indicated? *Best Pract Res Clin Obstet Gynaecol* **51:** 151–168. doi:10.1016/j.bpobgyn.2018.01.017

Wallin A, Orsini N, Wolk A. 2011. Red and processed meat consumption and risk of ovarian cancer: a dose-response meta-analysis of prospective studies. *Br J Cancer* **104:** 1196–1201. doi:10.1038/bjc.2011.49

Wang Y, Zhang Z, Wang J, Zhang X. 2020. Association between C-reactive protein level and subsequent risk of ovarian cancer: a meta-analysis of 13 cohorts in 1,852 ovarian cancer patients. *Medicine (Baltimore)* **99:** e18821. doi:10.1097/MD.0000000000018821

Wang T, Jake-Schoffman DE, Townsend MK, Vinci C, Willett WC, Tworoger SS. 2021a. Early life physical activity and risk of ovarian cancer in adulthood. *Int J Cancer* **149:** 2045–2051. doi:10.1002/ijc.33760

Wang T, Townsend MK, Vinci C, Jake-Schoffman DE, Tworoger SS. 2021b. Early life exposure to tobacco smoke and ovarian cancer risk in adulthood. *Int J Epidemiol* **50:** 965–974. doi:10.1093/ije/dyab018

Webb PM, Green AC, Jordan SJ. 2017. Trends in hormone use and ovarian cancer incidence in US white and Australian women: implications for the future. *Cancer Causes Control* **28:** 365–370. doi:10.1007/s10552-017-0868-0

Wentzensen N, Poole EM, Trabert B, White E, Arslan AA, Patel AV, Setiawan VW, Visvanathan K, Weiderpass E, Adami HO, et al. 2016. Ovarian cancer risk factors by histologic subtype: an analysis from the Ovarian Cancer Cohort Consortium. *J Clin Oncol* **34:** 2888–2898. doi:10.1200/JCO.2016.66.8178

Wheeler LJ, Desanto K, Teal SB, Sheeder J, Guntupalli SR. 2019. Intrauterine device use and ovarian cancer risk: a systematic review and meta-analysis. *Obstet Gynecol* **134:** 791–800. doi:10.1097/AOG.0000000000003463

Wilbur MA, Shih IM, Segars JH, Fader AN. 2017. Cancer implications for patients with endometriosis. *Semin Reprod Med* **35:** 110–116. doi:10.1055/s-0036-1597120

Wilson L, Pandeya N, Byles J, Mishra G. 2018. Hysterectomy and incidence of depressive symptoms in midlife women: the Australian longitudinal study on women's health. *Epidemiol Psychiatr Sci* **27:** 381–392. doi:10.1017/S2045796016001220

Xiao Q, Yang HP, Wentzensen N, Hollenbeck A, Matthews CE. 2013. Physical activity in different periods of life, sedentary behavior, and the risk of ovarian cancer in the NIH-AARP diet and health study. *Cancer Epidemiol Biomarkers Prev* **22:** 2000–2008. doi:10.1158/1055-9965.EPI-13-0154

Xie J, Poole EM, Terry KL, Fung TT, Rosner BA, Willett WC, Tworoger SS. 2014. A prospective cohort study of dietary indices and incidence of epithelial ovarian cancer. *J Ovarian Res* **7:** 112. doi:10.1186/s13048-014-0112-4

Xu H, Ding Y, Xin X, Wang W, Zhang D. 2018. Dietary fiber intake is associated with a reduced risk of ovarian cancer: a dose-response meta-analysis. *Nutr Res* **57:** 1–11. doi:10.1016/j.nutres.2018.04.011

Yammine S, Huybrechts I, Biessy C, Dossus L, Aglago EK, Naudin S, Ferrari P, Weiderpass E, Tjønneland A, Hansen L, et al. 2020. Dietary and circulating fatty acids and ovarian cancer risk in the European prospective investigation into cancer and nutrition. *Cancer Epidemiol Biomarkers Prev* **29:** 1739–1749. doi:10.1158/1055-9965.EPI-19-1477

Yang HP, Gierach GL, Danforth KN, Sherman ME, Park Y, Wentzensen N, Hollenbeck A, Schatzkin A, Brinton LA. 2011. Alcohol and endometrial cancer risk in the NIH-AARP diet and health study. *Int J Cancer* **128:** 2953–2961. doi:10.1002/ijc.25623

Yi QH, Ling SR, Chen KM, He WR, Li L, Yi CJ. 2012. Evaluation of the clinical value of simultaneous hysterectomy and bilateral salpingectomy in perimenopausal women. *Zhonghua Fu Chan Ke Za Zhi* **47:** 110–114.

Yoon SH, Kim SN, Shim SH, Kang SB, Lee SJ. 2016. Bilateral salpingectomy can reduce the risk of ovarian cancer in the general population: a meta-analysis. *Eur J Cancer* **55:** 38–46. doi:10.1016/j.ejca.2015.12.003

Yuan Z, Cao D, Bi X, Yu M, Yang J, Shen K. 2019. The effects of hysterectomy with bilateral salpingectomy on ovarian reserve. *Int J Gynaecol Obstet* **145:** 233–238. doi:10.1002/ijgo.12798

Zeng F, Wei H, Yeoh E, Zhang Z, Ren ZF, Colditz GA, Tworoger SS, Su X. 2016. Inflammatory markers of CRP, IL6, TNFα, and soluble TNFR2 and the risk of ovarian cancer: a meta-analysis of prospective studies. *Cancer Epidemiol Biomarkers Prev* **25:** 1231–1239. doi:10.1158/1055-9965.EPI-16-0120

Zerden ML, Castellano T, Doll KM, Stuart GS, Munoz MC, Boggess KA. 2018. Risk-reducing salpingectomy versus standard tubal sterilization: lessons from offering women options for interval sterilization. *South Med J* **111:** 173–177. doi:10.14423/SMJ.0000000000000779

Zhan X, Wang J, Pan S, Lu C. 2017. Tea consumption and the risk of ovarian cancer: a meta-analysis of epidemiological studies. *Oncotarget* **8:** 37796–37806. doi:10.18632/oncotarget.16890

Zhang M, Xie X, Lee AH, Binns CW. 2004. Sedentary behaviours and epithelial ovarian cancer risk. *Cancer Causes Control* **15:** 83–89. doi:10.1023/B:CACO.0000016633.47025.2a

Zhou Z, Zeng F, Yuan J, Tang J, Colditz GA, Tworoger SS, Trabert B, Su X. 2017. Pelvic inflammatory disease and the risk of ovarian cancer: a meta-analysis. *Cancer Causes Control* **28:** 415–428. doi:10.1007/s10552-017-0873-3

Early Detection of Ovarian Cancer

Naoko Sasamoto[1] and Kevin M. Elias[2]

[1]Obstetrics and Gynecology Epidemiology Center, Department of Obstetrics and Gynecology, Brigham and Women's Hospital and Harvard Medical School, Boston, Massachusetts 02115, USA

[2]Division of Gynecologic Oncology, Department of Obstetrics and Gynecology, Brigham and Women's Hospital, Dana-Farber Cancer Institute, Harvard Medical School, Boston, Massachusetts 02115, USA

Correspondence: kelias@bwh.harvard.edu

The risk of death from ovarian cancer is highly associated with the clinical stage at diagnosis. Efforts to implement screening for ovarian cancer have been largely unsuccessful, due to the low prevalence of the disease in the general population and the heterogeneity of the various cancer types that fall under the ovarian cancer designation. A practical test for early detection will require both high sensitivity and high specificity to balance reducing the number of cancer deaths with minimizing surgical interventions for false positive screens. The technology must be cost-effective to deliver at scale, widely accessible, and relatively noninvasive. Most importantly, a successful early detection test must be effective not only at diagnosing ovarian cancer but also in reducing ovarian cancer deaths. Stepwise or multimodal approaches among the various areas under investigation will likely be required to make early detection a reality.

The global burden of ovarian cancer is distinct from that of the other major gynecologic malignancies. Ovarian cancer incidence is highest in countries with high-income levels, but age-standardized mortality rates are roughly similar between highly developed and low- and middle-income countries (Cabasag et al. 2022; Huang et al. 2022). The reason for poor survival regardless of access to healthcare is that the majority of cases in both well-resourced and under-resourced countries continue to be diagnosed at late stage (Lowe et al. 2013). Traditionally, later stage at diagnosis has been attributed to early-stage disease being asymptomatic and the lack of a reliable screening test (US Preventive Services Task Force et al. 2018). However, while an approved screening test for both average-risk and high-risk women is still lacking, the idea that early-stage disease is asymptomatic has been challenged (Goff et al. 2007). In fact, a review of 419 women with high-risk, early-stage disease noted that 72% of patients reported one or more symptoms, with the most common being abdominal or pelvic pain (Chan et al. 2022). However, while increased awareness of ovarian cancer by patients and primary care physicians might prompt earlier recognition of disease, without better markers to identify disease below the resolution of standard imaging, it is not yet clear that symptom recognition will be enough to increase diagnoses at a sufficiently earlier disease stage to improve survival.

Cite this article as *Cold Spring Harb Perspect Med* doi: 10.1101/cshperspect.a041337

Recognizing and diagnosing early-stage cancer thus remains a pressing challenge. While age, histotype, grade, and extent of primary cytoreduction are all important prognostic factors for ovarian cancer, the anatomic stage at diagnosis remains the single largest predictor of ovarian cancer outcome (Gaitskell et al. 2022). Although 5-yr overall survival approaches 90% for those diagnosed at stage I, these rates fall to 25%–30% for stage III, and 10%–15% for stage IV (Fig. 1; Peres et al. 2019). Despite advances in cancer therapy, survival rates for advanced-stage ovarian cancer have improved only marginally in the past 20 yr for most patients (Knisely et al. 2020). Consequently, there have been considerable efforts to develop new diagnostic tests for ovarian cancer that might improve early detection of disease.

KEY CAVEATS TO DISCUSSING "EARLY DETECTION" OF OVARIAN CANCER

Early detection refers to diagnosis of ovarian cancer prior to the development of disseminated disease. Depending on the study design, this can be stage I (i.e., limited to the ovary or limited to the fallopian tube) or stage I/II (i.e., limited to the tubo-ovarian complex and the immediately adjacent structures) (Prat et al. 2015). The underlying rationale for early detection strategies is that the diagnosis of cancers at an earlier stage will lead to better disease outcomes, since earlier stage at diagnosis is associated with better long-term survival (Siegel et al. 2017; Henderson et al. 2018). For early diagnosis to impact health on a population level, however, requires that several caveats be acknowledged (Pinsky 2015).

First, "ovarian cancer" is a broad category of malignancies that includes epithelial, stromal, and germ-cell tumors. Even "epithelial ovarian cancer" is an overarching subtype that includes high- and low-grade serous carcinomas, high- and low-grade endometrioid carcinomas, clear-cell carcinomas, mucinous carcinomas, carcinosarcomas, and several rare histotypes. Clinically diagnosed stage I cancers are disproportionately either relatively indolent malignancies (e.g., mucinous carcinomas arising from a borderline tumor, low-grade serous or endometrioid carcinomas, or granulosa cell tumors) or nonepithelial tumors highly responsive to chemotherapy (e.g., dysgerminomas). Moreover, these tumors, which are both less aggressive and/or more responsive to treatment, are more likely to be diagnosed among adolescents and young women, who are likely to have better survival (Zapardiel et al. 2014). Thus, while stage I high-grade serous carcinomas, the target of most early detection efforts, no doubt fare better than advanced-stage tumors, the overall survival rate for stage I high-grade serous carcinoma is closer to 70%–75% than the ~90% seen for ovarian cancers overall. The gains in survival from diagnosing more high-grade serous ovarian cancers at an earlier stage will be more modest than when all stage I ovarian cancers are considered collectively.

Second, assessments of the impact of early detection on cancer outcomes must control for lead-time bias. One assumes that high-grade epithelial ovarian cancers currently diagnosed at an advanced stage, if detected earlier, will have the same favorable prognosis as stage I cancer, but any earlier diagnosis, irrespective of whether it impacts total life expectancy, will add to a patient's total survival time from diagnosis. While the survival proportion at any given time point is increased, there may be no true improvement in the patient's life expectancy (Andersson et al. 2017).

Third, early detection normally connotes the diagnosis of clinically asymptomatic disease. Indeed, ovarian cancer "screening" explicitly refers to the identification of disease among asymptomatic individuals (Henderson et al. 2018). However, many reports concerning purported biomarkers for ovarian cancer do not restrict the study population to subjects with occult disease. Thus, these studies tend to overestimate sensitivity for cancer detection. The need to focus on clinically asymptomatic disease is clear. Even when restricting the topic of early diagnosis to refer to only those tumor types that cause the majority of ovarian cancer deaths (i.e., high-grade serous carcinoma, high-grade endometrioid carcinoma, advanced stage clear-cell carcinoma, and carcinosarcoma), there can be a disconnect between anatomic disease stage and tumor volume. For example, a patient with a 30-

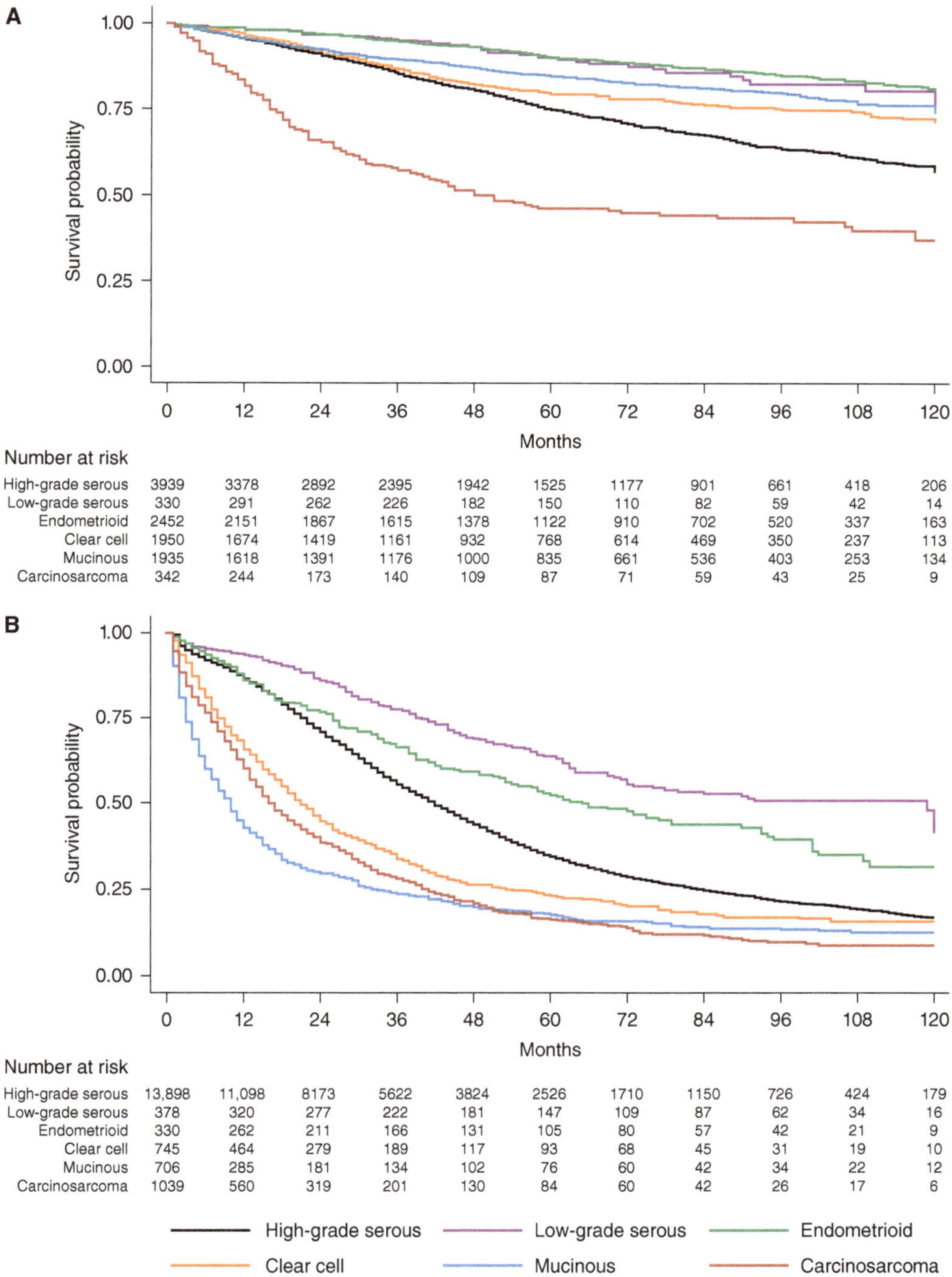

Figure 1. Kaplan–Meier survival curves of invasive epithelial ovarian cancer survival by stage and histotype, 2004–2014, SEER 18 registries. (*A*) Localized and regional-stage disease. (*B*) Distant-stage disease. Malignant Brenner tumors were excluded due to small sample size. (Figure reproduced from Peres et al. 2019, with permission from the author(s), © 2018 who hold the copyright; the paper was published by Oxford University Press.)

cm tumor limited to the ovary has a stage I malignancy, whereas the same patient with a 5-mm tumor in the fallopian tube and scattered 2–3-mm miliary deposits along the diaphragm and omentum has stage III disease. In this case, the stage I patient may be easily diagnosed by physical exam, whereas the stage III tumors may fall below the resolution of even the most advanced imaging techniques. One would expect very high levels of circulating biomarkers secreted from the 30-cm stage I tumor but perhaps very limited circulating biomarker quantities from the case with smaller volume disease. Thus, early detection approaches must consider both tumor size as well as disease burden when applied to clinical practice.

Finally, early detection of ovarian cancer should be considered separately from the problems of cancer risk reduction or interception. "Risk reduction" refers to the identification of individuals at increased relative risk of developing ovarian cancer (whether due to underlying genetic predisposition or family history) coupled with surgical prophylaxis (bilateral salpingectomy or salpingo-oophorectomy) to mitigate that risk (Zakhour et al. 2016). Risk-reducing surgery is highly effective, reducing the chances of developing ovarian cancer among high-risk individuals by more than 80% (De Felice et al. 2017). Although the success of risk reduction among high-risk individuals is widely accepted, more efforts are still needed to help identify high-risk individuals, as most patients with a genetic predisposition to ovarian cancer have no family history of the disease (Weitzel et al. 2007).

Furthermore, risk reduction is separate from "cancer interception." Interception refers to blocking the progression of carcinogenesis prior to the development of advanced disease (Beane et al. 2017). Indeed, the most effective screening programs, such as those for colorectal and cervical cancer, detect not only incident cancers but also precancerous lesions. Interception can be a temporizing measure prior to definitive risk reduction, or, if used to treat premalignant disease (e.g., cervical conization for high-grade cervical dysplasia), a curative intervention to prevent invasive cancer. Screening modalities that could recognize ovarian cancer precursors, for example, serous tubal intraepithelial carcinoma (STIC) lesions, would reduce ovarian cancer incidence and have a greater impact on disease mortality than detection of early-stage cancers alone (Folkins et al. 2008; Duffy 2015). While the recent identification of ovarian cancer precursor lesions in the fallopian tube has made the prospect of cancer interception feasible, these approaches are still in very early stages of clinical development (Mehrad et al. 2010; Chay et al. 2016; Singer 2021). Thus, for the following discussion, "early detection" will focus on the discovery of pelvic-confined, invasive, aggressive malignancies (high-grade serous carcinoma, etc.) among clinically asymptomatic individuals.

ASSESSING THE PERFORMANCE OF SCREENING TESTS

When discussing strategies for early detection of ovarian cancer, it helps to understand several different metrics that can be applied to describe test performance (Kampfrath and Levinson 2013). Sensitivity, sometimes called the "detection rate" or true positive rate (TPR), refers to the proportion of women with ovarian cancer with a positive test result. Conversely, specificity describes the proportion of women without ovarian cancer with a negative test result. The false positive rate (FPR) is equal to 1-specificity. When the sensitivity of a given test over a range of values is plotted against the FPR, the result is a receiver operating characteristic (ROC) curve (Hanley and McNeil 1982). A ROC curve displays tradeoffs between sensitivity and specificity. Often, ROC plots are summarized with the area under the curve (AUC), also known as the C-statistic. While reducing the performance of a diagnostic test to a single value can be helpful, this does come with a loss of granularity in the interpretation of the data. Two screening tests with very different sensitivity and specificity values can have the same C-statistic. Odds ratios (ORs) are another means of summarizing sensitivity and specificity. An OR gives the ratio of the odds of a true positive result versus the odds of a true negative result at a point along the ROC curve (Jaeschke et al. 1995). In low prevalence diseases, the OR approximates the true relative risk (Grimes and Schulz 2008).

The utility of any early detection test for ovarian cancer is highly influenced by the prevalence of the disease among the population being assessed. Prevalence is the total number of individuals among a defined population living with a given condition at a given time. With a 1.8% lifetime risk, ovarian cancer in the general population is a low prevalence disease; the clear majority of those being screened do not have and never will develop ovarian cancer but can be harmed by inappropriate surgical interventions (Henderson et al. 2018).

To ascertain the clinical utility of possible tests, positive predictive value (PPV) and negative predictive value (NPV) are more commonly used in practice. The PPV is the probability that a patient with a positive test has the cancer of interest, while the NPV is the probability that a patient with a negative test does not have this cancer. While sensitivity and specificity are fixed characteristics of a test, PPV and NPV depend on the disease prevalence (Pinsky 2015). Table 1 shows how the PPV and NPV vary based on the prevalence of the disease among the population being screened as well as the desired sensitivity and specificity of the test. In the United States in 2019, the prevalence of ovarian cancer (i.e., the number of women living with ovarian cancer) in the general population among all ages was about 1:714. If an early detection test were to be deployed to screen the general population, to attain a PPV of at least 10% with at least 75% sensitivity, a test would need extremely high specificity (99.06%). However, to achieve a similar sensitivity and PPV among a high-risk population with a disease prevalence of 1:100 (e.g., a *BRCA1* mutation carrier population over 40), only 93.3% specificity would be required. New tests for early detection should model performance characteristics within populations representative of the true prevalence of the disease among the proposed population to which the test will be applied. For example, a test modeled on cancer prevalence in postmenopausal women may not perform as well if directed at a premenopausal population or a population including both pre- and postmenopausal women.

DEVELOPMENT OF BIOMARKERS FOR EARLY DETECTION

A biomarker is "a characteristic that is objectively measured and evaluated as an indicator of normal biological processes, pathogenic processes, or pharmacologic responses to a therapeutic intervention" (Biomarkers Definitions Working Group 2001). Broadly speaking, biomarkers for ovarian cancer can be classified as imaging tests, circulating biomarkers, tumor-proximate biofluids, or some combination of these tools.

Clinical validation of biomarkers for early diagnosis can be divided into five phases (Pepe et al. 2001). Most published reports concern phase I studies. These often rely on various

Table 1. Effects of disease prevalence on test performance

Screening controls	Baseline test characteristics	High sensitivity	Testing higher risk population	Higher specificity	Ultrahigh specificity
Prevalence	1:714	1:714	1:100	1:714	1:714
Sensitivity	75%	97.5%	75%	75%	75%
Specificity	99.06%	98%	93.3%	99.8%	99.95%
PPV	10.06%	6.40%	10.16%	34.48%	67.77%
NPV	99.96%	100%	99.73%	99.96%	99.96%
Accuracy	96.87%	97.95%	91.64%	97.75%	97.68%
LR+	79.79	48.75	11.9	375	1500
LR−	0.25	0.03	0.27	0.25	0.25

(LR+) Positive likelihood ratio, (LR−) negative likelihood ratio, (NPV) negative predictive value, (PPV) positive predictive value.

"omics" approaches to create a model for distinguishing cases from controls. To avoid overfitting data, phase I studies should incorporate cross-validation and validation using independent data sets (Feng et al. 2004). Phase 2 studies evaluate the performance of a biomarker applied to a specific population; cases (individuals with cancer) and controls (individuals without cancer) are directly compared (Pepe et al. 2008). Phase 3 specimens are usually examined as a nested case-control study of prospectively collected specimens from a study cohort that is relevant to the clinical application (Baker et al. 2002). The biomarker is assessed for its performance at a time point when both cases and controls are asymptomatic. Examples include specimens from the Early Detection Research Network (EDRN) (Srivastava 2013). For phase 4 studies, biologic specimens are collected prospectively from a cohort that represents the target population that is envisioned for clinical application of the biomarker, such as the European Prospective Investigation into Cancer and Nutrition (EPIC) cohort (Riboli and Kaaks 1997; Pepe et al. 2008). Phase 5 studies, like the UK Collaborative Trial of Ovarian Cancer Screening (UKCTOCS), are randomized clinical trials that examine the impact of screening on reducing the burden of disease on the population (Jacobs et al. 2016).

EARLY DETECTION BIOMARKER RESEARCH IN PROSPECTIVE COHORT STUDIES

Many of the blood-based early detection biomarker studies on ovarian cancer to date have explored novel early detection biomarkers via a case-control design using samples collected from ovarian cancer cases at the time of diagnosis, which are usually late-stage disease, compared with hospital-based controls, who often are women admitted to the hospital for a benign pelvic mass or other gynecologic indication. The design of these studies might explain why most biomarkers identified thus far perform well in identifying women with ovarian cancer at later stage but do not validate when tested prospectively.

Cancer antigen 125 (CA125) is the single most utilized biomarker for ovarian cancer to date in discriminating ovarian cancer cases from controls (Cramer et al. 2011; Zhu et al. 2011). The name CA125 refers to the antigen recognized by a monoclonal antibody (OC125) identified by Bast and colleagues (1981) that is reactive against epithelial ovarian cancer cell lines and cryopreserved tumors, but not against benign tissue samples or nonovarian carcinomas. Later, this antibody was used for a radioimmunoassay that is highly prognostic for indicating the progression or regression of disease (Bast et al. 1983). At the molecular level, CA125 corresponds to the cleaved, circulating portion of mucin 16 (MUC16), an enormous, heavily *O*-glycosylated glycoprotein (22,152 amino acids) (Das and Batra 2015). Early studies suggested that CA125 might be useful for early diagnosis of ovarian cancer. However, two large, randomized screening trials comparing the combination of blood CA125 measurement and transvaginal ultrasound to usual care showed no significant differences in ovarian cancer mortality.

The Prostate, Lung, Colorectal and Ovarian (PLCO) cancer screening trial randomized 78,216 women aged 55 to 74 yr to undergo either annual screening ($n = 39{,}105$) or usual care ($n = 39{,}111$) at 10 screening centers across the United States between November 1993 and July 2001 (Buys et al. 2005). The intervention group was offered annual screening with CA125 for 6 yr and transvaginal ultrasound for 4 yr. Median follow-up was 12 yr. In the final analysis, there were 3.1 ovarian cancer deaths per 10,000 person-yr in the intervention group and 2.6 ovarian cancer deaths per 10,000 person-yr in the usual care group (mortality relative risk, 1.18; 95% CI, 0.82–1.71) (Buys et al. 2011). Moreover, of the 1080 women who underwent surgical evaluation for a false positive result, 163 women experienced at least one serious complication (15%).

The conclusion of PLCO was that a static CA125 level was insufficient to diagnose cancer, but there remained optimism that dynamic changes in CA125 might be more informative. UKCTOCS randomized a total of 202,638 postmenopausal women aged 50–74 yr to no treatment, annual CA125 screening (using an algorithm that focused on changes in CA125 compared to individual baseline levels) with transvaginal ultrasound scan as a second-line test (multimodal screening [MMS]), or annual screening with transvaginal ultrasound alone across 13 centers in England, Wales, and Northern Ireland (Menon et al. 2009). The initial results suggested a slight mortality benefit after 7 yr of screening if one excluded presumably cancer-prevalent cases at the time of study enrollment (Jacobs et al. 2016). However, in the final analysis with a median follow-up of 16 yr, despite a higher proportion of ovarian cancer cases diagnosed at stage I or II in the MMS arm, both the proportion of women diagnosed with ovarian cancer (1%) and the proportion of women dying from ovarian cancer (0.6%) were identical among the three groups (Menon et al. 2021).

The poor performance of CA125 in PLCO and UKCTOCS can be partially explained by another study examining blood values of four leading protein biomarkers, CA125, HE4, CA72.4, and CA15.3, in prospectively collected blood samples from 810 invasive epithelial ovarian cancer cases and 1939 controls in the prospective cohort of the EPIC study (Terry et al. 2016). CA125 remained the single best marker for the early detection of invasive epithelial ovarian cancer, with little additional benefit found from adding additional markers. However, the utility of CA125 was highly time-dependent, as CA125 was only able to detect stage III/IV ovarian cancer cases close to diagnosis (<6 mo) with limited ability to detect stage I/II disease. The performance in discriminating ovarian cancer cases from controls declined with longer time between blood draw to diagnosis.

EMERGING CIRCULATING BIOMARKERS

Recent advances in technology, including proteomics, transcriptomics, and metabolomics, allow measurement of a larger number of biomarkers at once with high sensitivity, accuracy, and reproducibility using low volume samples (Townsend et al. 2013; Kim et al. 2018; Liberto et al. 2022). These techniques have opened new research avenues for discovering early detection biomarkers in finite blood samples collected by existing large prospective cohort studies. This prospective study design, using blood samples collected months to years prior to clinical ovarian cancer diagnosis to discover novel early detection biomarkers, is ideal, because the samples are more likely to have been collected when the subjects had asymptomatic disease. Another advantage of using these population-based large prospective cohort studies for discovery of early detection biomarkers is that the controls are representative of the underlying population and not hospital-based controls who have reasons for being admitted to a hospital (e.g., those with benign pelvic mass or those who underwent gynecologic surgical procedures such as tubal ligation), which may erroneously result in null associations and limit the generalizability of the findings (Missmer 2019).

This approach has led to identification of several promising biomarkers. One recent study applied the Olink proteomics technology and measured 92 proteins simultaneously in 91 women who had blood collected up to 18 mo prior to ovarian cancer diagnosis and 182 matched controls (Mukama et al. 2022). This study identified nine biomarkers (CA125, HE4, FOLR1, KLK11, WISP1, MDK, CXCL13, MSLN, and ADAM8) that each showed an AUC $\geq$ 0.70 in discriminating ovarian cancer cases from controls. While these blood proteomic biomarkers showed good performance in distinguishing ovarian cancer cases from controls in blood collected up to 9 mo prior to clinical diagnosis, the performance of these biomarkers in discriminating ovarian cancer cases from controls was low in blood samples collected more than 9 mo prior to diagnosis. Another study examined tumor-associated autoantibodies (AAbs) against P53, CTAG1A, CTAG2, and NUDT11, in 194 ovarian cancer cases with blood collected up to 36 mo prior to their diagnosis and 705 matched controls in the EPIC cohort (Kaaks et al. 2018). However, the sensitivity of these markers in blood collected within 6 mo prior to clinical diagnosis was low, ranging from 0.19 to 0.33 at 0.98 specificity, and the discriminatory performance of these markers declined in blood samples collected more than 6 mo prior to diagnosis. Furthermore, when compared to CA125 alone, AAbs and CA125 combined did not improve the sensitivity of identifying ovarian cancer cases from controls. Consequently, the authors concluded that the additional values of these selected AAbs as early detection biomarkers of ovarian cancer was limited.

Because of the poor performance of new protein biomarkers in early diagnosis, cancer metabolites are emerging as alternative candidate biomarkers (Xiao et al. 2022). For example, a nested case-control study (157 cases/156 matched controls) from samples collected during the PLCO screening trial examined arachidonic acid/linoleic acid/α-linoleic acid (free fatty acid) metabolites (Hada et al. 2019). Increased levels of five fatty acid metabolites (8-HETE, 12,13-DHOME, 13-HODE, 9-HODE, and 9, 12,13-THOME) were associated with an increased risk of developing ovarian cancer in the ensuing decade. Several smaller studies have also confirmed that lipid metabolism appears to have discriminatory value for identifying ovarian cancer cases, suggesting a new class of molecule to incorporate into blood-based screening efforts (Gaul et al. 2015; Olkowicz et al. 2021).

Circulating nucleic acids are another emerging class of biomarkers. Both cell-free DNA (cfDNA) and circulating microRNA (miRNA) have attracted considerable interest (Hulstaert et al. 2021; Thusgaard et al. 2021). cfDNA techniques have generally focused on changes in DNA methylation (DNAme) patterns and the fragment size of DNA released from cancers compared to normal tissues (Cristiano et al. 2019; Guo et al. 2021; Markus et al. 2022). One study used the UKCTOCS cohort to examine samples predating a cancer diagnosis by up to 2 yr compared to matched controls (Widschwendter et al. 2017). A 3-DNAme panel had 96.9% specificity at 23.3% sensitivity overall. The authors noted a pronounced confounding effect, however, of DNA from white blood cells (WBCs) leaking into the serum during the sample transport time. If only "low-DNA" samples were included, the sensitivity improved to 57.9% at 88.1% specificity. Among RNA species, most attention has focused on miRNA. Unlike protein biomarkers, no single miRNA has sufficient diagnostic accuracy to be an ovarian cancer biomarker, but several groups have shown that combining small groups of miRNAs can produce models with high specificity and sensitivity (Elias et al. 2017; Yokoi et al. 2018). These analyses are facilitated by using machine-learning techniques (Reilly et al. 2022). For example, by training a neural network on 325 samples, a 7-miRNA model had a PPV of 91.3% and NPV of 78.6% when externally validated on an independent set from another center (Elias et al. 2017).

PROXIMATE TUMOR FLUIDS

Blood is not the only biological fluid being investigated as a source of biomarkers for ovarian cancer diagnosis. The anatomic continuity between the distal fallopian tube and the uterus has made cervical/vaginal secretions alternative sources of material for analysis (Žilovič et al. 2021). The collection techniques have included uterine lavage, tampons, and endocervical brushings (Kinde et al. 2013; Erickson et al. 2014; Wang et al. 2018; Salk et al. 2019). Several small studies have also demonstrated hysteroscopic techniques to cannulate and sample the fallopian tubes (Gizzo et al. 2017; Keenan et al. 2017; Powell et al. 2020). In one study, an antibody-functionalized carbon nanotube complex was even described that could incorporate an optical sensor into an intrauterine device (Williams et al. 2018).

Originally, most of these approaches were based on collecting shed cells for cytology or specific protein markers, but more recent efforts have focused on using either massively parallel sequencing or multiplex PCR to identify tumor-associated mutations, in particular *TP53* (Maritschnegg et al. 2015). The utility of this approach is based on the discovery that both early- and late-stage cancers have roughly similar patterns of somatic mutations and copy number alterations (Cheng et al. 2022). One study found that pathogenic *TP53* variants were even detectable in cervical smears more than 5 yr prior to an ovarian cancer diagnosis (Paracchini et al. 2020). Mutational analysis has been further augmented by examining the methylome of cervical brushings (Barrett et al. 2022).

One advantage of tumor-proximate analysis could be the possibility of testing for endometrial and ovarian cancers. In the study examining endocervical brushings from 656 patients with endometrial or ovarian cancers and 1002 healthy controls, Wang et al. (2018) reported 33% sensitivity at 99% specificity for ovarian cancer using a PCR panel of 18 mutations plus aneuploidy. However, using mutational analysis to detect cancers has also raised concerns because low-frequency mutations are detectable in virtually all women, regardless of the presence of cancer, and overly sensitive techniques might lead to high numbers of false positive results (Salk et al. 2019; Krimmel-Morrison et al. 2020).

TRANSVAGINAL ULTRASOUND FOR EARLY DETECTION

As noted above, both the PLCO and the UKCTOCS studies relied on transvaginal ultrasound (TVUS) as the imaging technique of choice for ovarian cancer screening. TVUS is the preferred clinical modality for imaging the adnexa as it provides superior detail regarding the internal composition of ovarian masses, allows for assessment of vascularity (via Doppler measurements), and provides a dynamic image, which can indicate surface papillary projects and adhesive disease.

Given the high NPV of imaging techniques, TVUS has been examined as a primary screening technique. A study at the University of Kentucky examined annual TVUS among 25,000 asymptomatic women from 1987 to 2005 (van Nagell et al. 2000, 2007). Eligible participants were either 50 yr or older with average risk or 25 yr or older with a family history of ovarian cancer. The initial screen focused on ovarian volume and the presence or absence of papillary or complex tissue projections. Study subjects with persistent abnormalities at 4–6 wk had a serum CA125 determination, tumor morphology indexing, and Doppler flow sonography, and were advised to undergo surgical evaluation. The study was not randomized; instead, the authors compared participants adherent to the annual screening to those receiving less than annual screening. TVUS screening had a sensitivity of 85.0%, specificity of 98.7%, PPV of 14.01%, and NPV of 99.9%. After 107,276 screening years, however, there were seven ovarian cancer deaths in the annually screened population and three ovarian cancer deaths among women not adhering to the screening protocol, suggesting a very high number of scans per case. These numbers are quite similar to the observations in the ultrasound-only arm of UKCTOCS. Following the initial baseline screen, 44,799 of the 50,639 women in the TVUS-only group went on to have a further 280,534 annual scans over the ensuing 9 yr (Kalsi et al. 2021). Based on the imaging, 960 women were referred for exploratory surgery; the PPV was 11.8% at 99.7% specificity. Again, no differences were seen in ovarian cancer deaths (Menon et al. 2021).

Both the Kentucky study and the UKCTOCS study highlight the high FPR of sonographic screening. For this reason, efforts have made to provide better risk assessment of incidental pelvic masses. Among women with a known pelvic mass, the International Ovarian Tumor Analysis (IOTA) group has issued guidelines to estimate the malignancy risk of ovarian tumors (Kaijser et al. 2013). The safety of conservative management according to the IOTA criteria is being evaluated by the IOTA5 study, an international, prospective cohort of 8519 patients with a low-risk pelvic mass (Froyman et al. 2019). Results reported at 2 yr of follow-up indicated that 20.2% of the masses had spontaneously resolved, while the incidence of invasive cancer was 0.4% and borderline tumor was 0.3%. In addition, 0.4% of patients experience ovarian torsion and 0.2% had cyst rupture. If ultrasound remains a part of early detection algorithms, validation of the IOTA guidelines may reduce the number of surgical interventions for false positive results.

EMERGING IMAGING MODALITIES

From a cost perspective, it is unlikely that other imaging techniques will supplant traditional TVUS as an initial imaging approach, but several tools are being developed for secondary screens. One approach is to improve the resolution of ultrasound using a contrast agent (Xun et al. 2021). For example, microbubbles, which combine a protein or lipid shell with a gaseous core, can improve the identification of abnormal vasculature within target lesions (Fleischer et al. 2010). Microbubbles appear to be especially useful for characterization of smaller tumors (Hu et al. 2022). Moreover, there is the potential to functionalize the microbubbles, for example, with antibodies to CA125, to improve the sensitivity of the image (Gao et al. 2017). Another approach is to use magnetic resonance imaging (MRI) as a second-line test following an abnormal ultrasound (Sadowski et al. 2018). Several novel MRI processing techniques have been described, including magnetic relaxometry (MRX), superconducting quantum interference detection (SQUID), and magnetic resonance spectroscopy (MRS), but applications to ovarian cancer diagnosis have been very limited to date; the high cost of these tests will likely limit widespread use (Belkic and Belkic 2017; Nebgen et al. 2019).

CONCLUSION

Early detection remains the best hope to reduce morbidity and mortality from ovarian cancer. However, the PLCO and UKCTOCS studies have shown that large-scale, population-level screening of unselected patients may not be feasible. Instead, a series of multimodal approaches will be required that triage patients into high- and low-risk groups, wherein the performance characteristics of screening tests became more favorable. For example, increased identification of *BRCA1/2* mutation carriers, better attention to family cancer histories, and use of polygenic risk scores may identify more individuals with increased propensity to develop ovarian cancer. These higher risk individuals could then be offered closer surveillance. Whether this is a sequential strategy progressing from blood-based biomarkers to tumor-proximate fluid sampling to more specialized imaging techniques or a series of reflex tests that concentrate interventions on the patients with the highest probability of having cancer remains to be seen. Large, prospectively collected cohorts will be key to testing and validating any of these approaches, and hopefully the combined results will make early detection and long-term survival a more common outcome for this disease.

ACKNOWLEDGMENTS

The authors thank the Honorable Tina Brozman Foundation, the Minnesota Ovarian Cancer Alliance, the Mighty Moose 5K Foundation, the Deborah and Robert First Family Fund, Greg and Peggy Strakosch, the Saltonstall Foundation, the Potter Foundation, the Brigham Ovarian Cancer Research Fund, and the V Foundation for supporting their early detection research efforts.

REFERENCES

Andersson TM, Rutherford MJ, Humphreys K. 2017. Assessment of lead-time bias in estimates of relative survival for breast cancer. *Cancer Epidemiol* **46:** 50–56. doi:10.1016/j.canep.2016.12.004

Baker SG, Kramer BS, Srivastava S. 2002. Markers for early detection of cancer: statistical guidelines for nested case-control studies. *BMC Med Res Methodol* **2:** 4. doi:10.1186/1471-2288-2-4

Barrett JE, Jones A, Evans I, Reisel D, Herzog C, Chindera K, Kristiansen M, Leavy OC, Manchanda R, Bjørge L, et al. 2022. The DNA methylome of cervical cells can predict the presence of ovarian cancer. *Nat Commun* **13:** 448. doi:10.1038/s41467-021-26615-y

Bast RC Jr, Feeney M, Lazarus H, Nadler LM, Colvin RB, Knapp RC. 1981. Reactivity of a monoclonal antibody with human ovarian carcinoma. *J Clin Invest* **68:** 1331–1337. doi:10.1172/JCI110380

Bast RC Jr, Klug TL, St John E, Jenison E, Niloff JM, Lazarus H, Berkowitz RS, Leavitt T, Griffiths CT, Parker L, et al. 1983. A radioimmunoassay using a monoclonal antibody to monitor the course of epithelial ovarian cancer. *N Engl J Med* **309:** 883–887. doi:10.1056/NEJM198310133091503

Beane J, Campbell JD, Lel J, Vick J, Spira A. 2017. Genomic approaches to accelerate cancer interception. *Lancet Oncol* **18:** e494–e502. doi:10.1016/S1470-2045(17)30373-X

Belkic K, Belkic D. 2017. The challenge of ovarian cancer: steps toward early detection through advanced signal processing in magnetic resonance spectroscopy. *Isr Med Assoc J* **19:** 517–525.

Biomarkers Definitions Working Group. 2001. Biomarkers and surrogate endpoints: preferred definitions and conceptual framework. *Clin Pharmacol Ther* **69:** 89–95. doi:10.1067/mcp.2001.113989

Buys SS, Partridge E, Greene MH, Prorok PC, Reding D, Riley TL, Hartge P, Fagerstrom RM, Ragard LR, Chia D, et al. 2005. Ovarian cancer screening in the Prostate, Lung, Colorectal and Ovarian (PLCO) cancer screening trial: findings from the initial screen of a randomized trial. *Am J Obstet Gynecol* **193:** 1630–1639. doi:10.1016/j.ajog.2005.05.005

Buys SS, Partridge E, Black A, Johnson CC, Lamerato L, Isaacs C, Reding DJ, Greenlee RT, Yokochi LA, Kessel B, et al. 2011. Effect of screening on ovarian cancer mortality: the Prostate, Lung, Colorectal and Ovarian (PLCO)

cancer screening randomized controlled trial. *JAMA* **305:** 2295–2303. doi:10.1001/jama.2011.766

Cabasag CJ, Fagan PJ, Ferlay J, Vignat J, Laversanne M, Liu L, van der Aa MA, Bray F, Soerjomataram I. 2022. Ovarian cancer today and tomorrow: a global assessment by world region and Human Development Index using GLOBOCAN 2020. *Int J Cancer* **151:** 1535–1541. doi:10.1002/ijc.34002

Chan JK, Tian C, Kesterson JP, Monk BJ, Kapp DS, Davidson B, Robertson S, Copeland LJ, Walker JL, Wenham RM, et al. 2022. Symptoms of women with high-risk early-stage ovarian cancer. *Obstet Gynecol* **139:** 157–162. doi:10.1097/AOG.0000000000004642

Chay WY, McCluggage WG, Lee CH, Köbel M, Irving J, Millar J, Gilks CB, Tinker AV. 2016. Outcomes of incidental fallopian tube high-grade serous carcinoma and serous tubal intraepithelial carcinoma in women at low risk of hereditary breast and ovarian cancer. *Int J Gynecol Cancer* **26:** 431–436. doi:10.1097/IGC.0000000000000639

Cheng Z, Mirza H, Ennis DP, Smith P, Morrill Gavarró L, Sokota C, Giannone G, Goranova T, Bradley T, Piskorz A, et al. 2022. The genomic landscape of early-stage ovarian high-grade serous carcinoma. *Clin Cancer Res* **28:** 2911–2922. doi:10.1158/1078-0432.CCR-21-1643

Cramer DW, Bast RC Jr, Berg CD, Diamandis EP, Godwin AK, Hartge P, Lokshin AE, Lu KH, McIntosh MW, Mor G, et al. 2011. Ovarian cancer biomarker performance in prostate, lung, colorectal, and ovarian cancer screening trial specimens. *Cancer Prev Res (Phila)* **4:** 365–374. doi:10.1158/1940-6207.CAPR-10-0195

Cristiano S, Leal A, Phallen J, Fiksel J, Adleff V, Bruhm DC, Jensen SO, Medina JE, Hruban C, White JR, et al. 2019. Genome-wide cell-free DNA fragmentation in patients with cancer. *Nature* **570:** 385–389. doi:10.1038/s41586-019-1272-6

Das S, Batra SK. 2015. Understanding the unique attributes of MUC16 (CA125): potential implications in targeted therapy. *Cancer Res* **75:** 4669–4674. doi:10.1158/0008-5472.CAN-15-1050

De Felice F, Marchetti C, Boccia SM, Romito A, Sassu CM, Porpora MG, Muzii L, Tombolini V, Benedetti Panici P. 2017. Risk-reducing salpingo-oophorectomy in BRCA1 and BRCA2 mutated patients: an evidence-based approach on what women should know. *Cancer Treat Rev* **61:** 1–5. doi:10.1016/j.ctrv.2017.09.005

Duffy MJ. 2015. Use of biomarkers in screening for cancer. *Adv Exp Med Biol* **867:** 27–39. doi:10.1007/978-94-017-7215-0_3

Elias KM, Fendler W, Stawiski K, Fiascone SJ, Vitonis AF, Berkowitz RS, Frendl G, Konstantinopoulos P, Crum CP, Kedzierska M, et al. 2017. Diagnostic potential for a serum miRNA neural network for detection of ovarian cancer. *eLife* **6:** 28932. doi:10.7554/eLife.28932

Erickson BK, Kinde I, Dobbin ZC, Wang Y, Martin JY, Alvarez RD, Conner MG, Huh WK, Roden RBS, Kinzler KW, et al. 2014. Detection of somatic TP53 mutations in tampons of patients with high-grade serous ovarian cancer. *Obstet Gynecol* **124:** 881–885. doi:10.1097/AOG.0000000000000484

Feng Z, Prentice R, Srivastava S. 2004. Research issues and strategies for genomic and proteomic biomarker discovery and validation: a statistical perspective. *Pharmacogenomics* **5:** 709–719. doi:10.1517/14622416.5.6.709

Fleischer AC, Lyshchik A, Andreotti RF, Hwang M, Jones HW III, Fishman DA. 2010. Advances in sonographic detection of ovarian cancer: depiction of tumor neovascularity with microbubbles. *AJR Am J Roentgenol* **194:** 343–348. doi:10.2214/AJR.09.3446

Folkins AK, Jarboe EA, Saleemuddin A, Lee Y, Callahan MJ, Drapkin R, Garber JE, Muto MG, Tworoger S, Crum CP. 2008. A candidate precursor to pelvic serous cancer (p53 signature) and its prevalence in ovaries and fallopian tubes from women with BRCA mutations. *Gynecol Oncol* **109:** 168–173. doi:10.1016/j.ygyno.2008.01.012

Froyman W, Landolfo C, De Cock B, Wynants L, Sladkevicius P, Testa AC, Van Holsbeke C, Domali E, Fruscio R, Epstein E, et al. 2019. Risk of complications in patients with conservatively managed ovarian tumours (IOTA5): a 2-year interim analysis of a multicentre, prospective, cohort study. *Lancet Oncol* **20:** 448–458. doi:10.1016/S1470-2045(18)30837-4

Gaitskell K, Hermon C, Barnes I, Pirie K, Floud S, Green J, Beral V, Reeves GK; Million Women Study Collaborators. 2022. Ovarian cancer survival by stage, histotype, and pre-diagnostic lifestyle factors, in the prospective UK Million Women Study. *Cancer Epidemiol* **76:** 102074. doi:10.1016/j.canep.2021.102074

Gao Y, Hernandez C, Yuan HX, Lilly J, Kota P, Zhou H, Wu H, Exner AA. 2017. Ultrasound molecular imaging of ovarian cancer with CA-125 targeted nanobubble contrast agents. *Nanomedicine* **13:** 2159–2168. doi:10.1016/j.nano.2017.06.001

Gaul DA, Mezencev R, Long TQ, Jones CM, Benigno BB, Gray A, Fernández FM, McDonald JF. 2015. Highly-accurate metabolomic detection of early-stage ovarian cancer. *Sci Rep* **5:** 16351. doi:10.1038/srep16351

Gizzo S, Noventa M, Quaranta M, Vitagliano A, Saccardi C, Litta P, Antona D. 2017. A novel hysteroscopic approach for ovarian cancer screening/early diagnosis. *Oncol Lett* **13:** 549–553. doi:10.3892/ol.2016.5493

Goff BA, Mandel LS, Drescher CW, Urban N, Gough S, Schurman KM, Patras J, Mahony BS, Andersen MR. 2007. Development of an ovarian cancer symptom index: possibilities for earlier detection. *Cancer* **109:** 221–227. doi:10.1002/cncr.22371

Grimes DA, Schulz KF. 2008. Making sense of odds and odds ratios. *Obstet Gynecol* **111:** 423–426. doi:10.1097/01.AOG.0000297304.32187.5d

Guo XM, Miller H, Matsuo K, Roman LD, Salhia B. 2021. Circulating cell-free DNA methylation profiles in the early detection of ovarian cancer: a scoping review of the literature. *Cancers (Basel)* **13:** 838. doi:10.3390/cancers13040838

Hada M, Edin ML, Hartge P, Lih FB, Wentzensen N, Zeldin DC, Trabert B. 2019. Prediagnostic serum levels of fatty acid metabolites and risk of ovarian cancer in the Prostate, Lung, Colorectal, and Ovarian (PLCO) Cancer Screening Trial. *Cancer Epidemiol Biomarkers Prev* **28:** 189–197. doi:10.1158/1055-9965.EPI-18-0392

Hanley JA, McNeil BJ. 1982. The meaning and use of the area under a receiver operating characteristic (ROC) curve. *Radiology* **143:** 29–36. doi:10.1148/radiology.143.1.7063747

Henderson JT, Webber EM, Sawaya GF. 2018. Screening for ovarian cancer: updated evidence report and systematic review for the US Preventive Services Task Force. *JAMA* **319:** 595–606. doi:10.1001/jama.2017.21421

Hu R, Shahai G, Liu H, Feng Y, Xiang H. 2022. Diagnostic value of two-dimensional transvaginal ultrasound combined with contrast-enhanced ultrasound in ovarian cancer. *Front Surg* **9:** 898365. doi:10.3389/fsurg.2022.898365

Huang J, Chan WC, Ngai CH, Lok V, Zhang L, Lucero-Prisno DE, Xu W, Zheng ZJ, Elcarte E, Withers M, et al. 2022. Worldwide burden, risk factors, and temporal trends of ovarian cancer: a global study. *Cancers (Basel)* **14:** 2230. doi:10.3390/cancers14092230

Hulstaert E, Morlion A, Levanon K, Vandesompele J, Mestdagh P. 2021. Candidate RNA biomarkers in biofluids for early diagnosis of ovarian cancer: a systematic review. *Gynecol Oncol* **160:** 633–642. doi:10.1016/j.ygyno.2020.11.018

Jacobs IJ, Menon U, Ryan A, Gentry-Maharaj A, Burnell M, Kalsi JK, Amso NN, Apostolidou S, Benjamin E, Cruickshank D, et al. 2016. Ovarian cancer screening and mortality in the UK Collaborative Trial of Ovarian Cancer Screening (UKCTOCS): a randomised controlled trial. *Lancet* **387:** 945–956. doi:10.1016/S0140-6736(15)01224-6

Jaeschke R, Guyatt G, Shannon H, Walter S, Cook D, Heddle N. 1995. Basic statistics for clinicians. 3: Assessing the effects of treatment: measures of association. *CMAJ* **152:** 351–357.

Kaaks R, Fortner RT, Hüsing A, Barrdahl M, Hopper M, Johnson T, Tjønneland A, Hansen L, Overvad K, Fournier A, et al. 2018. Tumor-associated autoantibodies as early detection markers for ovarian cancer? A prospective evaluation. *Int J Cancer* **143:** 515–526. doi:10.1002/ijc.31335

Kaijser J, Bourne T, Valentin L, Sayasneh A, Van Holsbeke C, Vergote I, Testa AC, Franchi D, Van Calster B, Timmerman D. 2013. Improving strategies for diagnosing ovarian cancer: a summary of the International Ovarian Tumor Analysis (IOTA) studies. *Ultrasound Obstet Gynecol* **41:** 9–20. doi:10.1002/uog.12323

Kalsi J, Gentry-Maharaj A, Ryan A, Singh N, Burnell M, Massingham S, Apostolidou S, Sharma A, Williamson K, Seif M, et al. 2021. Performance characteristics of the ultrasound strategy during incidence screening in the UK Collaborative Trial of Ovarian Cancer Screening (UKCTOCS). *Cancers (Basel)* **13:** 858. doi:10.3390/cancers13040858

Kampfrath T, Levinson SS. 2013. Brief critical review: statistical assessment of biomarker performance. *Clin Chim Acta* **419:** 102–107. doi:10.1016/j.cca.2013.02.006

Keenan M, Tate TH, Kieu K, Black JF, Utzinger U, Barton JK. 2017. Design and characterization of a combined OCT and wide field imaging falloposcope for ovarian cancer detection. *Biomed Opt Express* **8:** 124–136. doi:10.1364/BOE.8.000124

Kim CH, Tworoger SS, Stampfer MJ, Dillon ST, Gu X, Sawyer SJ, Chan AT, Libermann TA, Eliassen AH. 2018. Stability and reproducibility of proteomic profiles measured with an aptamer-based platform. *Sci Rep* **8:** 8382. doi:10.1038/s41598-018-26640-w

Kinde I, Bettegowda C, Wang Y, Wu J, Agrawal N, Shih Ie M, Kurman R, Dao F, Levine DA, Giuntoli R, et al. 2013. Evaluation of DNA from the Papanicolaou test to detect ovarian and endometrial cancers. *Sci Transl Med* **5:** 167ra164. doi:10.1126/scitranslmed.3004952

Knisely AT, St Clair CM, Hou JY, Collado FK, Hershman DL, Wright JD, Melamed A. 2020. Trends in primary treatment and median survival among women with advanced-stage epithelial ovarian cancer in the US from 2004 to 2016. *JAMA Netw Open* **3:** e2017517. doi:10.1001/jamanetworkopen.2020.17517

Krimmel-Morrison JD, Ghezelayagh TS, Lian S, Zhang Y, Fredrickson J, Nachmanson D, Baker KT, Radke MR, Hun E, Norquist BM, et al. 2020. Characterization of TP53 mutations in Pap test DNA of women with and without serous ovarian carcinoma. *Gynecol Oncol* **156:** 407–414. doi:10.1016/j.ygyno.2019.11.124

Liberto JM, Chen SY, Shih IM, Wang TH, Wang TL, Pisanic TR II. 2022. Current and emerging methods for ovarian cancer screening and diagnostics: a comprehensive review. *Cancers (Basel)* **14:** 2885. doi:10.3390/cancers14122885

Lowe KA, Chia VM, Taylor A, O'Malley C, Kelsh M, Mohamed M, Mowat FS, Goff B. 2013. An international assessment of ovarian cancer incidence and mortality. *Gynecol Oncol* **130:** 107–114. doi:10.1016/j.ygyno.2013.03.026

Maritschnegg E, Wang Y, Pecha N, Horvat R, Van Nieuwenhuysen E, Vergote I, Heitz F, Sehouli J, Kinde I, Diaz LA Jr, et al. 2015. Lavage of the uterine cavity for molecular detection of Müllerian duct carcinomas: a proof-of-concept study. *J Clin Oncol* **33:** 4293–4300. doi:10.1200/JCO.2015.61.3083

Markus H, Chandrananda D, Moore E, Mouliere F, Morris J, Brenton JD, Smith CG, Rosenfeld N. 2022. Refined characterization of circulating tumor DNA through biological feature integration. *Sci Rep* **12:** 1928. doi:10.1038/s41598-022-05606-z

Mehrad M, Ning G, Chen EY, Mehra KK, Crum CP. 2010. A pathologist's road map to benign, precancerous, and malignant intraepithelial proliferations in the fallopian tube. *Adv Anat Pathol* **17:** 293–302. doi:10.1097/PAP.0b013e3181ecdee1

Menon U, Gentry-Maharaj A, Hallett R, Ryan A, Burnell M, Sharma A, Lewis S, Davies S, Philpott S, Lopes A, et al. 2009. Sensitivity and specificity of multimodal and ultrasound screening for ovarian cancer, and stage distribution of detected cancers: results of the prevalence screen of the UK Collaborative Trial of Ovarian Cancer Screening (UKCTOCS). *Lancet Oncol* **10:** 327–340. doi:10.1016/S1470-2045(09)70026-9

Menon U, Gentry-Maharaj A, Burnell M, Singh N, Ryan A, Karpinskyj C, Carlino G, Taylor J, Massingham SK, Raikou M, et al. 2021. Ovarian cancer population screening and mortality after long-term follow-up in the UK Collaborative Trial of Ovarian Cancer Screening (UKCTOCS): a randomised controlled trial. *Lancet* **397:** 2182–2193. doi:10.1016/S0140-6736(21)00731-5

Missmer SA. 2019. Why so null? Methodologic necessities to advance endometriosis discovery. *Paediatr Perinat Epidemiol* **33:** 26–27. doi:10.1111/ppe.12540

Mukama T, Fortner RT, Katzke V, Hynes LC, Petrera A, Hauck SM, Johnson T, Schulze M, Schiborn C, Rostgaard-Hansen AL, et al. 2022. Prospective evaluation of

92 serum protein biomarkers for early detection of ovarian cancer. *Br J Cancer* **126:** 1301–1309. doi:10.1038/s41416-021-01697-z

Nebgen DR, Lu KH, Bast RC Jr. 2019. Novel approaches to ovarian cancer screening. *Curr Oncol Rep* **21:** 75. doi:10.1007/s11912-019-0816-0

Olkowicz M, Rosales-Solano H, Kulasingam V, Pawliszyn J. 2021. SPME-LC/MS-based serum metabolomic phenotyping for distinguishing ovarian cancer histologic subtypes: a pilot study. *Sci Rep* **11:** 22428. doi:10.1038/s41598-021-00802-9

Paracchini L, Pesenti C, Delle Marchette M, Beltrame L, Bianchi T, Grassi T, Buda A, Landoni F, Ceppi L, Bosetti C, et al. 2020. Detection of *TP53* clonal variants in Papanicolaou test samples collected up to 6 years prior to high-grade serous epithelial ovarian cancer diagnosis. *JAMA Netw Open* **3:** e207566. doi:10.1001/jamanetworkopen.2020.7566

Pepe MS, Etzioni R, Feng Z, Potter JD, Thompson ML, Thornquist M, Winget M, Yasui Y. 2001. Phases of biomarker development for early detection of cancer. *J Natl Cancer Inst* **93:** 1054–1061. doi:10.1093/jnci/93.14.1054

Pepe MS, Feng Z, Janes H, Bossuyt PM, Potter JD. 2008. Pivotal evaluation of the accuracy of a biomarker used for classification or prediction: standards for study design. *J Natl Cancer Inst* **100:** 1432–1438. doi:10.1093/jnci/djn326

Peres LC, Cushing-Haugen KL, Köbel M, Harris HR, Berchuck A, Rossing MA, Schildkraut JM, Doherty JA. 2019. Invasive epithelial ovarian cancer survival by histotype and disease stage. *J Natl Cancer Inst* **111:** 60–68. doi:10.1093/jnci/djy071

Pinsky PF. 2015. Principles of cancer screening. *Surg Clin North Am* **95:** 953–966. doi:10.1016/j.suc.2015.05.009

Powell CB, Littell RD, Landen CN Jr, Pramanik S, Hamilton IC, Suh-Burgmann EJ. 2020. Cytological sampling of fallopian tubes using a hysteroscopic catheter: a multi-center study. *Gynecol Oncol* **156:** 636–640. doi:10.1016/j.ygyno.2019.12.026

Prat J; FIGO Committee on Gynecologic Oncology. 2015. Abridged republication of FIGO's staging classification for cancer of the ovary, fallopian tube, and peritoneum. *Cancer* **121:** 3452–3454. doi:10.1002/cncr.29524

Reilly G, Bullock RG, Greenwood J, Ure DR, Stewart E, Davidoff P, DeGrazia J, Fritsche H, Dunton CJ, Bhardwaj N, et al. 2022. Analytical validation of a deep neural network algorithm for the detection of ovarian cancer. *JCO Clin Cancer Inform* **6:** e2100192. doi:10.1200/CCI.21.00192

Riboli E, Kaaks R. 1997. The EPIC Project: rationale and study design. European Prospective Investigation into Cancer and Nutrition. *Int J Epidemiol* **26** (Suppl 1): S6–S14. doi:10.1093/ije/26.suppl_1.S6

Sadowski EA, Robbins JB, Rockall AG, Thomassin-Naggara I. 2018. A systematic approach to adnexal masses discovered on ultrasound: the ADNEx MR scoring system. *Abdom Radiol (NY)* **43:** 679–695. doi:10.1007/s00261-017-1272-7

Salk JJ, Loubet-Senear K, Maritschnegg E, Valentine CC, Williams LN, Higgins JE, Horvat R, Vanderstichele A, Nachmanson D, Baker KT, et al. 2019. Ultra-sensitive TP53 sequencing for cancer detection reveals progressive clonal selection in normal tissue over a century of human lifespan. *Cell Rep* **28:** 132–144.e3. doi:10.1016/j.celrep.2019.05.109

Siegel RL, Miller KD, Jemal A. 2017. Cancer statistics, 2017. *CA Cancer J Clin* **67:** 7–30. doi:10.3322/caac.21387

Singer CF. 2021. Nonsurgical prevention strategies in *BRCA1* and *BRCA2* mutation carriers. *Breast Care (Basel)* **16:** 144–148. doi:10.1159/000507503

Srivastava S. 2013. The early detection research network: 10-year outlook. *Clin Chem* **59:** 60–67. doi:10.1373/clinchem.2012.184697

Terry KL, Schock H, Fortner RT, Hüsing A, Fichorova RN, Yamamoto HS, Vitonis AF, Johnson T, Overvad K, Tjønneland A, et al. 2016. A prospective evaluation of early detection biomarkers for ovarian cancer in the European EPIC Cohort. *Clin Cancer Res* **22:** 4664–4675. doi:10.1158/1078-0432.CCR-16-0316

Thusgaard CF, Korsholm M, Koldby KM, Kruse TA, Thomassen M, Jochumsen KM. 2021. Epithelial ovarian cancer and the use of circulating tumor DNA: a systematic review. *Gynecol Oncol* **161:** 884–895. doi:10.1016/j.ygyno.2021.04.020

Townsend MK, Clish CB, Kraft P, Wu C, Souza AL, Deik AA, Tworoger SS, Wolpin BM. 2013. Reproducibility of metabolomic profiles among men and women in 2 large cohort studies. *Clin Chem* **59:** 1657–1667. doi:10.1373/clinchem.2012.199133

US Preventive Services Task Force; Grossman DC, Curry SJ, Owens DK, Barry MJ, Davidson KW, Doubeni CA, Epling JW Jr, Kemper AR, Krist AH, et al. 2018. Screening for ovarian cancer: US Preventive Services Task Force recommendation statement. *JAMA* **319:** 588–594. doi:10.1001/jama.2017.21926

van Nagell JR Jr, DePriest PD, Reedy MB, Gallion HH, Ueland FR, Pavlik EJ, Kryscio RJ. 2000. The efficacy of transvaginal sonographic screening in asymptomatic women at risk for ovarian cancer. *Gynecol Oncol* **77:** 350–356. doi:10.1006/gyno.2000.5816

van Nagell JR Jr, DePriest PD, Ueland FR, DeSimone CP, Cooper AL, McDonald JM, Pavlik EJ, Kryscio RJ. 2007. Ovarian cancer screening with annual transvaginal sonography: findings of 25,000 women screened. *Cancer* **109:** 1887–1896. doi:10.1002/cncr.22594

Wang Y, Li L, Douville C, Cohen JD, Yen TT, Kinde I, Sundfelt K, Kjaer SK, Hruban RH, Shih IM, et al. 2018. Evaluation of liquid from the Papanicolaou test and other liquid biopsies for the detection of endometrial and ovarian cancers. *Sci Transl Med* **10:** eaap8793. doi:10.1126/scitranslmed.aap8793

Weitzel JN, Lagos VI, Cullinane CA, Gambol PJ, Culver JO, Blazer KR, Palomares MR, Lowstuter KJ, MacDonald DJ. 2007. Limited family structure and BRCA gene mutation status in single cases of breast cancer. *JAMA* **297:** 2587–2595. doi:10.1001/jama.297.23.2587

Widschwendter M, Zikan M, Wahl B, Lempiäinen H, Paprotka T, Evans I, Jones A, Ghazali S, Reisel D, Eichner J, et al. 2017. The potential of circulating tumor DNA methylation analysis for the early detection and management of ovarian cancer. *Genome Med* **9:** 116. doi:10.1186/s13073-017-0500-7

Williams RM, Lee C, Galassi TV, Harvey JD, Leicher R, Sirenko M, Dorso MA, Shah J, Olvera N, Dao F, et al.

2018. Noninvasive ovarian cancer biomarker detection via an optical nanosensor implant. *Sci Adv* **4:** eaaq1090. doi:10.1126/sciadv.aaq1090

Xiao Y, Bi M, Guo H, Li M. 2022. Multi-omics approaches for biomarker discovery in early ovarian cancer diagnosis. *EBioMedicine* **79:** 104001. doi:10.1016/j.ebiom.2022.104001

Xun L, Zhai L, Xu H. 2021. Comparison of conventional, Doppler and contrast-enhanced ultrasonography in differential diagnosis of ovarian masses: a systematic review and meta-analysis. *BMJ Open* **11:** e052830. doi:10.1136/bmjopen-2021-052830

Yokoi A, Matsuzaki J, Yamamoto Y, Yoneoka Y, Takahashi K, Shimizu H, Uehara T, Ishikawa M, Ikeda SI, Sonoda T, et al. 2018. Integrated extracellular microRNA profiling for ovarian cancer screening. *Nat Commun* **9:** 4319. doi:10.1038/s41467-018-06434-4

Zakhour M, Danovitch Y, Lester J, Rimel BJ, Walsh CS, Li AJ, Karlan BY, Cass I. 2016. Occult and subsequent cancer incidence following risk-reducing surgery in BRCA mutation carriers. *Gynecol Oncol* **143:** 231–235. doi:10.1016/j.ygyno.2016.08.336

Zapardiel I, Diestro MD, Aletti G. 2014. Conservative treatment of early stage ovarian cancer: oncological and fertility outcomes. *Eur J Surg Oncol* **40:** 387–393. doi:10.1016/j.ejso.2013.11.028

Zhu CS, Pinsky PF, Cramer DW, Ransohoff DF, Hartge P, Pfeiffer RM, Urban N, Mor G, Bast RC Jr, Moore LE, et al. 2011. A framework for evaluating biomarkers for early detection: validation of biomarker panels for ovarian cancer. *Cancer Prev Res (Phila)* **4:** 375–383. doi:10.1158/1940-6207.CAPR-10-0193

Žilovič D, Čiurliene R, Sabaliauskaite R, Jarmalaite S. 2021. Future screening prospects for ovarian cancer. *Cancers (Basel)* **13:** 3840. doi:10.3390/cancers13153840

The Emerging Role of the Single-Cell and Spatial Tumor Microenvironment in High-Grade Serous Ovarian Cancer

Inga-Maria Launonen,[1] Anna Vähärautio,[1,2] and Anniina Färkkilä[1,3,4]

[1]Research Program in Systems Oncology, University of Helsinki, 00014 Helsinki, Finland

[2]Foundation for the Finnish Cancer Institute, 00290 Helsinki, Finland

[3]FIMM and HiLlfe, 00014 Helsinki, Finland

[4]Department of Obstetrics and Gynecology, Helsinki University Hospital, 00290 Helsinki, Finland

Correspondence: anniina.farkkila@helsinki.fi

The development of single-cell and spatial technologies has enabled a more detailed understanding of the tumor microenvironment and its role in therapy response and clinical outcome of high-grade serous ovarian cancer (HGSC). Interestingly, emerging evidence suggests that HGSCs with different genetic drivers harbor distinct tumor-immune microenvironments. Further, spatial cell–cell interactions have been shown to shape the $CD8^+$ T-cell phenotypes and responses to immune checkpoint blockade therapies. The heterogeneous stroma consisting of cancer-associated fibroblast (CAF) subtypes, endothelia, and site-specific stromal types such as mesothelium modulates treatment responses via increasing stiffness and by producing ligands that promote drug resistance, angiogenesis, or immune escape. Chemotherapy itself shifts CAFs toward an inflammatory phenotype that associates with poor survival and immune-suppressive signaling. New emerging immunotherapies include combinational approaches and agents targeting, for example, the tumor-intrinsic endoplasmic reticulum pathway. A more detailed understanding of the spatial interplay of tumor, immune, and stromal cells in the tumor microenvironment is needed to develop more efficient immunotherapeutic strategies for HGSC.

Tumorigenesis and cancer progression are dependent on the ability of malignant cells to escape the recognition and attack by the host immune system (Kim et al. 2007). Antitumor immunity and immune escape involve a complex interplay of host-dependent and tumor-intrinsic processes (Fig. 1).

Two main mechanisms of immune escape have been recognized: (1) innate escape, in which T cells and other relevant immune cells are excluded from the tumor microenvironment (TME) (Zhang et al. 2003; Danilova et al. 2016), and (2) adaptive escape, where tumor progresses despite the presence of T cells via up-regulation of immune resistance mechanisms (Tumeh et al. 2014). To elicit antitumor immunity, tumor-derived novel peptides called neoantigens arising from somatic mutations are

Cite this article as *Cold Spring Harb Perspect Med* doi: 10.1101/cshperspect.a041314

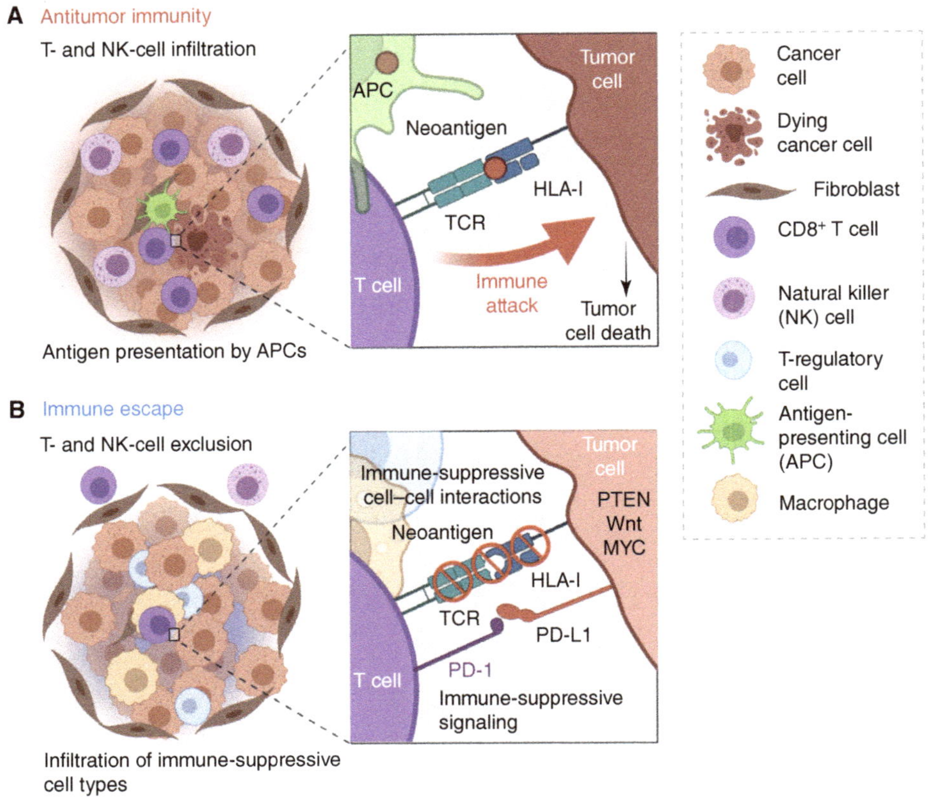

Figure 1. Mechanisms of antitumor immunity and immune escape. (*A*) Critical components of the antitumor immune response include the presence of T and natural killer (NK) cells in the tumor microenvironment (TME), presentation of neoantigens to T cells by dendritic cells, and recognition of neoantigens on human leukocyte antigen (HLA) molecules by T-cell receptors (TCRs), resulting in immune attack and tumor cell death. (*B*) Currently known immune escape mechanisms include exclusion of T and NK cells, infiltration of suppressive cell types such as macrophages and T-regulatory cells, decreased neoantigen expression, ineffective TCR repertoire, the host HLA-class, immune-suppressive signals, and cellular interactions in the TME. (APC) Antigen-presenting cell.

presented to T cells by antigen-presenting cells. Host T cells are activated via their T-cell receptors (TCRs), which recognize the neoantigens presented by the human leukocyte antigens (HLAs) on the membranes of tumor cells and subsequently kick off an antitumor immune response (Fig. 1; Waldman et al. 2020). Accumulating evidence suggests that tumor cell–intrinsic molecular aberrations contribute to defective T-cell infiltration or activation in the TME, thereby leading to immune escape (Kalbasi and Ribas 2020; Nguyen and Spranger 2020). For instance, lack of T-cell infiltration and immunotherapy resistance have been associated with loss-of-function mutations of *PTEN* (Peng et al. 2016), enhanced WNT/β-catenin signaling (Spranger et al. 2015; Luke et al. 2019; Jiménez-Sánchez et al. 2020), or MYC activation (Casey et al. 2016; Jiménez-Sánchez et al. 2020; Dhanasekaran et al. 2021). Further, key tumor cell–intrinsic components of immunogenicity such as the host HLA class (Chowell et al. 2018) or the presence of HLA allele-specific loss of heterozygosity (HLA-LOH) (McGranahan et al. 2017) can lead to immune escape. Tumor cells can also dynamically develop adaptive immune escape mechanisms via, for example, loss of neoantigen expression (Rosenthal et al. 2019) or increased expression of immune-suppressive factors such as PD-L1 (Dong et al. 2002) or IDO1

(Prendergast et al. 2014). Cancer immunotherapies targeting mostly the adaptive mechanisms using immune checkpoint blockade (ICB) have been widely adopted in the clinical setting (Robert et al. 2015; Robert 2020) with >1000 clinical trials ongoing (www.clinicaltrials.gov). However, immune escape mechanisms are highly heterogeneous across different tumors, and most tumors fail to respond to current immunotherapies (Sharma et al. 2017).

Recent developments in single-cell technologies have enabled the investigation of cellular phenotypes in tumors at an unprecedented resolution. Further, advances in spatial tissue–based technologies have enabled investigation of the dynamics of the cells within their local TME niches. Both intrinsic and adaptive immune escape involve spatial mechanisms: spatial localization dictates the cellular phenotypes in T-cell exclusion (Duraiswamy et al. 2021; Launonen et al. 2021), and spatial interactions define how the tumor cells avoid immune attack using adaptive mechanisms (Schürch et al. 2020). The emergence of high-dimensional, tissue-imaging technologies has recently enabled analysis of the TME in situ at single-cell resolution (Lin et al. 2018; Keren et al. 2019; Black et al. 2021). The implementation of these novel technologies on fixed tumor tissues of clinical samples and the development of analytical methods has made it feasible to detect, classify, and profile single cells in their spatial niches in the TME.

TUMOR GENOTYPES SHAPE THE TUMOR MICROENVIRONMENT AND THERAPY RESPONSES IN OVARIAN CANCER

Molecularly, HGSC is characterized by ubiquitous deleterious mutations in *TP53* (Cancer Genome Atlas Research Network 2011). In addition to *TP53*, HGSCs harbor a plethora of genetic drivers, and these genotypes show distinct molecular phenotypes and clinical behavior. The most common genotype of HGSCs, accounting for 20% of the tumors, is characterized by defects in the *BRCA1/2* genes (Konstantinopoulos et al. 2015). *BRCA1/2*-deficient tumors are markedly sensitive to DNA-damaging therapies such as platinum-based chemotherapy and poly-ADP ribose polymerase (PARP) inhibitors (Lord and Ashworth 2017). By contrast, HGSCs with other genotypic drivers, such as *CCNE1* amplification, show poor responses to therapies (Nakayama et al. 2010). In recent years, it has become increasingly evident that antitumor immunity plays a critical role in HGSC therapy responses and clinical outcomes (Li et al. 2017; Yuan et al. 2017). Unfortunately, single-agent ICB therapies in unselected HGSC patient populations have failed to produce clinical benefits (Matulonis et al. 2019). Much of this is due to the lack of mechanistic understanding of the immune escape mechanisms to enable efficient patient stratification. Interestingly, emerging evidence suggests that HGSC genotypes harbor distinct immune escape mechanisms; *BRCA1/2*-deficient HGSCs have been associated with a higher neoantigen load and immune cell infiltration (Strickland et al. 2016). Further, single-cell spatial profiling identified a phenotypically distinct TME with evidence of increased spatial immunosurveillance and distinct prognostication in the *BRCA1/2*-deficient tumors (Launonen et al. 2021). First, *BRCA1/2*-mutated tumors were enriched in proliferating epithelial tumor cells, while tumor cells without mutations in any genes of the homologous recombination (HR) pathway (HRwt) predominantly showed characteristics of an epithelial–mesenchymal transition (EMT)-like phenotype. M2-like macrophages formed the largest immune cell subpopulation, followed by $CD8^+$ T cells. These cell types were more abundant in *BRCA1/2*-mutated tumors as compared with HRwt tumors, and the ratio of $CD8^+$ T cells to M1-like $IBA1^+CD11c^+$ and $IBA1^+CD163^+CD11c^+$ macrophages was higher in *BRCA1/2* mutant tumors as well. In addition, the receptor protein PD-1 showed higher expression in the $CD4^+$, $CD8^+$, and $FOXP3^+CD4^+$ T cells of the *BRCA1/2*-mutated tumors compared with the HRwt tumors. Interestingly, increased proportions of $CD8^+$ and $CD4^+$ T cells associated with better prognosis, and in the *BRCA1/2*-mutated tumors, proximity of $CD8^+$ and $CD4^+$ T cells to proliferating epithelial cells was associated with increased platinum-free interval (PFI) independent of cell abundances, underscoring the importance of spatial cell–cell interactions for tumor cell eradication. Furthermore, Ki67 expression in tumor cells was associated with a longer PFI specifically in *BRCA1/2*-mutated tumors; however, this relationship was not independent of proximity to $CD8^+$ and $CD4^+$ T cells. Together, these data suggest that highly proliferating epithelial cells in *BRCA1/2*-mutated tumors attract T cells, possibly via increased presentation of neoantigens, leading to the increased spatial immune surveillance and prolonged PFI. By contrast, tumors without mutations in any of the genes belonging to the HR pathway had a higher stromal-to-tumor ratio, enrichment of EMT-like cancer cells, and decreased immune cell infiltration likely contributing to their worse prognosis (see Porter and Matulonis 2023).

Emerging preclinical data also suggests distinct STING-dependent TME in the BRCA-mutated HGSCs (Ding et al. 2018), and that these inherent differences in the TME composition also contribute to the potential responses to immunotherapies (Iyer et al. 2021; Zhang et al. 2021). Using genetically engineered, syngeneic mouse models, Iyer et al. demonstrated that homologous recombination deficiency (HRD) genotypes elicited distinct immune landscapes; the HRD tumors were most heavily infiltrated with immune cells with the highest proportions of CD3-positive T cells, highly exhausted $CD8^+$ T cells, M2-like macrophages, and the lowest proportion of T-regulatory cells (Tregs). Similarly, Zhang et al. (2021) described distinct immunotherapy combinations for CCNE1-amplified organoids. These differences correlated with elevated levels of cytokines known to drive T-cell suppression and myeloid cell infiltration. The HRD tumors showed long-term responses to ICB in combination with olaparib, and the HR-proficient genotypes were widely resistant to immunotherapy and DNA-damaging agents. Consistently, promising activity was shown in a phase I/II clinical study combining PARP inhibitor and a PD-1 inhibitor in HGSC patients (Konstantinopoulos et al. 2019), and several large clinical phase III studies have since been launched with expected results in the next 2–3 years. Importantly, subsequent translational work indicated that tumor mutational profiles related to HRD are associated with the spatial immune microenvironment and responses to this combination (Färkkilä et al. 2020). More specifically, the presence of mutational signature 3 (Sig3) as a surrogate of HRD and gene-expression profiles indicating interferon (IFN)-primed, $CD8^+$, and PD-$L1^+$ T cells in the TME was associated with significantly prolonged progression-free survival (PFS) (hazard ratio [HR] = 0.32), while absence of these biomarkers was associated with resistance to niraparib/pembrolizumab (overall response rate [ORR] 0%). Additionally, tCycIF single-cell imaging showed that Sig3-positive tumors exhibited higher PD-L1 expression in tumor cells and in macrophages. Single-cell imaging revealed an IFN-activated state of exhausted and effector $CD8^+$ T cells, and prominent spatial interactions of exhausted $CD8^+$ T cells with macrophages and tumor cells in the responders. Importantly, proximity of PD-L1-positive tumor cells and exhausted $CD8^+$ T cells was enriched specifically in the Sig3-positive tumors, strengthening the notion that differences in spatial relationships within the TME also contributes to enhanced responses to the combination of PARP plus PD-1 inhibition in the HRD tumors. More recently, a lysophosphatidic acid (LPA)-controlled myeloid cell–derived gene signature was also associated with resistance to the niraparib/pembrolizumab combination (Chae et al. 2022). Ablation of the LPA-generating enzyme autotaxin (ATX) in ovarian cancer cells reprogrammed the tumor-immune microenvironment, extended host survival, and improved the effects of immunotherapies via the type I IFN pathway. These results implicate the LPA pathway as a critical regulator of dendritic cell function and immune suppression in the ovarian cancer TME. The role of myeloid cells in regulating the activation and suppression of tumor-infiltrating $CD8^+$ T cells was also highlighted recently (Duraiswamy et al. 2021). These investigators showed that tumor-specific, polyfunctional $CD8^+$ T cells accumulate in tumor islets, where they engage antigen and up-regulate PD-1. The activation of these $CD8^+$ T cells and responses to ICBs are dependent on CD28 costimulation by antigen-presenting cells in intraepithelial tumor myeloid niches, further strengthening the role of the spatial cell–cell interactions in the regulation of the immune microenvironment and therapy responses in ovarian cancer.

STROMAL CELLS SHAPE THERAPY RESPONSES AND ARE ALSO MODULATED BY CHEMOTHERAPY

In addition to the cancer and immune cells, HGSCs contain highly variable proportions of nonimmune stroma, composed of fibroblasts, adipocytes, extracellular matrix (ECM), and endothelia, among others (referred to simply as stroma from here on). In line with results from other solid cancers, higher stromal content is associated with poor prognosis of HGSC (Lou et al. 2019), suggesting that stroma may modulate the treatment response or aggressiveness of the tumors. The key cell type within stroma is the CAF, an activated fibroblast type that is widely found across solid cancers. Lately, single-cell RNA-sequencing (scRNA-seq) analyses have enabled a deeper, unbiased subtyping of CAFs based on inferred main functions. Myofibroblasts, expressing the smooth-muscle cell marker *ACTA2* encoding α-SMA, are the prototypic CAF subtype, producing various ECM proteins to the TME (Chen et al. 2021). Other CAF subtypes that were originally discovered in pancreatic cancer have been found in HGSC, namely, inflammatory CAFs (iCAFs) that secrete inflammatory mediators such as IL-6 and LIF, and antigen-presenting CAFs (apCAFs) that express type II HLAs (Hornburg et al. 2021; Zhang et al. 2022). In addition to these populations, an increasing number of CAF subtypes have been reported in individual studies, as the subtypes are not strictly distinct, and cell-type definition by scRNA-seq is based on clustering algorithms that inherently lack a ground truth.

HGSCs contain tissue-specific stromal cell types, creating distinct niches to each primary or metastatic cancer cell population. Primary tumors in the adnexa contain ovarian-specific steroidogenic stromal types expressing *STAR* (Qian et al. 2020; Olbrecht et al. 2021). Omentum is primarily composed of adipocytes that fuel metastatic cancer growth by providing lipids and adipokines (Nieman et al. 2011; Motohara et al. 2019). Metastases in the abdominal cavity such as peritoneum and omentum also contain mesothelial cells (Natarajan et al. 2019), which may display CAF-like phenotypes with expression of FAP as well as ACTA2 and/or inflammatory mediators (Zhang et al. 2022). Mesothelial cells were found to drive HGSC chemoresistance via production of osteopontin, the inhibition of which improved platinum sensitivity in xenograft models (Qian et al. 2021).

CAFs can be derived from multiple different cell types: tissue-resident fibroblasts, mesenchymal stem cells, adipocytes, endothelial cells, and, as speculated, even epithelial cells through EMT (Bu et al. 2019). Recently, mesothelial cells were found to be the cell of origin for apCAFs, which induce Treg cell generation (Huang et al. 2022). CAFs do not contain genetic aberrations above the baseline found in normal fibroblasts (Qiu et al. 2008) yet are transcriptionally heterogeneous. Their heterogeneity is thought to be derived from their various cells of origin and external signals—such as secreted factors or distinct stressors—that drive CAFs to various states (Chen et al. 2021). Recent evidence suggests that genetic drivers may modulate the CAF phenotypes at least in pancreatic cancer, where loss of BRCA function leads to a shift from myofibroblastic toward immune-regulatory CAFs marked by clusterin expression (Shaashua et al. 2022). The roles of CAFs in treatment resistance are as variable as their phenotypes. CAFs produce ECM and the resulting increased stiffness, along with substrates provided by ECM such as *COL6*, have been shown to contribute to chemoresistance (Pietilä et al. 2021). CAFs also produce a variety of signaling molecules with protumorigenic functions, such as TGF-β, which promotes immunosuppressive phenotypes in T cells, macrophages, and neutrophils, CXCL12 and VEGFA, which promote angiogenesis, as well as cytokines or growth factors, such as LIF, IGF1, HGF, or IL6, which directly promote tumor growth and progression, as well as modify immune cell states (Chen et al. 2021). On the other hand, depletion of CAFs in PDAC mouse models by direct elimination of α-SMA$^+$ myofibroblasts (Özdemir et al. 2014) or suppression of

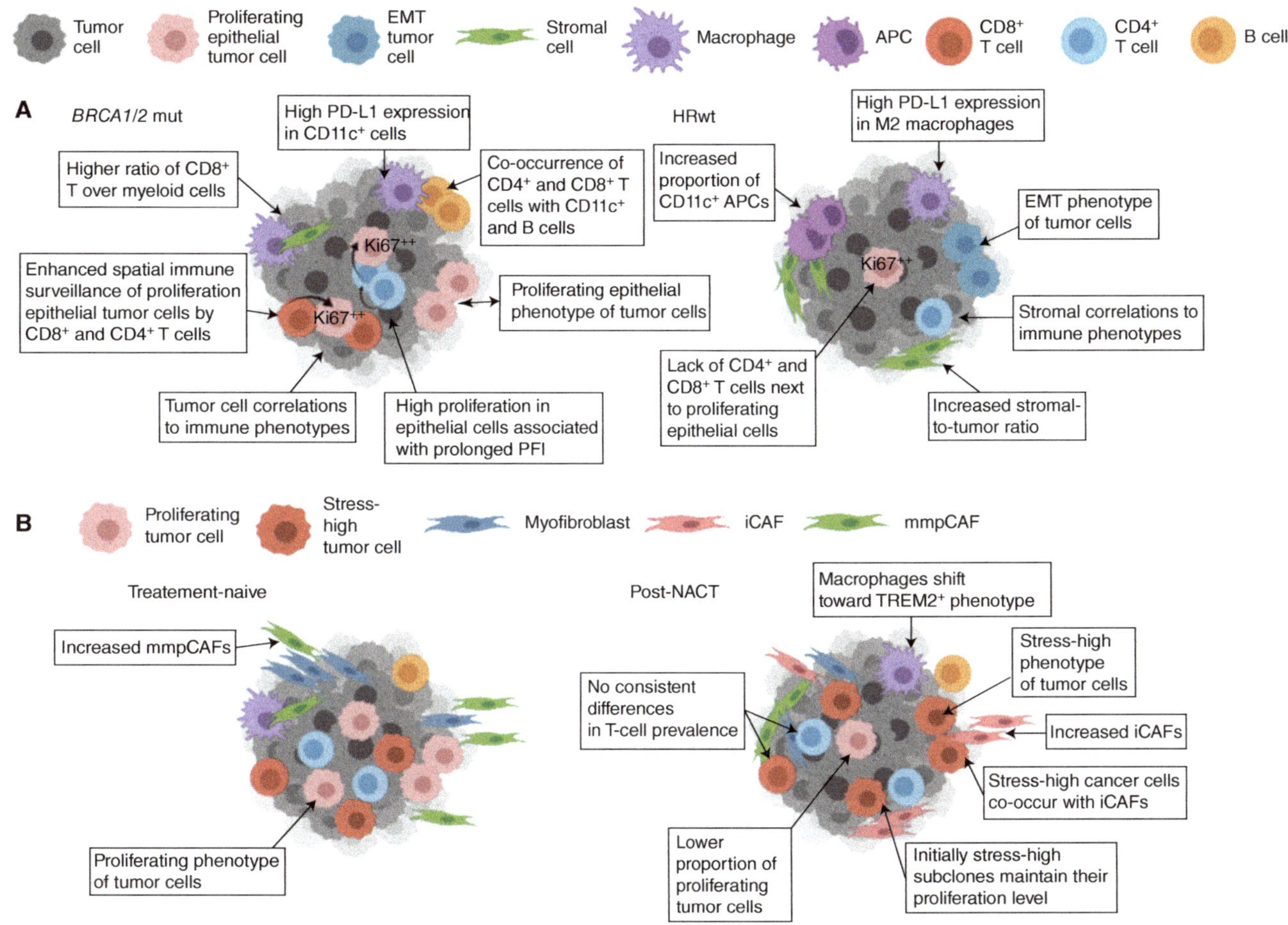

Figure 2. Distinct tumor microenvironments according to the tumor genotype (*A*) or treatment phase (*B*) in high-grade serous ovarian cancer (HGSOC). Single-cell analyses reveal enhanced spatial immune surveillance features in the tumor microenvironment of *BRCA1/2*-mutated HGSCs (*A*), and chemotherapy-induced changes in cancer-associated fibroblast (CAF) subtypes (*B*). (iCAF) Inflammatory cancer-associated fibroblast, (mmpCAF) matrix-metalloproteinase-high cancer-associated fibroblast. (EMT) Epithelial–mesenchymal transition, (APC) antigen-presenting cell, (PFI) platinum-free interval.

Hedgehog signaling (Rhim et al. 2014) led to increased immunosuppression and cancer growth, which demonstrates that some types of CAFs have tumor-suppressive roles.

Stroma, while modulating the treatment response, is also affected by treatments, as shown by a single-cell transcriptomic analysis of paired, metastatic HGSC tumors before and after neoadjuvant chemotherapy (Zhang et al. 2022). While chemotherapy somewhat reduced the proportion of CAFs expressing matrix metalloproteinases (mmpCAFs), it strongly increased the prevalence of iCAFs that were significantly associated with an inflammatory stress-high cancer cell subpopulation. This subpopulation was highly increased after chemotherapy, at least partially by subclonal enrichment, and was associated with poor response when present in treatment-naive samples. Stress-high inflammatory cancer cells and iCAFs had high ligand–receptor interaction potentials, suggesting a vicious cycle of paracrine feedforward loops that further induce these states in cancer cells and stroma. As many of the ligands produced are known to limit immune response, such as M2 polarization driven by LIF and IL-6 (Duluc et al. 2007), enhanced understanding of this interaction could improve treatment responses of combined chemo- and immune therapies.

CONCLUDING REMARKS AND FUTURE DIRECTIONS

As the spatial and functional interplay of the tumor genotypes, immune cells, and stromal cells is starting to be unraveled, a more detailed understanding of the spatial interplay of the tumor genotypes and immune microenvironment will be critical to develop biomarkers and novel, more efficient immunotherapeutic strategies for HGSC (Fig. 2). With the development of new tissue-imaging technologies applicable to pathology-grade tumor samples (Färkkilä et al. 2020), the discovered single-cell spatial features can be further developed into clinical biomarkers to guide patient selection and enable precision oncology in ovarian cancer.

REFERENCES

**Reference is also in this subject collection.*

Black S, Phillips D, Hickey JW, Kennedy-Darling J, Venkataraaman VG, Samusik N, Goltsev Y, Schürch CM, Nolan GP. 2021. CODEX multiplexed tissue imaging with DNA-conjugated antibodies. *Nat Protoc* **16:** 3802–3835. doi:10.1038/s41596-021-00556-8

Bu L, Baba H, Yoshida N, Miyake K, Yasuda T, Uchihara T, Tan P, Ishimoto T. 2019. Biological heterogeneity and versatility of cancer-associated fibroblasts in the tumor microenvironment. *Oncogene* **38:** 4887–4901. doi:10.1038/s41388-019-0765-y

Cancer Genome Atlas Research Network. 2011. Integrated genomic analyses of ovarian carcinoma. *Nature* **474:** 609–615. doi:10.1038/nature10166

Casey SC, Tong L, Li Y, Do R, Walz S, Fitzgerald KN, Gouw AM, Baylot V, Gütgemann I, Eilers M, et al. 2016. MYC regulates the antitumor immune response through CD47 and PD-L1. *Science* **352:** 227–231. doi:10.1126/science.aac9935

Chae CS, Sandoval TA, Hwang SM, Park ES, Giovanelli P, Awasthi D, Salvagno C, Emmanuelli A, Tan C, Chaudhary V, et al. 2022. Tumor-derived lysophosphatidic acid blunts protective type I interferon responses in ovarian cancer. *Cancer Discov* **12:** 1904–1921. doi:10.1158/2159-8290.CD-21-1181

Chen Y, McAndrews KM, Kalluri R. 2021. Clinical and therapeutic relevance of cancer-associated fibroblasts. *Nat Rev Clin Oncol* **18:** 792–804. doi:10.1038/s41571-021-00546-5

Chowell D, Morris LGT, Grigg CM, Weber JK, Samstein RM, Makarov V, Kuo F, Kendall SM, Requena D, Riaz N, et al. 2018. Patient HLA class I genotype influences cancer response to checkpoint blockade immunotherapy. *Science* **359:** 582–587. doi:10.1126/science.aao4572

Danilova L, Wang H, Sunshine J, Kaunitz GJ, Cottrell TR, Xu S, Esandrio J, Anders RA, Cope L, Pardoll DM, et al. 2016. Association of PD-1/PD-L axis expression with cytolytic activity, mutational load, and prognosis in melanoma and other solid tumors. *Proc Natl Acad Sci* **113:** E7769–E7777. doi:10.1073/pnas.1607836113

Dhanasekaran R, Deutzmann A, Mahauad-Fernandez WD, Hansen AS, Gouw AM, Felsher DW. 2021. The MYC oncogene—the grand orchestrator of cancer growth and immune evasion. *Nat Rev Clin Oncol* **19:** 23–36. doi:10.1038/s41571-021-00549-2

Ding L, Kim HJ, Wang Q, Kearns M, Jiang T, Ohlson CE, Li BB, Xie S, Liu JF, Stover EH, et al. 2018. PARP inhibition elicits STING-dependent antitumor immunity in Brca1-deficient ovarian cancer. *Cell Rep* **25:** 2972–2980.e5. doi:10.1016/j.celrep.2018.11.054

Dong H, Strome SE, Salomao DR, Tamura H, Hirano F, Flies DB, Roche PC, Lu J, Zhu G, Tamada K, et al. 2002. Tumor-associated B7-H1 promotes T-cell apoptosis: a potential mechanism of immune evasion. *Nat Med* **8:** 793–800. doi:10.1038/nm730

Duluc D, Delneste Y, Tan F, Moles MP, Grimaud L, Lenoir J, Preisser L, Anegon I, Catala L, Ifrah N, et al. 2007. Tumor-associated leukemia inhibitory factor and IL-6 skew monocyte differentiation into tumor-associated macrophage-like cells. *Blood* **110:** 4319–4330. doi:10.1182/blood-2007-02-072587

Duraiswamy J, Turrini R, Minasyan A, Barras D, Crespo I, Grimm AJ, Casado J, Genolet R, Benedetti F, Wicky A, et al. 2021. Myeloid antigen-presenting cell niches sustain antitumor T cells and license PD-1 blockade via CD28 costimulation. *Cancer Cell* **39:** 1623–1642.e20. doi:10.1016/j.ccell.2021.10.008

Färkkilä A, Gulhan DC, Casado J, Jacobson CA, Nguyen H, Kochupurakkal B, Maliga Z, Yapp C, Chen YA, Schapiro D, et al. 2020. Immunogenomic profiling determines responses to combined PARP and PD-1 inhibition in ovarian cancer. *Nat Commun* **11:** 1459. doi:10.1038/s41467-020-15315-8

Hornburg M, Desbois M, Lu S, Guan Y, Lo AA, Kaufman S, Elrod A, Lotstein A, DesRochers TM, Munoz-Rodriguez JL, et al. 2021. Single-cell dissection of cellular components and interactions shaping the tumor immune phenotypes in ovarian cancer. *Cancer Cell* **39:** 928–944.e6. doi:10.1016/j.ccell.2021.04.004

Huang H, Wang Z, Zhang Y, Pradhan RN, Ganguly D, Chandra R, Murimwa G, Wright S, Gu X, Maddipati R, et al. 2022. Mesothelial cell-derived antigen-presenting cancer-associated fibroblasts induce expansion of regulatory T cells in pancreatic cancer. *Cancer Cell* **40:** 656–673.e7. doi:10.1016/j.ccell.2022.04.011

Iyer S, Zhang S, Yucel S, Horn H, Smith SG, Reinhardt F, Hoefsmit E, Assatova B, Casado J, Meinsohn MC, et al. 2021. Genetically defined syngeneic mouse models of ovarian cancer as tools for the discovery of combination immunotherapy. *Cancer Discov* **11:** 384–407. doi:10.1158/2159-8290.CD-20-0818

Jiménez-Sánchez A, Cybulska P, Mager KL, Koplev S, Cast O, Couturier DL, Memon D, Selenica P, Nikolovski I, Mazaheri Y, et al. 2020. Unraveling tumor-immune heterogeneity in advanced ovarian cancer uncovers immunogenic effect of chemotherapy. *Nat Genet* **52:** 582–593. doi:10.1038/s41588-020-0630-5

Kalbasi A, Ribas A. 2020. Tumour-intrinsic resistance to immune checkpoint blockade. *Nat Rev Immunol* **20:** 25–39. doi:10.1038/s41577-019-0218-4

Keren L, Bosse M, Thompson S, Risom T, Vijayaragavan K, McCaffrey E, Marquez D, Angoshtari R, Greenwald NF, Fienberg H, et al. 2019. MIBI-TOF: a multiplexed imaging platform relates cellular phenotypes and tissue structure. *Sci Adv* **5:** eaax5851. doi:10.1126/sciadv.aax5851

Kim R, Emi M, Tanabe K. 2007. Cancer immunoediting from immune surveillance to immune escape. *Immunology* **121:** 1–14. doi:10.1111/j.1365-2567.2007.02587.x

Konstantinopoulos PA, Ceccaldi R, Shapiro GI, D'Andrea AD. 2015. Homologous recombination deficiency: exploiting the fundamental vulnerability of ovarian cancer. *Cancer Discov* **5:** 1137–1154. doi:10.1158/2159-8290.CD-15-0714

Konstantinopoulos PA, Waggoner S, Vidal GA, Mita M, Moroney JW, Holloway R, Van Le L, Sachdev JC, Chapman-Davis E, Colon-Otero G, et al. 2019. Single-arm phases 1 and 2 trial of niraparib in combination with pembrolizumab in patients with recurrent platinum-resistant ovarian carcinoma. *JAMA Oncol* **5:** 1141–1149. doi:10.1001/jamaoncol.2019.1048

Launonen IM, Lyytikäinen N, Casado J, Anttila E, Szabó A, Haltia UM, Jacobson C, Lin JR, Maliga Z, Santagata S, et al. 2021. Single-cell tumor-immune microenvironment of *BRCA1/2* mutated high-grade serous ovarian cancer. *Nat Commun* **3:** 835.

Li J, Wang J, Chen R, Bai Y, Lu X. 2017. The prognostic value of tumor-infiltrating T lymphocytes in ovarian cancer. *Oncotarget* **8:** 15621–15631. doi:10.18632/oncotarget.14919

Lin JR, Izar B, Wang S, Yapp C, Mei S, Shah PM, Santagata S, Sorger PK. 2018. Highly multiplexed immunofluorescence imaging of human tissues and tumors using t-CyCIF and conventional optical microscopes. *eLife* **7:** e31657. doi:10.7554/eLife.31657

Lord CJ, Ashworth A. 2017. PARP inhibitors: synthetic lethality in the clinic. *Science* **355:** 1152–1158. doi:10.1126/science.aam7344

Lou E, Vogel RI, Hoostal S, Klein M, Linden MA, Teoh D, Geller MA. 2019. Tumor-stroma proportion as a predictive biomarker of resistance to platinum-based chemotherapy in patients with ovarian cancer. *JAMA Oncol* **5:** 1222–1224. doi:10.1001/jamaoncol.2019.1943

Luke JJ, Bao R, Sweis RF, Spranger S, Gajewski TF. 2019. WNT/β-catenin pathway activation correlates with immune exclusion across human cancers. *Clin Cancer Res* **25:** 3074–3083. doi:10.1158/1078-0432.CCR-18-1942

Matulonis UA, Shapira-Frommer R, Santin AD, Lisyanskaya AS, Pignata S, Vergote I, Raspagliesi F, Sonke GS, Birrer M, Provencher DM, et al. 2019. Antitumor activity and safety of pembrolizumab in patients with advanced recurrent ovarian cancer: results from the phase II KEYNOTE-100 study. *Ann Oncol* **30:** 1080–1087. doi:10.1093/annonc/mdz135

McGranahan N, Rosenthal R, Hiley CT, Rowan AJ, Watkins TBK, Wilson GA, Birkbak NJ, Veeriah S, Van Loo P, Herrero J, et al. 2017. Allele-specific HLA loss and immune escape in lung cancer evolution. *Cell* **171:** 1259–1271.e11. doi:10.1016/j.cell.2017.10.001

Motohara T, Masuda K, Morotti M, Zheng Y, El-Sahhar S, Chong KY, Wietek N, Alsaadi A, Carrami EM, Hu Z, et al. 2019. An evolving story of the metastatic voyage of ovarian cancer cells: cellular and molecular orchestration of the adipose-rich metastatic microenvironment. *Oncogene* **38:** 2885–2898. doi:10.1038/s41388-018-0637-x

Nakayama N, Nakayama K, Shamima Y, Ishikawa M, Katagiri A, Iida K, Miyazaki K. 2010. Gene amplification CCNE1 is related to poor survival and potential therapeutic target in ovarian cancer. *Cancer* **116:** 2621–2634. doi:10.1002/cncr.24987

Natarajan S, Foreman KM, Soriano MI, Rossen NS, Shehade H, Fregoso DR, Eggold JT, Krishnan V, Dorigo O, Krieg AJ, et al. 2019. Collagen remodeling in the hypoxic tumor-mesothelial niche promotes ovarian cancer metastasis. *Cancer Res* **79:** 2271–2284. doi:10.1158/0008-5472.CAN-18-2616

Nguyen KB, Spranger S. 2020. Modulation of the immune microenvironment by tumor-intrinsic oncogenic signaling. *J Cell Biol* **219:** e201908224. doi:10.1083/jcb.201908224

Nieman KM, Kenny HA, Penicka CV, Ladanyi A, Buell-Gutbrod R, Zillhardt MR, Romero IL, Carey MS, Mills GB, Hotamisligil GS, et al. 2011. Adipocytes promote ovarian cancer metastasis and provide energy for rapid tumor growth. *Nat Med* **17:** 1498–1503. doi:10.1038/nm.2492

Olbrecht S, Busschaert P, Qian J, Vanderstichele A, Loverix L, Van Gorp T, Van Nieuwenhuysen E, Han S, Van den Broeck A, Coosemans A, et al. 2021. High-grade serous tubo-ovarian cancer refined with single-cell RNA sequencing: specific cell subtypes influence survival and determine molecular subtype classification. *Genome Med* **13:** 111. doi:10.1186/s13073-021-00922-x

Özdemir BC, Pentcheva-Hoang T, Carstens JL, Zheng X, Wu CC, Simpson TR, Laklai H, Sugimoto H, Kahlert C, Novitskiy SV, et al. 2014. Depletion of carcinoma-associated fibroblasts and fibrosis induces immunosuppression and accelerates pancreas cancer with reduced survival. *Cancer Cell* **25:** 719–734. doi:10.1016/j.ccr.2014.04.005

Peng W, Chen JQ, Liu C, Malu S, Creasy C, Tetzlaff MT, Xu C, McKenzie JA, Zhang C, Liang X, et al. 2016. Loss of PTEN promotes resistance to T cell-mediated immunotherapy. *Cancer Discov* **6:** 202–216. doi:10.1158/2159-8290.CD-15-0283

Pietilä EA, Gonzalez-Molina J, Moyano-Galceran L, Jamalzadeh S, Zhang K, Lehtinen L, Turunen SP, Martins TA, Gultekin O, Lamminen T, et al. 2021. Co-evolution of matrisome and adaptive adhesion dynamics drives ovarian cancer chemoresistance. *Nat Commun* **12:** 3904. doi:10.1038/s41467-021-24009-8

*Porter RL, Matulonis U. 2023. Ovarian cancer therapy. *Cold Spring Harb Perspect Med* doi:10.1101/cshperspect.a038232

Prendergast GC, Smith C, Thomas S, Mandik-Nayak L, Laury-Kleintop L, Metz R, Muller AJ. 2014. Indoleamine 2,3-dioxygenase pathways of pathogenic inflammation and immune escape in cancer. *Cancer Immunol Immunother* **63:** 721–735. doi:10.1007/s00262-014-1549-4

Qian J, Olbrecht S, Boeckx B, Vos H, Laoui D, Etlioglu E, Wauters E, Pomella V, Verbandt S, Busschaert P, et al. 2020. A pan-cancer blueprint of the heterogeneous tumor microenvironment revealed by single-cell profiling. *Cell Res* **30:** 745–762. doi:10.1038/s41422-020-0355-0

Qian J, LeSavage BL, Hubka KM, Ma C, Natarajan S, Eggold JT, Xiao Y, Fuh KC, Krishnan V, Enejder A, et al. 2021. Cancer-associated mesothelial cells promote ovarian cancer chemoresistance through paracrine osteopontin signaling. *J Clin Invest* **131:** e146186. doi:10.1172/JCI146186

Qiu W, Hu M, Sridhar A, Opeskin K, Fox S, Shipitsin M, Trivett M, Thompson ER, Ramakrishna M, Gorringe KL, et al. 2008. No evidence of clonal somatic genetic alterations in cancer-associated fibroblasts from human breast and ovarian carcinomas. *Nat Genet* **40:** 650–655. doi:10.1038/ng.117

Rhim AD, Oberstein PE, Thomas DH, Mirek ET, Palermo CF, Sastra SA, Dekleva EN, Saunders T, Becerra CP, Tattersall IW, et al. 2014. Stromal elements act to restrain, rather than support, pancreatic ductal adenocarcinoma. *Cancer Cell* **25:** 735–747. doi:10.1016/j.ccr.2014.04.021

Robert C. 2020. A decade of immune-checkpoint inhibitors in cancer therapy. *Nat Commun* **11:** 3801. doi:10.1038/s41467-020-17670-y

Robert C, Schachter J, Long GV, Arance A, Grob JJ, Mortier L, Daud A, Carlino MS, McNeil C, Lotem M, et al. 2015. Pembrolizumab versus ipilimumab in advanced melanoma. *N Engl J Med* **372:** 2521–2532. doi:10.1056/NEJMoa1503093

Rosenthal R, Cadieux EL, Salgado R, Bakir MA, Moore DA, Hiley CT, Lund T, Tanić M, Reading JL, Joshi K, et al. 2019. Neoantigen-directed immune escape in lung cancer evolution. *Nature* **567:** 479–485. doi:10.1038/s41586-019-1032-7

Schürch CM, Bhate SS, Barlow GL, Phillips DJ, Noti L, Zlobec I, Chu P, Black S, Demeter J, McIlwain DR, et al. 2020. Coordinated cellular neighborhoods orchestrate antitumoral immunity at the colorectal cancer invasive front. *Cell* **182:** 1341–1359.e19. doi:10.1016/j.cell.2020.07.005

Shaashua L, Ben-Shmuel A, Pevsner-Fischer M, Friedman G, Levi-Galibov O, Nandakumar S, Barki D, Nevo R, Brown LE, Zhang W, et al. 2022. BRCA mutational status shapes the stromal microenvironment of pancreatic cancer linking clusterin expression in cancer associated fibroblasts with HSF1 signaling. *Nat Commun* **13:** 6513. doi:10.1038/s41467-022-34081-3

Sharma P, Hu-Lieskovan S, Wargo JA, Ribas A. 2017. Primary, adaptive, and acquired resistance to cancer immunotherapy. *Cell* **168:** 707–723. doi:10.1016/j.cell.2017.01.017

Spranger S, Bao R, Gajewski TF. 2015. Melanoma-intrinsic β-catenin signalling prevents anti-tumour immunity. *Nature* **523:** 231–235. doi:10.1038/nature14404

Strickland KC, Howitt BE, Shukla SA, Rodig S, Ritterhouse LL, Liu JF, Garber JE, Chowdhury D, Wu CJ, D'Andrea AD, et al. 2016. Association and prognostic significance of BRCA1/2-mutation status with neoantigen load, number of tumor-infiltrating lymphocytes and expression of PD-1/PD-L1 in high grade serous ovarian cancer. *Oncotarget* **7:** 13587–13598. doi:10.18632/oncotarget.7277

Tumeh PC, Harview CL, Yearley JH, Shintaku IP, Taylor EJ, Robert L, Chmielowski B, Spasic M, Henry G, Ciobanu V, et al. 2014. PD-1 blockade induces responses by inhibiting adaptive immune resistance. *Nature* **515:** 568–571. doi:10.1038/nature13954

Waldman AD, Fritz JM, Lenardo MJ. 2020. A guide to cancer immunotherapy: from T cell basic science to clinical practice. *Nat Rev Immunol* **20:** 651–668. doi:10.1038/s41577-020-0306-5

Yuan X, Zhang J, Li D, Mao Y, Mo F, Du W, Ma X. 2017. Prognostic significance of tumor-associated macrophages in ovarian cancer: a meta-analysis. *Gynecol Oncol* **147:** 181–187. doi:10.1016/j.ygyno.2017.07.007

Zhang L, Conejo-Garcia JR, Katsaros D, Gimotty PA, Massobrio M, Regnani G, Makrigiannakis A, Gray H, Schlienger K, Liebman MN, et al. 2003. Intratumoral T cells, recurrence, and survival in epithelial ovarian cancer. *N Engl J Med* **348:** 203–213. doi:10.1056/NEJMoa020177

Zhang S, Iyer S, Ran H, Dolgalev I, Gu S, Wei W, Foster CJR, Loomis CA, Olvera N, Dao F, et al. 2021. Genetically defined, syngeneic organoid platform for developing combination therapies for ovarian cancer. *Cancer Discov* **11:** 362–383. doi:10.1158/2159-8290.CD-20-0455

Zhang K, Erkan EP, Jamalzadeh S, Dai J, Andersson N, Kaipio K, Lamminen T, Mansuri N, Huhtinen K, Carpén O, et al. 2022. Longitudinal single-cell RNA-seq analysis reveals stress-promoted chemoresistance in metastatic ovarian cancer. *Sci Adv* **8:** eabm1831. doi:10.1126/sciadv.abm1831

Ovarian Cancer Therapy

Diana Miao, Ursula A. Matulonis, and Rebecca L. Porter

Division of Gynecologic Oncology, Department of Medical Oncology, Dana-Farber Cancer Institute, Boston, Massachusetts 02215, USA

Correspondence: Rebecca_porter@dfci.harvard.edu

Significant advances in basic and translational research have improved our understanding of the molecular alterations and biological vulnerabilities of the different histologic subsets of epithelial ovarian cancer (EOC). This has led to clinical trials that have incorporated novel agents based on molecular aspects into the treatment paradigm for both newly diagnosed and recurrent disease. The past decade has witnessed several regulatory approvals in the United States and Europe for the treatment of EOC, including the antiangiogenic agent, bevacizumab, poly(ADP-ribose) polymerase inhibitors in various therapeutic settings, and the antibody–drug conjugate (ADC), mirvetuximab soravtansine. Immune checkpoint inhibitors do not demonstrate substantial activity as single agents in ovarian cancer, except for the rare entity of microsatellite instability (MSI) high ovarian cancer. Current research is focused on new treatment paradigms such as ADCs, genetically specific therapies, and other novel immunotherapies such as bispecific antibodies, radioligand therapies, cellular therapies, and vaccines. In addition, combination efforts are focused on incorporating conventional chemotherapy, targeted therapies, immune-oncology drugs, and/or novel agents to improve outcomes for patients with newly diagnosed as well as recurrent EOC. This review will focus on the management of high-grade serous ovarian cancer, the most common type of EOC, accounting for ~75% of cases. Recent advances in the management of rarer histologic subtypes with distinct molecular and clinical characteristics, including clear cell, mucinous, endometrioid, and low-grade serous, will be briefly discussed. Non-EOCs, including germ cell and sex cord stromal tumors and their treatment, have been reviewed elsewhere [see Ray-Coquard et al. (2019). *N Engl J Med* **381:** 2416–2428. doi:10.1056/NEJMoa1911361].

TREATMENT OF NEWLY DIAGNOSED OVARIAN CANCER

Surgical Management

The goals for surgery for a suspected new diagnosis of ovarian cancer include confirmation of diagnosis via pathology, surgical staging via the International Federation of Gynecology and Obstetrics (FIGO) system (Mutch and Prat 2014), cytoreduction to remove potentially poorly perfused cancer tissue, and allow improved chemotherapy access and symptom control.

For apparently pelvis-confined ovarian cancer (stage I or II), complete surgical staging includes a total hysterectomy with bilateral salpingo-oophorectomy to remove the primary site of the tumor, as well as possible lymph node assessment, omentectomy, collection of pelvic washings, and peritoneal biopsies to ex-

Cite this article as *Cold Spring Harb Perspect Med* doi: 10.1101/cshperspect.a038232

clude microscopic metastatic spread. For advanced stage (stage III or IV) disease, the goal of surgery is to remove all visible cancer cells leading to R0. This includes total hysterectomy with bilateral salpingo-oophorectomy and other procedures as needed, including omentectomy, diaphragm stripping, splenectomy, bowel resection, removal of enlarged and thus suspicious lymph nodes containing cancer, and peritonectomy.

For advanced-stage disease, completeness of cytoreduction is a major prognostic factor for clinical outcomes. Achieving a complete (no macroscopic residual tumor or R0) or optimal (<1 cm of maximum residual disease diameter) cytoreduction is associated with improved survival (Chi et al. 2006; Chang et al. 2013; Tseng et al. 2018) compared to suboptimal (>1 cm residual disease) cytoreduction. However, retrospective and secondary analyses have also shown that initial disease burden and distribution may also be prognostic for survival even when similar degrees of cytoreduction are achieved (Horowitz et al. 2015), suggesting that the inherent tumor biology may be distinct and more aggressive in patients presenting with extensive disease. Given the critical importance of achieving at least optimal cytoreduction if primary cytoreductive surgery (PCS) is attempted, diagnostic laparoscopy has been used to predict the feasibility of optimal PCS (Fagotti et al. 2006, 2008). For patients who are deemed by a gynecologic oncologist unable to undergo primary debulking, neoadjuvant chemotherapy (NACT) followed by interval cytoreductive surgery (ICS) is an alternative for initial management of newly diagnosed ovarian cancer.

Neoadjuvant Chemotherapy

High-grade serous ovarian cancer (HGSOC) is very frequently (>80%) highly sensitive to platinum and taxane-based chemotherapy, making NACT an attractive approach when initial disease distribution is not amenable to optimal cytoreduction or when patient comorbidities make pursuing an extensive surgical procedure excessively risky. However, when PCS is feasible, it is generally the preferred treatment approach to maximize long-term outcomes. Consequently, all patients newly diagnosed with ovarian cancer should have a referral to a gynecologic oncologist (Table 1).

Several randomized controlled trials have compared a PCS approach (cytoreductive surgery followed by adjuvant carboplatin and paclitaxel) to an NACT approach (carboplatin and paclitaxel followed by ICS and then the completion of platinum-based chemotherapy) in patients who are deemed to be good candidates for PCS. Three of these have demonstrated equivalent outcomes for progression-free survival (PFS) and overall survival (OS) for the two strategies (Vergote et al. 2010; Kehoe et al. 2015; Fagotti et al. 2020), while one study could not confirm noninferiority of the NACT approach (OS 49 mo for PCS vs. 44 mo for NACT) (Onda et al. 2020). However, these trials have been criticized due to relatively low rates of optimal cytoreduction and poorer-than-expected survival outcomes overall, which have partially been attributed to the high numbers of patients with stage IIIC and IV disease included. Retrospective analyses using national databases have also demonstrated conflicting results regarding PCS versus NACT/ICS (Vergote et al. 1998; Schwartz et al. 1999; Kayikcioglu et al. 2001; Everett et al. 2006; Bristow et al. 2007). Overall, studies generally find that NACT results in complete cytoreduction more frequently than primary debulking surgery (PDS) and has lower risks of perioperative complications (lower blood loss, mortality, operative time, duration of hospitalization, intensive care unit [ICU] admission, bowel surgery), but OS with NACT is either unchanged or slightly worse. The mechanism explaining the lack of OS benefit with NACT despite higher rates of optimal cytoreduction remains unclear. Some retrospective studies have suggested that the NACT approach is associated with a higher risk of platinum-resistant (PR) recurrence and shorter time to development of platinum resistance (Rauh-Hain et al. 2013; da Costa et al. 2015; Petrillo et al. 2015), although these findings have not been assessed prospectively. Patients receiving NACT in nonrandomized studies tend to have lower performance status at baseline, which may

Table 1. Key ongoing clinical trials in newly diagnosed high-grade epithelial ovarian cancer

Study name	Study drug(s)	Patient population	Study arms
NCT05009082 AGO-OVAR-28 (Heitz et al. 2023)	Niraparib + bevacizumab maintenance	Stage III, IV newly diagnosed high-grade epithelial ovarian cancer (EOC)	Standard of care (SOC), niraparib maintenance; SOC + bevacizumab; niraparib + bevacizumab maintenance
NCT03522246 ATHENA (Monk et al. 2021b)	Rucaparib + nivolumab maintenance	Stage III, IV; complete response (CR)/partial response (PR) to platinum-based adjuvant chemotherapy (C/T)	Rucaparib, nivolumab
			Rucaparib, placebo
			Placebo, nivolumab
			Placebo, placebo
NCT03740165 ENGOT-ov43 KEYLYNK-001 (Fujiwara et al. 2019)	Pembrolizumab concurrent + pembrolizumab + olaparib maintenance	Stage III, IV, *BRCAwt*	C/T
			C/T + pembro, pembro maintenance; C/T + pembro, pembro + olaparib maintenance
NCT03602859 ENGOT-ov44 FIRST (Hardy-Bessard et al. 2019)	Niraparib + dostarlimab maintenance	Stage III suboptimally cytoreduced, stage IV	SOC, placebo + placebo maintenance; SOC, niraparib + placebo maintenance; SOC + dostarlimab, niraparib + dostarlimab maintenance
NCT04111978 ENGOT-ov54/ MATAO (Heinzelmann-Schwarz et al. 2021)	Letrozole maintenance	Stage II–IV estrogen-receptor (ER)-positive EOC after receipt of SOC platinum C/T	Placebo maintenance
			Letrozole maintenance

independently contribute to poorer survival outcomes (Rauh-Hain et al. 2017). Subgroup analyses of the above trials have suggested that patients with IIIC disease with relatively small metastatic tumors (<45 mm) benefited more from PCS, while patients with stage IV disease had better OS with NACT (van Meurs et al. 2013).

Thus, controversy remains surrounding the efficacies of NACT versus PCS in patients who are candidates for PCS predicted to have a high probability of achieving optimal cytoreduction, and predictive measures to guide these decisions are an active area of current investigation. An expert panel convened by the Society of Gynecologic Oncology (SGO) and the American Society of Clinical Oncology (ASCO) has published guidelines for clinicians to navigate this decision (Wright et al. 2016). Overall, PCS is favored over NACT when a high likelihood of optimal cytoreduction is present, with NACT being an alternative for patients with medical comorbidities, extensive bowel involvement, or stage IV disease (Bartels et al. 2019).

Adjuvant Chemotherapy

The combination of intravenous (IV) carboplatin and paclitaxel for six cycles has been the standard of care (SOC) since several trials demonstrated its noninferiority and favorable side effect profile compared with the historically used combinations such as cisplatin and cyclophosphamide or cisplatin and paclitaxel (McGuire et al. 1996; Neijt et al. 2000; Ozols et al. 2003).

Attempts to improve upon the carboplatin and paclitaxel regimen by incorporating additional chemotherapy agents (e.g., gemcitabine, liposomal doxorubicin, topotecan) did not demonstrate improved PFS or OS of any combination compared with the doublet alone (Bookman et al. 2009). Substitution of docetaxel for paclitaxel in combination with carboplatin in the SCOTROC trial revealed equivalent PFS and OS, but did report decreased neuropathy with docetaxel (Vasey et al. 2004). Similarly, substitution of pegylated liposomal doxorubicin (PLD) for paclitaxel was found to have comparable efficacy in the MITO-2 study (Pignata et al. 2011). Therefore, these combinations remain options for patients with significant peripheral neuropathy or other contraindications to paclitaxel.

IP Chemotherapy

Intraperitoneal (IP) chemotherapy has been tested in several randomized phase III studies for patients with advanced ovarian cancer and with disease confined to the abdominal cavity (stage III). IP chemotherapy is hypothesized to improve treatment of small-volume IP disease by exposing the peritoneal cavity to high and prolonged concentrations of chemotherapy while limiting plasma absorption (Markman and Walker 2006). GOG-172 was a randomized study comparing IV paclitaxel (135 mg/m^2) over a 24-hour period followed by either IV cisplatin (75 mg/m^2) on day 2 (IV group) or IP cisplatin (100 mg/m^2) on day 2 and IP paclitaxel (60 mg/m^2) on day 8 (IP group) (Armstrong et al. 2006). Both treatments were given every 3 weeks for six cycles. Overall, the IP group had significantly improved PFS (23.8 vs. 18.3 mo) and OS (65.6 vs. 49.7 mo) compared to the IV group. This survival benefit was observed despite only 42% of patients completing all six cycles of IP therapy (compared to 83% in the IV group). Patients in the IP group had higher rates of toxicities and also reported significantly worse quality of life during and for 3–6 weeks after treatment, but this difference resolved by 1 year posttreatment. Thus, subsequent trials were designed to assess whether the survival benefits seen with IP therapy in GOG-172 could be reproduced with more convenient and tolerable regimens.

GOG-252 decreased the dose of IP cisplatin to 75 mg/m^2 and substituted IP cisplatin for IP carboplatin (Walker et al. 2019). This trial included three arms: (1) IV carboplatin: IV paclitaxel 80 mg/m^2 once per week with IV carboplatin (area under the curve [AUC] 6), (2) IP carboplatin: IV paclitaxel 80 mg/m^2 once per week with IP carboplatin (AUC 6), and (3) IP cisplatin: IV paclitaxel 135 mg/m^2 once every 3 weeks on day 1 plus IP cisplatin 75 mg/m^2 once every 3 weeks on day 2 plus IP paclitaxel 60 mg/m^2 once every 3 weeks on day 8. All arms included six cycles of chemotherapy and IV bevacizumab (15 mg/kg) administered in cycles 2–22. Notably, a "dose-dense" regimen for paclitaxel was used in the IV therapy only arm. Ultimately, no difference in PFS or OS was seen among the three arms. Grade 3 and higher hypertension was significantly worse in the IP cisplatin arm at 20.5% compared to 11.9% and 14.3% in the IV carboplatin and IP carboplatin arms, respectively; the authors concluded that the interaction between IP cisplatin and bevacizumab leads to increased hypertension, and overall fewer cycles of chemotherapy were administered in the IP cisplatin arm.

The Japanese IPOCC randomized trial thus allocated patients to receive either IV carboplatin (AUC 6) or IP carboplatin (AUC 6) every 3 weeks with weekly paclitaxel (80 mg/m^2) without bevacizumab for six cycles following debulking surgery. Patients undergoing both primary and interval debulking surgeries were included; ∼55% of patients in both arms had suboptimal debulking (>2 cm residual disease). This trial reported a modest improvement in PFS with IP chemotherapy (20.7 vs. 23.5 mo) but no difference in OS (Nagao et al. 2023). Rates of adverse events were similar in both groups, and most patients (60% in IP vs. 68% in IV groups) were able to complete all six cycles of therapy.

Only one study on IV versus IP chemotherapy has included information on *BRCA* mutational status. GOG 9923 randomized patients to IV carboplatin/paclitaxel/bevacizumab every 3 weeks, IV carboplatin weekly with every 3-week paclitaxel and bevacizumab, or IV paclitaxel and bevacizumab with IP cisplatin (Gillen et al. 2021). A post hoc analysis demonstrated no difference in median PFS between patients with positive and negative *BRCA* testing. All patients received a poly(ADP-ribose) polymerase inhibitors (PARPi) during chemotherapy. The benefit of IP versus IV chemotherapy in the setting of PARPi maintenance remains an unanswered question.

Overall, comparison of results across the trials is difficult as the treatment regimens for both the IV and IP arms have varied substantially. The logistical challenges and increased toxicity of IP chemotherapy combined with simultaneous improvements in other aspects of ovarian cancer treatment, including maintenance therapy, have limited widespread adoption of IP chemotherapy into the present treatment landscape. Nonetheless, long-term follow-up of patients receiving IP chemotherapy has demonstrated OS benefits extending past 10 years, especially in patients with high-grade serous histology, no gross residual disease, and completion of more cycles of IP chemotherapy (Tewari et al. 2015); thus, IP chemotherapy may still be a valuable part of the treatment plan for select patients with stage III disease who are likely to tolerate IP chemotherapy following a primary cytoreduction to no gross residual disease at centers with experience in managing IP protocols.

HIPEC

Another approach to IP delivery of chemotherapy is hyperthermic IP chemotherapy (HIPEC), founded on the hypothesis that heating the chemotherapy increases penetration at the peritoneum and impairs DNA repair by cancer cells. A multicenter phase 3 clinical trial (OVHIPEC-1) found that patients undergoing HIPEC (cisplatin 100 mg/m^2 for 90 min at 40°C) at the time of optimal ICS compared to optimal cytoreductive surgery alone experienced substantially prolonged PFS (14.2 vs. 10.7 mo) and OS (45.7 vs. 33.9 mo) with similar rates of severe adverse events and similar rates of complete cytoreduction in both groups (van Driel et al. 2018), with similar findings at 10-year follow-up (Aronson et al. 2023). Of note, patients in the HIPEC group ultimately received one more dose of chemotherapy total compared to the non-HIPEC group; the contribution of this to the survival benefit remains unknown. While *BRCA* mutational status was not reported initially in OVHIPEC-1, a subsequent exploratory secondary analysis of *BRCA* status and homologous recombination deficiency (HRD) status in the OVHIPEC-1 tumor samples found that clinical benefit seemed most significant in patients with *BRCA* wild-type (*BRCAwt*), HRD-positive tumors (compared to *BRCA* mutant [*BRCAm*] or HRD-proficient tumors) (Koole et al. 2022). Outside of the clinical trial setting, HIPEC also increases ICU use, cost of treatment, and risks of renal toxicity, although this can be mitigated with the addition of sodium thiosulfate (Dellinger and Han 2021). Thus, HIPEC can currently be considered at the time of ICS if optimal cytoreduction can be achieved at centers and with surgeons who have experience in administering HIPEC and postoperative care. Further ongoing prospective trials evaluating HIPEC at the time of primary or ICS (discussed in the "Investigational Approaches in the First Line and Maintenance Setting" section) will provide additional clarity on the optimal implementation of HIPEC in ovarian cancer.

Dose-Dense Chemotherapy

In addition to questions surrounding the role of IP therapy, the optimal regimen for IV therapy has also been investigated in several studies. Weekly administration of paclitaxel (80 mg/m^2), termed "dose-dense," has been compared to every 3-week paclitaxel (175 mg/m^2) in combination with carboplatin (AUC 6) every 3 weeks in the Japanese GOG-3016 trial. In this study of patients with stage II–IV epithelial ovarian cancer (EOC), an improvement in PFS and OS was reported with dose-dense therapy (28.2 vs. 17.5 mo and 100.5 vs. 62.2 mo, respectively), with especially large benefit in patients with suboptimal cytoreduction (Katsumata et al. 2013).

Subsequently, GOG-262 compared dose-dense to conventional paclitaxel therapy in patients with suboptimally cytoreduced stages III and IV disease, stratified by whether patients received bevacizumab (Chan et al. 2016). In the overall cohort, no difference in PFS was seen. However, in patients who did not receive bevacizumab, weekly paclitaxel was associated with a PFS benefit of 3.9 months (14.2 vs. 10.3 mo). Additionally, the ICON8 trial compared three arms in stage IC–IV ovarian cancer including (1) standard every 3-week dosing of carboplatin and paclitaxel (175 mg/m^2), (2) every 3-week carboplatin and dose-dense paclitaxel (80 mg/m^2 weekly), and (3) weekly carboplatin (AUC 2) and dose-dense paclitaxel (80 mg/m^2 weekly). PFS and OS were similar in all three arms (Clamp et al. 2019). Specifically, at 10-year follow-up, median PFS was 17.7 months in group 1, 20.8 months in group 2, and 21.0 months in group 3, with median OS of 24–25 months in all three groups (Clamp et al. 2022). Thus, IV carboplatin and paclitaxel administered every 3 weeks are generally considered SOC, although dose-dense paclitaxel is an acceptable alternative in certain circumstances, such as patients with poor performance status or significant comorbidities. A modified dose-dense regimen of weekly carboplatin (AUC 2) and weekly paclitaxel (60 mg/m^2) assessed in the MITO-7 trial can be considered for patients with major comorbidities as it demonstrated equivalent PFS and improved quality of life compared to every 3-week carboplatin (AUC 6) and paclitaxel (175 mg/m^2) with lower rates of myelosuppression and neuropathy (Pignata et al. 2014).

MAINTENANCE THERAPY

The continuation of anticancer therapy with the goal of maintaining a response following upfront adjuvant carboplatin and paclitaxel has been extensively studied in ovarian cancer. This was initially attempted with single-agent chemotherapy, including with paclitaxel (Markman et al. 2009; Copeland et al. 2022) or topotecan (De Placido et al. 2004; Pfisterer et al. 2006b). While there was a PFS benefit associated with paclitaxel maintenance (Markman et al. 2003), maintenance chemotherapies did not demonstrate an OS benefit and/or were associated with unacceptable levels of toxicity (for review, see Markman 2015). Today, antiangiogenesis agents and PARPi in specific subsets of patients have acceptable toxicity as maintenance therapy.

Angiogenesis Inhibitors

Angiogenesis, and in particular the vascular endothelial growth factor (VEGF), plays an important role in tumor growth and metastasis in many human malignancies, including ovarian cancer (Wong et al. 2003; Hanahan and Weinberg 2011). Bevacizumab is a humanized monoclonal antibody that disrupts angiogenesis by inhibiting VEGF-A. The phase III GOG-218 trial evaluated the addition of bevacizumab (15 mg/kg every 3 wk) to chemotherapy and as maintenance therapy versus placebo in first-line therapy for women with advanced ovarian cancer after PDS. This was a three-arm, double-blind, placebo-controlled superiority trial that compared carboplatin/paclitaxel plus bevacizumab followed by 12 months of bevacizumab maintenance (bevacizumab-throughout) to carboplatin/paclitaxel plus bevacizumab with placebo maintenance (bevacizumab-initiation) to carboplatin/paclitaxel plus placebo with placebo maintenance (control) (Burger et al. 2011). The initial analysis of PFS saw an improvement in PFS from 10.3 months in the control to 11.2 in the bevacizumab-initiation group and 14.1 months in the bevacizumab-throughout group. This result led to the Food and Drug Administration (FDA) approval of bevacizumab for first-line treatment and for maintenance therapy of ovarian cancer. However, the final analysis of GOG-218 did not reveal a benefit in OS for patients treated with bevacizumab compared with chemotherapy alone (Tewari et al. 2019).

ICON7, which was a nonblinded, non-placebo-controlled trial, testing half the dose of bevacizumab, randomized patients with high-risk, early stage (stage I or IIA and clear-cell or grade 3 tumors), and advanced (stage IIB–IV) ovarian cancers after optimal or suboptimal debulking to carboplatin and paclitaxel every 3 weeks or carboplatin and paclitaxel plus bevacizumab at a dose half of that used in GOG-218 (7.5 mg/kg every 3 wk) as maintenance. The median PFS was 19.0 months in the bevacizumab group versus 17.3 months in the chemotherapy alone group (Perren et al. 2011), with long-term results also showing no significant difference in the mPFS between the two groups (Oza et al. 2015). The final results failed to demonstrate a difference in OS in the population as a whole; however, an OS benefit was seen in a retrospectively defined subgroup with poor prognosis, including stage IV disease or inoperable or suboptimally cytoreduced stage III (Oza et al. 2015). Lastly, the BOOST trial compared maintenance therapy with bevacizumab (15 mg/kg every 3 wk) for 15 or 30 months, finding no difference in PFS or OS with prolonged administration of bevacizumab beyond 15 months (Pfisterer et al. 2023). Thus, bevacizumab is considered a possible maintenance therapy for patients with advanced (stage III or IV) ovarian cancer for a maximum duration of 15 months with a careful risk and benefit discussion with the patient.

Although bevacizumab is well tolerated overall, it can lead to toxicities such as hypertension, proteinuria, thrombotic events (i.e., myocardial infarction, cerebrovascular accident), wound healing complications, hemorrhage, or gastrointestinal perforation. The half-life of bevacizumab is 20 days; therefore, physicians must be mindful of toxicities even after cessation of therapy, and surgical planning must also take this into account, holding bevacizumab for at least one cycle of treatment before and after surgery.

Besides bevacizumab, other agents targeting angiogenesis have also been investigated in combination with carboplatin and paclitaxel in up-front and maintenance therapy in ovarian cancer. Addition of nintedanib, an oral VEGF receptor 1–3 inhibitor, to carboplatin and paclitaxel following PDS did not result in a statistically significant improvement in PFS or OS in stage IIB–IV ovarian cancer (du Bois et al. 2016). Inhibiting the interaction of angiopoietin-1 (ANG-1) and ANG-2 with their receptor, the tyrosine kinase receptor TIE2, using IV trebaninib (15 mg/kg) was tested in the TRINOVA-3 trial and also failed to demonstrate improvement in PFS compared to placebo when combined with carboplatin and paclitaxel (Vergote et al. 2019).

Overall, while GOG-218 and ICON7 demonstrated a PFS benefit with the addition of bevacizumab, the lack of OS benefit, potential adverse events, and substantial financial toxicity (Mehta and Hay 2014) have limited the widespread routine use of bevacizumab in the first-line maintenance setting, with practice patterns varying widely. In a real-world analysis of 1498 patients with newly diagnosed advanced ovarian cancer in Europe and the United States, bevacizumab was used by 20% of patients in the United States and 11% in Europe in a nonuniform fashion (Monberg et al. 2019). Patterns of use have also fluctuated over time, likely due in part to changes in approvals and reimbursement as well as evolving data with PARPi as maintenance (discussed in the next section). In addition, bevacizumab has also proven beneficial in the treatment of recurrent disease (discussed later in this review), potentially arguing for reserving this agent for later lines of therapy (Table 2).

PARPi

Approximately 50% of HGSOC possess genetic or epigenetic alterations in the homologous recombination (HR) DNA repair pathway, most commonly caused by germline or somatic mutations or epigenetic silencing of *BRCA1* or *BRCA2* (Cancer Genome Atlas Research Network 2011; Konstantinopoulos et al. 2015). PARPi have been studied intensively in ovarian cancer since the initial observation in 2005 of their antitumor activity in vitro against *BRCAm* embryonic stem cell lines (Farmer et al. 2005). Several mechanisms have been proposed to explain the effects of PARPi in HR-deficient cells, including the inhibition of base excision repair, PARP-DNA complex trapping at the replication forks, enhancement of toxic nonhomologous end joining (NHEJ) in PARP1-deficient cells, and inhibition of PARP1/Pol-mediated alternative end joining (Konstantinopoulos et al. 2015; D'Andrea 2018). A large body of preclinical work and clinical trials (discussed in the "Treatment of Recurrent Ovarian Cancer" section) led to the first FDA approval of a PARPi, olaparib, for the treatment of individuals with a germline

Table 2. Key ongoing clinical trials in recurrent ovarian cancer

Study name	Study drug(s)	Patient population	Study arms
NCT05092360 ARTISTRY-7 GOG-3063 ENGOT-ov68 KETYNOTE-C71 (Herzog et al. 2023)	Nemvaleukin + pembrolizumab	Platinum-sensitive recurrent ovarian cancer (PS-ROC), or precision recall (PR)-ROC with up to five prior lines; prior bevacizumab required	Nemvaleukin + pembrolizumab Nemvaleukin Pembrolizumab Physician's choice chemotherapy
NCT05281471 OnPrime/GOG-3076 (Holloway et al. 2022)	Olvimulogene nanivacirepvec (Olvi-Vec) oncolytic immunotherapy	PR-ROC	Olvi-Vec followed by platinum-doublet chemotherapy + bevacizumab Platinum-doublet chemotherapy + bevacizumab
NCT05445778 GLORIOSA (O'Malley et al. 2023)	Mirvetuximab maintenance	PS-ROC without progression after second-line platinum-based chemotherapy with bevacizumab FRα >75% by PS2	Mirvetuximab + bevacizumab maintenance Bevacizumab maintenance
NCT05255471 MITO 35b (Schettino et al. 2022)	Olaparib	PS-ROC with progression during or after first-line PARPi maintenance	Olaparib Platinum-based chemotherapy
NCT04679064 NItCHE-MITO33 (Musacchio et al. 2021)	Niraparib + dostarlimab	Recurrent ovarian cancer, platinum ineligible	Niraparib + dostarlimab Physician's choice chemotherapy
NCT05870748 REFRaME-01 GOG-3086 (Naumann et al. 2023)	Luveltamab tazevibulin —ADC targeting FRα	PR-ROC FRα TPS ≥25%	Luveltamab tazevibulin Physician's choice chemotherapy
NCT06161025 REJOICE-Ovarian01 (Ray-Coquard et al. 2024)	Raludotatug deruxtecan (R-DXd)—ADC targeting CDH6	PR-ROC, prior mirvetuximab required for patients with high FRα expression	Raludotatug deruxtecan Physician's choice chemotherapy

(ADC) Antibody–drug conjugate, (FRα) folate receptor α, (PARPi) poly(ADP-ribose) polymerase inhibitors.

BRCA mutation (*gBRCAm*) and recurrent ovarian cancer (ROC) following at least three lines of prior chemotherapy. Based upon the success of PARPi in the recurrent setting, their role in maintenance treatment after up-front chemotherapy has now also been established, and it is one of the most significant advances in the field in recent years. However, several FDA approvals have been withdrawn for recurrent cancer, which is discussed below.

The landmark SOLO-1 trial randomized individuals with *BRCAm* (either germline or somatic *BRCAm*) stage III or IV high-grade serous or endometrioid ovarian cancer who had a complete or partial response to up-front platinum-based chemotherapy to receive olaparib (300 mg twice daily) maintenance for 24 months or placebo (Moore et al. 2018a). At median follow-up of 41 months, the risk of disease progression or death was 70% lower with olaparib compared to placebo. These findings led to the approval of olaparib for maintenance therapy in women with *BRCAm* advanced ovarian cancer who experienced a complete or partial response to first-line chemotherapy. At 7-year OS follow-up, 67% of olaparib patients versus 47% of placebo patients were alive (DiSilvestro et al. 2023), which is not statistically significant but is clinically significant.

Given the high prevalence of HRD in HGSOC even in the absence of *BRCA1/2* germline or somatic mutations, other trials have assessed the efficacy of PARPi in patients with *BRCAwt* tumors. The PRIMA/ENGOT-OV26/GOG-3012 trial (NCT02655016) tested the efficacy of 3 years of niraparib maintenance (300 mg daily) following up-front chemotherapy in women with advanced high-grade serous or endometrioid ovarian cancers (González-Martín et al. 2019). It is noteworthy that the patient population in this trial was selected for those at high risk for recurrence, including women with inoperable stage III/IV disease, who required NACT, or who were left with residual disease. In the overall population, niraparib maintenance significantly prolonged PFS from 8.2 to 13.8 months (hazard ratio [HR] 0.62, 95% confidence interval [CI] 0.50–0.76; $P < 0.001$), with the effect being more pronounced in patients with *BRCAm* (HR 0.40, 95% CI 0.27–0.62) or positive HRD testing (HR 0.43, 95% CI 0.31–0.59). A diminished but statistically significant benefit for niraparib maintenance was detected in the *BRCAwt* and HR-proficient group (HR 0.68, 95% CI 0.49–0.94). Based on this, niraparib has FDA approval as maintenance therapy in the first-line setting regardless of *BRCA* status. Importantly, the final OS data at a median follow-up of 73.9 months revealed no benefit of niraparib over placebo, with an OS HR of 1.01 (95% CI 0.84–1.23; $P = 0.8834$) in the overall population and 0.95 (95% CI 0.70–1.29) and 0.93 (95% CI 0.69–1.26) in the HRD and HR-proficient populations, respectively (Monk et al. 2024b).

Additionally, the ATHENA/GOG-3020 study randomized patients with newly diagnosed stages III and IV high-grade EOC following completion of first-line platinum-doublet chemotherapy and surgery to receive maintenance with the PARPi rucaparib (600 mg twice daily) plus placebo (MONO arm), rucaparib plus nivolumab (COMBO arm; discussed in later sections), and nivolumab plus placebo or double placebo. Similar to other first-line PARPi studies, ATHENA-MONO reported a PFS benefit in the overall study population, with a more robust benefit seen in the HRD population (median PFS 28.7 vs. 11.3 mo for rucaparib vs. placebo) compared to the HRD-negative population (PFS 12.1 vs. 9.1 mo) (Monk et al. 2022). The updated PFS data at 4-year follow-up revealed that the median PFS was consistently longer or not reached with rucaparib compared with placebo maintenance in the intention-to-treat (ITT) populations as well as in the HRD subgroup (Kristeleit et al. 2024a). Although not mature, updated OS data in the ITT population found the median OS not reached in the rucaparib arm versus 46.2 months in the placebo arm (HR 0.83, 95% CI 0.58–1.17). The medial OS was not reached in either arm in the HRD population (HR 0.84, 95% CI 0.44–1.58) (Kristeleit et al. 2024b).

Given the activity of both bevacizumab and PARPi independently for maintenance therapy in ovarian cancer, the PAOLA-1 trial tested olaparib versus placebo in combination with bevacizumab following up-front chemotherapy in women with either high-grade serous or endometrioid ovarian cancer, regardless of degree of surgical debulking or *BRCA* mutation status. The combination resulted in a HR for disease progression or death of 0.59 overall (95% CI 0.49–0.72; $P < 0.0001$); the HR was 0.31 (95% CI 0.20–0.47) in the *BRCAm* population and 0.33 (95% CI 0.25–0.45) in all patients testing positive for HRD (including *BRCA* mutant) (Ray-Coquard et al. 2019). In *BRCAwt* patients with HRD-negative tumors, there was no benefit with the combination of PARPi and bevacizumab (HR 0.92, 95% CI 0.72–1.17) over bevacizumab alone. As both arms received bevacizumab, it is not possible to distinguish whether bevacizumab provided additional clinical benefit beyond that of olaparib in the *BRCAm* and HRD-positive groups. Based on these data, the combination of bevacizumab and olaparib received FDA approval as first-line maintenance therapy for patients with *BRCAm* or *BRCAwt*/HRD-positive disease; there is no approval for homologous recombination proficiency (HRP) patients. Of note, different methods to define HRD status have been used across trials. PAOLA-1, VELIA, and PRIMA used the Myriad myChoice HRD assay, with a positive test being defined by a tumor *BRCAm* or a genomic instability score ≥42. ATHENA-MONO used the FoundationOne CDx next-generation sequencing assay, which defines positive HRD status as *BRCA* mutations detected in the tumor (which may be germline or somatic) or high loss-of-heterozygosity.

Taken together, the results from SOLO-1, PRIMA, ATHENA-MONO, and PAOLA-1 clearly support the use of PARPi in the maintenance setting following response to first-line platinum-based chemotherapy in patients with *BRCAm* or HRD-deficient tumors. The benefit of PARPi in the *BRCAwt*, HRD-negative disease is much less clear and should include a risk/benefit discussion with the patient to review the PFS results, lack of OS benefit, and toxicity profile. Across all studies, PARPi therapy is associated with frequent development of bone marrow suppression (thrombocytopenia, anemia, and neutropenia), as well as fatigue and nausea. Myelodysplastic syndrome (MDS) and acute myeloid leukemia (AML), referred to collectively as therapy-related myeloid neoplasia (TMN), have been identified with the use of PARPi. Development of TMN portends extremely poor prognosis, with almost half of reported cases resulting in death (Morice et al. 2021). Rates of TMN were reported at up to 6%–8% in the recurrent maintenance setting in SOLO2, NOVA, and ARIEL3, but are lower in the primary maintenance setting at 0.5%–1.5% across the major studies (González-Martín et al. 2019; Ray-Coquard et al. 2019; DiSilvestro et al. 2023; Monk et al. 2023), likely related to lower cumulative chemotherapy exposure and shorter and predefined duration of PARPi. These data further support the use of PARPi in the first-line setting rather than later in their disease course and use in appropriate molecularly defined populations.

In summary, germline and somatic genetic testing along with HRD testing have become crucial in the initial management of newly diagnosed ovarian cancer, as PARPi maintenance therapy in *BRCAm* and HRD-positive patients leads to a substantial prolongation of PFS and OS. Germline genetic testing for *BRCA1/2* and other ovarian cancer susceptibility genes is recommended as part of the initial workup for all patients newly diagnosed with EOC (Konstantinopoulos et al. 2020). For patients without *BRCAm* or HRD positivity, niraparib and bevacizumab are both FDA-approved options for maintenance therapy, but the lack of OS benefit with bevacizumab and shorter PFS extension with niraparib should be carefully weighed against the risks of side effects and financial toxicity in this population. Furthermore, concern exists that acquired resistance to PARPi when used in the up-front setting could limit treatment options for recurrent disease.

Endocrine

Low-grade serous ovarian cancers (LGSOCs) demonstrate ER positivity and sensitivity to endocrine therapy. Commonly used agents include the selective estrogen receptor modulator (SERM) tamoxifen, the aromatase inhibitors letrozole and anastrozole, and the selective estrogen receptor antagonist fulvestrant.

In a retrospective study of patients with LGSOC, patients receiving hormonal suppression (mostly aromatase inhibitors) following up-front chemotherapy experienced a median PFS that was nearly double that in the observation group (64.9 vs. 26.4 mo; $P < 0.001$) (Gershenson et al. 2017). While no difference was seen in OS in the population as a whole, there was an improvement in OS detected with maintenance hormonal therapy in a subgroup that had persistent disease following initial chemotherapy. The phase III trial GY019 is testing the efficacy of letrozole with or without chemotherapy as first-line treatment following surgical cytoreduction in advanced LGSOC and is ongoing (NCT04095364).

Nevertheless, the treatment of LGSOC is primarily surgical, and numerous studies have confirmed that degree of residual disease is the most important prognostic feature (Nickles Fader et al. 2013; Gershenson et al. 2015), with systemic chemotherapy, hormonal therapy, or targeted agents used for maintenance therapy or palliative control of recurrent disease, which is discussed in further detail in the "Targeted Therapies for Specific Histological Epithelial Ovarian Cancer Subtypes" section. When patients present with unresectable disease at diagnosis, combining hormonal therapy with CDK4/6 inhibition, which has been shown to synergistically enhance sensitivity to estrogen receptor blockade (Finn et al. 2009), can improve rates of complete or optimal cytoreduction at ICS (Cobb et al. 2022).

INVESTIGATIONAL APPROACHES IN THE FIRST LINE AND MAINTENANCE SETTING

Despite the progress in ovarian cancer treatment described above, only about half of newly diagnosed women live beyond 5 years (Pavlidis et al. 2021), highlighting a great need for further investigational approaches.

VEGFi

A major area of research interest is improving the rates of optimal debulking during initial surgery. The addition of bevacizumab to NACT has been investigated in the phase II ANTHALYA and GEICO 1205 trials. Both trials randomized patients to four cycles of NACT plus bevacizumab (15 mg/kg every 3 wk) versus chemotherapy alone; after surgery, all patients received three cycles of chemotherapy and bevacizumab for 15 months. The primary end point was complete macroscopic response at interval debulking surgery. In GEICO 1205, there was no difference in the proportion of patients with complete cytoreduction or optimal surgery (Garcia Garcia et al. 2019). Grade 3 or greater adverse events were less common in the bevacizumab group during neoadjuvant cycles. In ANTHALYA, the complete resection rate at interval debulking surgery for the bevacizumab group was 58.6%, exceeding the predefined reference rate of 45% (Rouzier et al. 2017). The group that did not receive bevacizumab had a 51.4% complete resection rate, but the study was not designed for comparative analyses. Patients had similar rates of severe adverse events both pre- and postoperatively. Overall, these trials demonstrated acceptable safety of the addition of bevacizumab to NACT, but mixed effects on surgical operability and complete resection rate. The use of bevacizumab in the neoadjuvant setting has become more common, especially in patients with stage IV disease or symptomatic ascites, although more effective agents are needed to further improve surgical resectability.

PARPi

While PARPi are presently indicated only for maintenance therapy after the completion of chemotherapy, interest exists in using PARP inhibition earlier in the treatment course, especially in the *BRCAm* population. This approach may facilitate the ability to perform an optimal cytoreductive surgery or in some cases and/or reduce chemotherapy exposure; however, this is an area still in early stages of clinical investigation.

The NOW trial was a small feasibility study in which 15 patients with germline *BRCA1/2*, *RAD51C/D*, or *PALB2* mutations and newly diagnosed advanced high-grade EOC not amenable to primary cytoreduction received two cycles of olaparib (300 mg twice daily) followed by reassessment with CA-125 and imaging to determine whether surgery was possible. Ultimately, 13/15 patients underwent interval surgery after olaparib only, with optimal cytoreduction in all 13 cases and one pathologic complete response (Westin et al. 2023). Other trials have attempted to combine PARPi with NACT, although this requires a dose reduction of the PARPi for tolerability. The phase II NUVOLA trial administered olaparib in an intermittent fashion (150 mg twice daily, days 1–3) with NACT (weekly carboplatin AUC2 and paclitaxel 60 mg/m^2 every 3 wk) to patients with *BRCAm* and stage III and IV high-grade serous or endometrioid ovarian cancer not amenable to PCS. Ultimately, 4/35 (11.4%) of patients achieved pathologic complete response, not meeting the trial end point of 20% pathologic complete response and with higher hematologic toxicity compared to chemotherapy alone (Salutari et al. 2023). The phase II OPAL-C trial is evaluating the use of neoadjuvant niraparib in a randomized fashion compared to standard platinum-taxane chemotherapy in patients with stage III/IV ovarian cancer with HRD-deficient tumors (assessed by the Myriad myChoice CDx PLUS assay) (Belotte et al. 2024). Ultimately, the success of PARPi prior to surgery for patients with *gBRCAm* depends on the ability to obtain timely genetic testing following a diagnosis of ovarian cancer, as this approach is unlikely to be sufficiently active in an unselected patient population. A multicenter, prospective, phase II window-of-opportunity (WoO) trial of olaparib alone or olaparib with the PD-1 inhibitor, durvalumab, for 3–4 weeks prior to front-line surgery in patients with advanced EOC is ongoing (NCT04644289).

The addition of olaparib to an IP/IV chemotherapy regimen has been investigated in a phase I trial in which 29% of patients had a germline *BRCA* mutation. The maximum tolerated dose of olaparib was 100 mg twice daily when administered with IV/IP paclitaxel, IP cisplatin, and IV bevacizumab (Cadoo et al. 2020). Efficacy was encouraging, with a median PFS of 32.9 months, although further studies in larger cohorts are needed, and this should not be considered SOC.

ADCs

Antibody–drug conjugates (ADCs) are an emerging drug class combining a monoclonal antibody targeting a tumor-associated antigen joined to a payload of a cytotoxic chemotherapy molecule with a linker. This design allows for the delivery of cytotoxic chemotherapy directly to target cancer cells and has shown promising activity in a number of tumor types, including in gynecologic cancers (Karpel et al. 2023). The approval of the folate receptor α (FRα)-targeting ADC, mirvetuximab soravtansine, for the treatment of recurrent PR ovarian cancer with FRα overexpression is discussed in detail in the "Antibody–Drug Conjugates" section. Based on the favorable results of mirvetuximab in the PR-ROC, exploratory studies are also underway testing its efficacy in the first-line setting. A single-arm phase II trial is ongoing using carboplatin and mirvetuximab as neoadjuvant and adjuvant chemotherapy in patients with newly diagnosed advanced EOC with FRα-positive HGSOC (NCT04606914). Numerous other ADCs are in development for recurrent EOC and are likely to be investigated in earlier line settings in the future.

Immunotherapy

Immune checkpoint inhibitors (ICIs) have revolutionized the treatment of certain solid and hematologic malignancies (Postow et al. 2015). However, ICIs have proved minimally active as single agents in the vast majority of patients with ovarian cancer, despite the known correlation between the presence of intratumoral $CD3^+$ T cells in ovarian cancer tumors and improved clinical outcomes (Zhang et al. 2003; Sato et al. 2005; Hwang et al. 2012). Across several trials, the overall response rate (ORR) to single-agent ICI has been <15% (Disis et al. 2019; Matulonis et al. 2019; Varga et al. 2019; Hamanishi et al. 2021) for recurrent disease. At present, except for pembrolizumab, which is approved for use in microsatellite instability-high (MSI-H) ovarian tumors through its tumor-agnostic label, the use of other immunotherapy agents is currently limited to clinical trials in EOC.

Attempts to sensitize ovarian cancer to immunotherapy have been made by combining ICIs with other agents in numerous clinical trials. For example, it was hypothesized that anti-angiogenesis agents could potentiate the effects of ICIs by promoting T-cell infiltration into the tumor microenvironment and reducing local immunosuppression. Unfortunately, the addition of ICIs to chemotherapy with or without bevacizumab in the first-line setting for advanced ovarian cancer in the IMagyn050 trial did not demonstrate significantly improved outcomes (Monk et al. 2021a; Moore et al. 2021).

The combination of PARPi and ICI is also of interest given interactions between DNA damage and tumor immunogenicity, including the upregulation of PD-L1 expression by PARPi (Jiao et al. 2017; Césaire et al. 2018). Combining immunotherapy with both VEGFi and PARPi in the maintenance setting was tested in the DUO-O trial (NCT03737643). In this trial, patients with newly diagnosed non-*BRCAm* advanced ovarian cancer received adjuvant carboplatin, paclitaxel, and bevacizumab with or without durvalumab, and then received maintenance bevacizumab with placebo (arm 1), durvalumab (arm 2), or durvalumab and olaparib (arm 3). The study met its coprimary end points with improved PFS in arm 3 compared with arm 1 in both the ITT population (HR 0.63; $P < 0.0001$) and the HRD population (HR 0.49; $P < 0.0001$) (Harter et al. 2023b). However, parsing out the individual contributions of each of these agents remains challenging, given that there was no treatment arm receiving olaparib without durvalumab. The ATHENA-COMBO study (NCT03522246) is investigating rucaparib 600 mg twice daily and nivolumab 480 mg every 4 weeks compared to rucaparib monotherapy as maintenance therapy following platinum-based chemotherapy in newly diagnosed stage III and IV high-grade ovarian cancer (Monk et al. 2022). At a median follow-up of 48 months, the addition of nivolumab to rucaparib was not associated with a PFS benefit in the ITT population, with median PFS for 15 months for the combination versus 20.2 months for rucaparib (HR 1.3, 95% CI 1.1, 1.5) or in HRD or PD-L1 subsets (Monk et al. 2024a). In addition, the FIRST trial (NCT03307785) is underway, testing the combination of dostarlimab with niraparib in newly diagnosed stage III disease with high-risk features (suboptimal debulking, planned NACT) or stage IV nonmucinous EOC. Following adjuvant chemotherapy with or without bevacizumab, patients are randomized to maintenance therapy with niraparib, niraparib plus dostarlimab, or placebo for up to 3 years, stratified by the *BRCA*/HRD status. The ENGOT-ov43/KEYLYNK-001 trial (NCT03740 165) is testing the benefit of adding pembrolizumab to chemotherapy with or without bevacizumab and as maintenance with and without olaparib in patients with *BRCAwt* advanced ovarian cancer (NCT03740165). Identifying biomarkers of response to ICI combinations will be critical for incorporating these agents into the management of ovarian cancer.

HIPEC

Given the promising results of HIPEC with interval debulking surgery in OVHIPEC-1, interest exists in expanding HIPEC to primary cytoreduction. A randomized controlled trial of HIPEC at the time of primary or interval cytoreduction for stage III/IV ovarian cancer patients in South Korea found no benefit to HIPEC in the overall population (Lim et al. 2022), although this trial has been criticized for having a highly heterogeneous patient population. Other ongoing studies of HIPEC (OVHIPEC-2, CHIPPI-1808, HOTT/GOG-3068) at the time of primary or ICS are also incorporating bevacizumab and PARPi use into the planned treatment protocol (Koole et al. 2020; El Hajj et al. 2021) (NCT05659381).

HIPEC has also been investigated for ROC with some phase II studies showing promising findings (Spiliotis et al. 2015) and others showing minimal benefits (Zivanovic et al. 2021; Classe et al. 2023). Most recently, two phase III trials of HIPEC at the time of secondary cytoreduction have yielded conflicting results. The CHIPOR study involving 415 patients randomized to HIPEC or no HIPEC after six cycles of platinum-based chemotherapy followed by secondary cytoreductive surgery to no gross residual or <2.5 mm residual disease demonstrated comparable median PFS in both groups (10.2 mo with HIPEC vs. 9.5 mo without HIPEC) but significantly prolonged median OS in the HIPEC group (54.3 vs. 45.8 mo) (Classe et al. 2024). Meanwhile, the HORSE/MITO18 study, which randomized 167 patients to HIPEC or no HIPEC at time of secondary cytoreductive surgery to no gross residual or <2.5 mm residual disease followed by six cycles of platinum-based chemotherapy, observed no difference in median PFS between groups (25 mo with HIPEC vs. 23 mo without HIPEC), with median OS not reached (Fagotti et al. 2025). Overall, defining the optimal role of HIPEC in the management of ovarian cancer remains an active area of research (Della Corte et al. 2023).

TREATMENT OF EARLY-STAGE AND RARE HISTOLOGY CANCERS

The previous sections have focused on advanced ovarian cancer, given that only ~25% of patients with EOC are diagnosed with stage I or stage II disease. In rare cases of histological grade 1 cancer confined to the ovary (stage IA or IB), surgery alone is sufficient for treatment with a 5-year OS of >90% (Young et al. 1990). However, for patients with positive peritoneal washings (stage IC), tumor involving the pelvis (stage II), or high-risk features such as high tumor grade or clear cell histology, adjuvant therapy is warranted, given significantly higher recurrence risk. ICON1 and ACTION were parallel randomized controlled trials comparing adjuvant platinum-based chemotherapy to observation following surgery for early-stage ovarian cancer, finding that adjuvant chemotherapy improves PFS, with a marginal improvement in OS. These trials had different inclusion criteria —a large number of patients with incomplete staging and heterogeneous platinum-based chemotherapy regimens (Trimbos et al. 2003); thus, uncertainty exists in the optimal management of these patients. Retrospective analyses have suggested that suboptimally staged patients with presumed unrecognized occult disease and those with known residual disease may be driving the clinical benefit of adjuvant therapy (Collinson et al. 2014).

In an effort to decrease treatment intensity among this relatively low-risk group of patients, GOG-157 tested whether three cycles of carboplatin and paclitaxel were sufficient in early-stage disease, which was defined as high-grade stage IA-B, stage IC EOC or any stage I clear cell, or completely resected stage II tumors. While there was a nonsignificant trend toward increased survival with six cycles, there was also increased toxicity (Bell et al. 2006). However, a subsequent exploratory analysis of the GOG-157 data revealed a survival advantage for six cycles in patients with serous tumors, so this remains the preferred adjuvant therapy in most cases (Chan et al. 2016).

Mucinous tumors comprise 3%–5% of EOCs and are mostly diagnosed at an early stage with a low risk of lymph node metastasis or recurrence, especially when tumors have an expansile pattern of invasion. Patients with infiltrative mucinous ovarian carcinomas are more likely to present with advanced disease and have occult lymph node involvement. Thus, lymph node assessment should be considered for apparently ovary-confined infiltrative mucinous ovarian cancers but can be omitted for expansile mucinous carcinomas. Adjuvant chemotherapy for three to six cycles is recommended for stage II or above disease, and can be considered for stage IC, although the ultimate impact on OS remains unclear (Morice et al. 2019). Response to platinum/taxane chemotherapy is relatively poor; however, attempts to identify superior adjuvant treatments, including gastrointestinal-based regimens, have not been successful. The GOG-241 trial comparing gastrointestinal chemotherapy regimen to standard platinum/taxane chemotherapy in mucinous ovarian cancers was terminated prematurely due to poor accrual (Gore et al. 2015).

Clear cell carcinomas of the ovary comprise ~4%–12% of EOCs (Tan and Kaye 2007), with a higher incidence among Asian women, and have distinct clinical and molecular features compared to serous ovarian cancers. For example, clear cell carcinomas more frequently present in early stages are associated with a history of endometriosis, carry a substantial risk of thromboembolic events, and tend to present in younger women. Molecularly, *BRCA1/2* mutations and p53 alterations are uncommon, while tumors more frequently harbor mutations in *ARID1A* and *PIK3CA* (Gadducci et al. 2021). Because these cancers are often diagnosed in younger women with clinically pelvic-confined disease and tend to be chemotherapy-resistant (Sugiyama et al. 2000), much interest exists in fertility-sparing management and treatment de-escalation. While all stages of clear cell cancer were considered high risk in the subgroup analysis of ICON1/ACTION, which seemed to have the greatest benefit from adjuvant chemotherapy, subsequent analyses have questioned the therapeutic benefit of chemotherapy for stage I ovarian clear cell cancers. Retrospective analyses of the ACTION trial and retrospective single-institution and national database studies suggest that adjuvant chemotherapy does not improve survival for stage IA-B ovarian clear cell carcinoma, but may increase OS for stage IC (Bogani et al. 2020; Manning-Geist et al. 2022; Shuqing and Zhiling 2023). However, patients for whom omission of chemotherapy is being considered should undergo full staging lymphadenectomy due to a risk of 4%–15% of occult lymph node metastases (Mahdi et al. 2013). Lymphadenectomy may not influence survival if adjuvant chemotherapy is planned.

Lastly, endometrioid ovarian cancers represent ~10% of EOCs and are often diagnosed in conjunction with endometriosis or with endometrioid endometrial carcinomas. High-grade endometrioid ovarian cancer is treated like HGSOC, but low-grade cancers, like endometrioid uterine cancers, harbor frequent mutations in *CTNNB1* and *PTEN*, and are more often mismatch repair-deficient (MMRd) and are frequently ER^+/PR^+ (Pierson et al. 2020). Thus, observation is recommended for stage IA/B grade 1 endometrioid endometrial cancers, while systemic therapy should be considered for stage IC and above and for all grade 2/3 disease. For patients with ER^+/PR^+ tumors, maintenance hormonal therapy with letrozole or similar agents can be considered after the completion of chemotherapy, although prospective data supporting this approach is limited (Tyulyandina et al. 2019). An ongoing randomized controlled trial (MATAO) comparing letrozole maintenance to placebo in patients with newly diagnosed stage II–IV low or high-grade endometrioid or serous ovarian cancer following standard platinum-based chemotherapy will be illuminating on this issue (McLaughlin et al. 2022).

Overall, given the relative rarity of nonserous histology EOCs, specific prospective data concerning their management are limited (Table 3). While all patients diagnosed with HGSOCs should receive adjuvant chemotherapy, the impact of adjuvant chemotherapy on survival in other histological subtypes of EOC is more unclear. The ongoing phase III JGOG-3020 trial (NCT04063527) will address some questions about the role of adjuvant chemotherapy in these patients, randomizing newly diagnosed patients with either stage IA/IB, grade 2 and 3, or clear cell carcinoma or with stage IC of any histologic type EOC to adjuvant chemotherapy or observation after complete surgical staging, including full lymph node dissection.

SURVEILLANCE FOLLOWING PRIMARY TREATMENT

Following treatment of either early-stage or advanced EOC, patients should be closely monitored for disease recurrence (Salani et al. 2017). The majority of patients with advanced disease experience relapse, with the typical time frame between 12 and 18 months. Most guidelines agree that surveillance should consist of symptom review and physical examination every 2–4 months for the first 2–3 years after the completion of adjuvant therapy, with radiographic imaging as needed. The recommendations for CA125 measurements remain less clear. In one randomized trial, early treatment of relapsed disease based on CA125 concentration as compared with radiographic or symptomatic relapse did not alter survival (Rustin and Van Der Burg 2009). Notably, this study was conducted prior to the use of newer agents such as bevacizumab and PARPi. When recurrent disease is suspected on the basis of exam, symptoms, or CA125 elevation, it should be confirmed by radiographic imaging, and if uncertainty persists, biopsy.

More recently, numerous studies have demonstrated that the presence of circulating tumor DNA (ctDNA) postoperatively or in the surveillance setting is highly prognostic for cancer recurrence (Hou et al. 2022; Zhu et al. 2023). Whether changing strategies for maintenance

Table 3. Clinical trials in nonserous high-grade epithelial ovarian cancers

Study name	Study drug(s)	Patient population	Study arms
NCT05296512	Lenvatinib Pembrolizumab	Recurrent clear cell ovarian cancer after prior platinum-based therapy	Lenvatinib + pembrolizumab
NCT06065462	LB-100 Dostarlimab	Recurrent clear cell ovarian cancer	Dostarlimab + LB-100

therapy or chemotherapy for recurrence based on the measurement of ctDNA can meaningfully improve survival in ovarian cancer remains to be seen.

Treatment of Recurrent Ovarian Cancer

Once a diagnosis of ROC has been established, the treatment plan must take into account several factors, including biological and clinical characteristics of the patient's disease, as well as patient-specific psychosocial elements. More specifically, the magnitude and pattern of disease burden, as well as current or impending clinical symptoms and prior and persistent toxicities from previous lines of therapy, are important to consider. In addition, the platinum-sensitivity and *BRCA* mutational status of the tumor, prior lines of therapy used, and patient eligibility for available clinical trials are essential considerations. Finally, the specific values and preferences of each individual patient and their performance status and social support mechanisms should strongly influence decisions surrounding a treatment plan.

PLATINUM-SENSITIVE RECURRENCE

In considering the optimal management of ROC, patients are commonly stratified based on the duration of their response to first-line platinum-based chemotherapy. The platinum-free interval (PFI) is defined as the time elapsed between completion of platinum-based chemotherapy and detection of recurrent disease. Historically, disease recurrence has been defined as platinum-sensitive when the PFI is at least 6 months; a cancer that initially responds to platinum but recurs in <6 months has been considered PR. In contrast, platinum-refractory cancers grow during platinum-based chemotherapy or within 4 weeks of stopping therapy. However, more recently, the Ovarian Cancer Consensus Conference recommended that additional factors should be considered when defining patient populations for clinical trials and choosing next lines of therapy. These include assessment of treatment-free interval (TFI), not only with platinum agents (TFIp) but also with nonplatinum (TFInp) and biological agents (TFIb), as well as histological subtype, *BRCA* status, number and types of prior lines of therapy, current tumor burden, and presence or absence of symptoms (Wilson et al. 2017). Regardless of the definition, platinum-sensitive ROC (PS-ROC) eventually transforms into PR disease with repeated exposure to platinum-containing agents (Markman et al. 2004). Treatment considerations for PS-ROC include secondary cytoreductive surgery in select circumstances, clinical trials, systemic chemotherapy with and without biological and targeted therapy, and maintenance therapy (Table 4).

Secondary Cytoreduction

As with the decision for primary cytoreduction versus ICS, the clinical benefit from secondary cytoreduction followed by adjuvant chemotherapy versus adjuvant chemotherapy alone for ROC has been difficult to assess due to differences in the extent of patient disease and surgical effort, as well as confounding effects from subsequent lines of therapy. The completeness of secondary cytoreduction has been shown to be a major predictor of longer subsequent OS in retrospective studies (Harter et al. 2006). The DESKTOP III (NCT01166737) trial in Germany randomized patients with a first recurrence of platinum-sensitive ROC to chemotherapy alone or debulking surgery followed by chemotherapy (Harter et al. 2021). Only patients with a high likelihood of complete resection were eligible; specifically, patients had to have undergone a complete cytoreduction at their primary surgery, have an Eastern Cooperative Oncology Group (ECOG) performance status of 0, and ascites of 500 mL or less. Ultimately, complete resection was achieved in 76% of patients and a PFS and OS benefit from undergoing secondary cytoreduction (median PFS 18.4 vs. 10.4 mo, median OS 53.6 vs. 46.0 mo) was reported, with no deaths within 30 days of surgery. Notably, patients who did not achieve a complete resection had relatively poor outcomes (median OS 27.7 mo, 95% CI 23.5–38.7) compared to those with complete resections (median OS 61.9 mo, 95% CI 55.3–78.9). About three-quarters of patients in both groups received at least

Table 4. Surgical clinical trials for ovarian cancer

Study name	Study intervention	Patient population	Study arms
NCT04575935 LANCE	Minimally invasive ICS	ICS for stage IIIC and IV EOC	Minimally invasive surgery (MIS) Laparotomy
NCT05659381 GOG-3068 HOTT	HIPEC at ICS Niraparib	Newly diagnosed stage IIIC and IV high-grade serous or endometrioid ovarian cancer with ≤1.0 cm residual disease undergoing ICS	HIPEC (cisplatin 100 mg/m^2) + chemotherapy + niraparib Chemotherapy + niraparib
NCT03772028 OVHIPEC-2	HIPEC at PCS	Newly diagnosed stage III EOC following PCS with ≤2.5 mm residual disease	HIPEC (cisplatin 100 mg/m^2) No HIPEC
NCT03842982 CHIPPI-1808	HIPEC at PCS or ICS	Newly diagnosed stage III EOC following PCS with ≤2.5 mm residual disease	HIPEC (cisplatin) No HIPEC
NCT05827523 KOV-HIPEC-04 (Lim et al. 2024)	HIPEC at ICS	Newly diagnosed stage III/IV EOC following PCS with ≤2.5 mm residual disease	HIPEC (cisplatin 75 mg/m^2) No HIPEC
NCT05123807 HI-MOC	HIPEC at secondary cytoreduction	Recurrent mucinous ovarian cancer undergoing secondary cytoreduction	HIPEC (cisplatin)
NCT04415944	HIPEC at time of second look laparoscopy	Newly diagnosed stage I–IVA EOC undergoing second look laparoscopy after optimal cytoreduction and systemic chemotherapy	HIPEC (carboplatin)

(EOC) Epithelial ovarian cancer, (HIPEC) hyperthermic intraperitoneal chemotherapy, (ICS) interval cytoreductive surgery, (PCS) primary cytoreductive surgery.

five cycles of platinum-containing chemotherapy, with small numbers receiving subsequent bevacizumab or PARPi.

Similarly, the SOC-1 trial in China (NCT016111766) randomized patients with a platinum-sensitive first recurrence of ovarian cancer to cytoreductive surgery followed by chemotherapy or chemotherapy alone inclusion (Shi et al. 2021; Jiang et al. 2024). Again, patients were preselected to have a high likelihood of successful complete resection; specifically, initial disease stage, completeness of cytoreduction at primary surgery, PFI, ECOG performance status, CA125 level, and the presence of ascites were incorporated into a logistic regression model. This information was combined with positron emission tomography (PET)-computed tomography (CT) imaging to assess the distribution of recurrent disease to determine eligibility. The rate of complete cytoreduction was 77%, and the vast majority of patients in both groups received platinum-based IV chemotherapy and rarely received PARPi or bevacizumab maintenance. There was a significant PFS benefit associated with surgery, with a median PFS of 17.4 months in the surgery versus 11.9 months in the no surgery group ($P < 0.0001$). However, no benefit was seen in OS with median OS 58.1 months in the surgery group versus 53.9 months in the no surgery group (HR 0.82, 95% CI 0.56–1.19). The authors attributed the lack of OS benefit to multiple factors, including a high crossover of 37% to subsequent surgery at next relapse in the no surgery group.

The GOG-213 trial (NCT00565851), which enrolled patients in the United States and South Korea, was designed to assess the potential benefit of bevacizumab added to chemotherapy and continued as maintenance therapy in relapsed ovarian cancer, as well as the impact of secondary cytoreduction in platinum-sensitive ROC (Coleman et al. 2019). Eligibility for surgery was determined by CT scan, and excluded if not medically fit for surgery or if they had diffuse carcinomatosis, ascites, or extra-abdominal disease. In contrast to SOC-1 and DESKTOP III, the authors found no difference in PFS or OS (mPFS 18.9 vs. 16.2 mo and mOS 50.6 vs. 64.7 mo in the surgery vs. no surgery groups, respectively). This finding extended even to patients who experienced complete resection. The complete cytoreduction rate was 67%. In contrast to the other two studies, the vast majority of patients in GOG-213 received bevacizumab with their subsequent chemotherapy. *BRCA* mutational status was not recorded, and subsequent PARPi treatment was unknown.

All three trials had long accrual times despite enrolling patients at multiple, high-volume centers, emphasizing the difficulty in conducting surgical randomized controlled trials. Two similar trials (SOCceR and EORTC 55963) were closed prematurely due to insufficient enrollment. Given the mixed results from SOC-1, DESKTOP III, and GOG-213, the decision to pursue secondary cytoreductive surgery remains controversial. Overall, it should only be considered for patients with platinum-sensitive disease and good performance status when complete gross resection seems likely. Consensus guidelines from the SGO on secondary cytoreductive surgery suggest that laparoscopic exploration may be useful to augment assessment of disease distribution, as ultimately about a quarter to a third of patients in all three trials had substantial unresectable disease despite favorable preoperative imaging and/or clinical characteristics (Harrison et al. 2021). Data for subsequent cytoreduction (tertiary, quaternary) are limited to retrospective series, but could be of clinical benefit for patients with oligometastatic recurrences with long TFIs following secondary cytoreduction (Shih et al. 2010; Fotopoulou et al. 2013; Manning-Geist et al. 2021).

Chemotherapy

Many treatment options exist for patients with a first platinum-sensitive recurrence who are candidates for systemic therapy. Outside of a clinical trial, patients with PS-ROC are commonly treated with a platinum-containing regimen based on the results of the MITO-8 study. This trial randomized patients with platinum-sensitive disease to platinum-based or nonplatinum agents, finding a significantly longer PFS with platinum-based chemotherapy (Pignata et al. 2017). Most patients are treated with a platinum doublet, given that this approach has been shown to extend survival when compared with single-agent platinum (Parmar et al. 2003). Paclitaxel, gemcitabine, and PLD are all options with demonstrated efficacy in a clinical trial setting (Parmar et al. 2003; Pfisterer et al. 2006a; Pujade-Lauraine et al. 2010), with choice of therapy often being guided by differing toxicity profiles, schedule of administration, and patient preferences. Compared to primary chemotherapy, the accumulated dose of platinum with treatment for recurrence disease does entail significant additional toxicity, including risk of life-threatening allergic reactions, additional bone marrow suppression and neurotoxicity, and a small but significant risk of secondary MDS and AML (Travis et al. 1999). Chemotherapy desensitization protocols, although somewhat cumbersome logistically, have allowed many patients to safely continue receiving platinum-based chemotherapy after acquiring a drug allergy (Li et al. 2014).

When patients are unable to tolerate platinum-based doublet therapy, single-agent chemotherapy with gemcitabine (Ferrandina et al. 2008), PLD (Gordon et al. 2001), topotecan (Mitchell et al. 2005; Morris et al. 2008), etoposide (Rose et al. 1998), or nanoparticle albumin-bound paclitaxel (nab-paclitaxel) (Teneriello et al. 2009) can be considered, with ORRs ranging from 25% to 64%.

Bevacizumab Maintenance

Bevacizumab carries an FDA approval in combination with either carboplatin/paclitaxel or carboplatin/gemcitabine and as maintenance therapy until disease progression in PS-ROC. These approvals are based on the results of two randomized phase III trials, GOG-213 (Coleman et al. 2017b) and OCEANS (Aghajanian et al. 2012, 2015). GOG-213 randomized women with PS-ROC to carboplatin and paclitaxel or carboplatin, paclitaxel, and bevacizumab plus bevacizumab maintenance with OS as the primary end point. In GOG-213, a PFS benefit was seen (mPFS 13.8 mo in the bevacizumab group vs. 10.4 mo with chemotherapy alone), with a marginal OS benefit of 5 months with bevacizumab (median OS 42.6 vs. 37.3 mo; HR 0.82, 95% CI 0.69–0.996) following reanalysis due to initial incorrect stratification (Coleman et al. 2017b). In OCEANS, the addition of bevacizumab to carboplatin and gemcitabine was tested with the primary end point being PFS and secondary end point OS. The bevacizumab group had a superior PFS of 12.4 versus 8.4 months (HR 0.46, 95% CI 0.39–0.61; $P < 0.0001$); OS was not significantly improved, although the study was not powered for this outcome (Aghajanian et al. 2012, 2015). Of note, patients with prior bevacizumab exposure were excluded from OCEANS and comprised only 5%–10% of patients in GOG-213. Given increasing use of bevacizumab in the first-line setting, MITO16b was a randomized, phase III trial designed to assess the addition of bevacizumab to a carboplatin-based doublets in patients with ROC who had previously received bevacizumab with first-line treatment. Again, this study found a PFS benefit with bevacizumab (11.8 vs. 8.8 mo), but no OS benefit (Pignata et al. 2021). High rates of crossover as well as differences in subsequent lines of therapy patients receive after coming off trial likely limit the evaluation of OS in these trials.

PARPi Maintenance

Starting in March of 2017, three PARPi's—olaparib, niraparib, and rucaparib—obtained FDA approval for maintenance therapy in PS-ROC disease regardless of *BRCA* mutational status based on initial PFS data. More recently, approvals have been withdrawn based on updated OS data. Currently, in the United States, PARPi indications are limited only to patients with *BRCA* mutations who have PS-ROC and who are in response to their most recent platinum regimen. The data supporting this evolution will be briefly reviewed, given the major impact these trials have had on the field.

In the recurrent disease setting, PARPi were first evaluated and approved for the treatment of recurrent disease. Olaparib was the first to obtain FDA approval for the treatment of ROC in December 2014 for patients with *gBRCA* mutations following three prior lines of therapy, based on the results of Kaufman et al. (2015). Thereafter, rucaparib (600 mg twice daily) was approved for patients with germline or somatic *BRCA* mutations after at least two prior lines of therapy based on the results of ARIEL2 (Swisher et al. 2017) and niraparib (300 mg once daily) was approved for HRD-positive ROC after at least three prior lines of therapy based on the results of the QUADRA trial (Moore et al. 2019). The international, multicenter phase III ARIEL4 trial of rucaparib (600 mg twice daily) versus chemotherapy in ROC again found a PFS benefit with rucaparib (7.4 vs. 5.4 mo) (Kristeleit et al. 2022). However, an updated analysis presented at the 2022 IGSC conference demonstrated worse survival for olaparib compared to nonplatinum chemotherapy for patients with three or more prior lines of chemotherapy (Leath et al. 2022). Based on these results, the pharmaceutical companies that manufacture olaparib, rucaparib, and niraparib voluntarily withdrew their indications for treatment of third-line or higher ovarian cancer. Currently, there is no indication for the use of PARPi as a treatment for ROC in the United States.

Olaparib (300 mg twice daily), niraparb (300 mg once daily), and rucaparib (600 mg twice daily) also gained approvals for maintenance therapy following response to platinum-based chemotherapy regardless of the *BRCA* status based on the initial results of Study-19 (Ledermann et al. 2012, 2016), SOLO-2 (Pujade-Lauraine et al. 2017), NOVA (Mirza et al. 2016), and ARIEL3 (Coleman et al. 2017a). Of note, the primary outcome measure for these studies was PFS or ORR. Subsequently, the final OS analysis in the NOVA study, which was a nonanalytical end point, found no significant difference in median OS for niraparib versus placebo in the *gBRCAm* cohort (median OS 40.9 vs. 38.1 mo) or the non-*gBRCAm* cohort (median OS 31.0 vs. 34.8 mo) (Matulonis et al. 2023b). This led to the withdrawal of the indication for maintenance niraparib for patients with platinum-sensitive ROC other than those with *gBRCAm*. Similarly, final OS data from the ARIEL3 trial of rucaparib versus placebo maintenance in PS-ROC reported a median OS of 45.9 versus 47.8 months with rucaparib versus placebo in the *BRCAm* cohort (HR 0.83, 95% CI 0.58–1.19), 40.5 versus 47.8 months in the HRD^+ cohort (HR 1.01, 95% CI 0.77–1.32), and 36.0 versus 43.2 months in the overall population (HR 1.00, 95% CI 0.81–1.22) (Coleman et al. 2022). This led to the restriction of rucaparib only for PS-ROC patients who harbor *gBRCA* mutations.

In summary, based on the above data as well as the known higher rates of TMN associated with PARPi use in the recurrent maintenance across several trials (González-Martín et al. 2019; Ray-Coquard et al. 2019; Matulonis et al. 2023b), PARPi are no longer indicated for maintenance therapy of ROC for patients with *BRCAwt* cancer and should not be prescribed for the treatment of ROC in any patient population. They remain an option for maintenance therapy for patients with PS-ROC with *gBRCA* mutations based on favorable results from the *BRCAm* cohorts of SOLO2, NOVA, Study 19, and ARIEL3. Notably, subsequent analyses of patients treated on the SOLO-2 and PAOLA-1 trials revealed a shorter benefit of second-line platinum-based chemotherapy in patients who progressed on PARPi maintenance therapy compared with those who progressed after or were not treated with PARPi maintenance (Frenel et al. 2022; Harter et al. 2023a). This has raised concern that prior PARPi therapy may induce resistance to future therapies, further underscoring the importance of careful selection of appropriate patients for PARPi maintenance.

Limited data exist on the use of PARPi for maintenance after previous PARPi exposure. Retrospective data suggest that re-exposure to PARPi could be safe and of clinical benefit, even in patients with prior progression on PARPi (Essel et al. 2021; Moubarak et al. 2022). The phase III, double-blind, multicenter OReO trial enrolled patients with prior exposure to PARPi for at least 12–18 months, including *BRCAm* and non-*BRCAm* cohorts (Pujade-Lauraine et al. 2023). Only a small portion of patients (7% of *BRCAm* cohort and 14% of non-*BRCAm* cohort) were enrolled at first recurrence after maintenance PARPi following first-line chemotherapy. Most patients were heavily pretreated, with more than 85% having received at least three prior lines of chemotherapy. The trial found a small but statistically significant increase in PFS with olaparib regardless of *BRCA* status. In the *BRCAm* cohort, mPFS was 4.3 versus 2.8 months with 1-year PFS rates of 19% versus 0%. In the non-*BRCAm* cohort, mPFS was 5.3 versus 2.8 months and 1-year PFS rates were 14% versus 0%. These results suggest that some patients may derive benefit from PARPi after prior PARPi, but a better understanding of how to identify those patients is needed.

The CAPRI trial was designed to address acquired resistance to PARP inhibition and enrolled patients with recurrent, platinum-sensitive *BRCAm* or HRD HGSOC who had demonstrated prior clinical benefit from PARPi and had no intervening chemotherapy (Wethington et al. 2023). Most patients received their initial PARPi course for treatment of recurrent disease. In the single-arm study, patients received the ataxia telangiectasia and Rad3-related kinase inhibitor (ATRi) ceralasertib (160 mg daily) with olaparib (300 mg twice daily) based on preclinical evidence that adding ATRi to PARPi could overcome PARPi resistance in cell lines and murine models (Kim et al. 2020; Zimmermann et al. 2022). The combination regimen exhibited an ORR of 50% with acceptable toxicity (Wethington et al. 2023), supporting consideration of combinatorial approaches to overcome acquired PARPi resistance. Overall, more data will be needed to guide decision-making about PARPi use in the likely increasingly common scenario of ROC, following first-line PARPi maintenance therapy.

Summary of Treatment for PS-ROC

The backbone of therapy in PS-ROC remains platinum-based chemotherapy, with secondary cytoreductive surgery considered in a select group of patients. PARPi maintenance is an option in patients with a *gBRCAm*; clinical benefit of adding PARPi maintenance is seen in a subset of patients, who remain poorly defined at present. The addition of bevacizumab for maintenance is also an option for all patients, although the effect on OS is unclear, especially in patients with prior bevacizumab exposure. While there have been no clinical trials to directly compare PARPi and bevacizumab maintenance strategies, a network meta-analysis was performed to determine differences in efficacy between bevacizumab and PARPi maintenance in patients with PS-ROC with respect to *BRCA* mutation status (Bartoletti et al. 2020). In all comers, there was an improvement in PFS with PARPi compared to bevacizumab (HR 0.70, 95% CI 0.54–0.91), which was more significant in the *BRCAm* group (HR 0.46, 95% CI 0.36–0.59). In the *BRCAwt* group, there was no statistically significant difference in PFS between the two therapeutic strategies (HR 0.87, 95% CI 0.63–1.20). Bevacizumab or PARPi combinations each showed superior PFS compared with chemotherapy alone in all three cohorts, arguing for at least one of these strategies to be employed in all patients with PS-ROC. Although these data are hypothesis generating, direct comparisons are lacking, and the decision therefore remains individualized. Considerations should include *BRCA* status, previous therapies, preexisting or prior toxicities, and the individual when determining a treatment course.

PLATINUM-RESISTANT RECURRENCE

Disease recurrence <6 months after conclusion of platinum-based chemotherapy has historically been categorized as PR-ROC. Multiple mechanisms of platinum resistance have been identified, including decreased accumulation and/or inactivation of the drug in the cell, increased DNA repair, altered proapoptotic signaling and execution of cell death in response to DNA damage, as well as resistance conferred by the tumor microenvironment and immune system (for review, see Binju et al. 2019). In patients with PR-ROC, goals of treatment should focus on controlling and preventing symptoms from cancer, avoiding toxicities, and maintaining quality of life. In general, treatment options consist of clinical trials, ADCs, or single-agent nonplatinum chemotherapy with or without bevacizumab.

Chemotherapy/Surgery

Sequential, single-agent chemotherapy remains the mainstay of treatment for PR-ROC. There are many chemotherapy agents available, and the optimal sequence is unknown. Options commonly used as initial therapies include weekly paclitaxel (Markman et al. 2002), PLD (Mutch et al. 2007), topotecan (Safra et al. 2007), gemcitabine (Mutch et al. 2007), pemetrexed (Miller et al. 2009), and oral etoposide (Rose et al. 1998). Each is associated with relatively low response rates (5%–25%) and short PFS intervals.

Surgery has traditionally not been recommended for PR-ROC except for palliative intent, given the overall poor survival in this population. Palliative intestinal diversion to relieve intractable nausea and vomiting via surgical, endoscopic, or interventional radiology approaches due to recurrent small or large bowel obstruction is especially common. However, given advancements in the medical and surgical management of ovarian cancer, a number of trials are re-exploring the utility of secondary cytoreductive surgery with or without HIPEC in PR-ROC. These include HIPOVA-1, which is a phase III randomized trial comparing NACT and bevacizumab followed by ICS with HIPEC and additional chemotherapy and bevacizumab with SOC chemotherapy and bevacizumab (NCT03220932). The phase I/II PARROT study administered pressurized IP aerosol chemotherapy with doxorubicin and cisplatin every 28–42 days via diagnostic laparoscopy for PR-ROC, finding a clinical benefit rate of 82% with good safety and tolerability (Vizzielli et al. 2024), but further study in larger patient populations is needed.

Antibody–Drug Conjugates

ADCs are an expanding class of therapeutics that aim to specifically target cancer cells while minimizing systemic toxicity. ADCs with various payloads and targets are under intense investigation across many areas of oncology, and several have shown promise in the field of ovarian cancer (for review, see Lee and Liu 2019). Mirvetuximab soravtansine is an ADC consisting of a humanized FRα-binding monoclonal antibody attached via a cleavable linker to the tubulin-targeting maytansinoid payload, DM4. FRα is overexpressed in ~80% of EOCs, most notably in HGSOC (Kalli et al. 2008; O'Shannessy et al. 2013), and is correlated with worse prognosis (Bax et al. 2023). Initial promising activity of mirvetuximab soravtansine was seen in phase I trials in heavily pretreated patients with PR-ROC whose tumors have FRα overexpression (Moore et al. 2014, 2017a,b). These results led to the randomized phase III FORWARD I trial (NCT02631876), which compared mirvetuximab soravtansine to standard chemotherapy (weekly paclitaxel, PLD, or topotecan) in PR-ROC with medium (50%–74%) or high (75% of greater) FRα expression (Moore et al. 2021). Key findings from FORWARD I included a higher ORR for mirvetuximab compared with chemotherapy (22% vs. 12%; $P = 0.015$) in the overall population with no significant difference in PFS or OS. Common side effects included nausea, diarrhea, and fatigue, as well as ocular disorders such as blurred vision and keratopathy, which were low grade and manageable with dose modification or delays with no long-term sequelae. Notably, FORWARD I used a different method of FRα quantification, specifically a simplified scoring system (10X), from the PS2$^+$ scoring method used in the phase 1 trials (Moore et al. 2021). In the prespecified FRα-high subgroup, the mirvetuximab group had a longer PFS (HR 0.69; $P = 0.049$) and OS (HR 0.62; $P = 0.033$) and higher ORR (24% vs. 10%; $P = 0.014$) compared with the chemotherapy group. Retrospective analyses of FRα staining using the prior PS2$^+$ method revealed that FORWARD I included patients with lower FRα levels, with a signal of benefit in patients with strong PS2$^+$ staining (Moore et al. 2021).

Subsequently, the SORAYA and MIRASOL trials investigated the efficacy of mirvetuximab in FRα-high disease assessed using the PS2$^+$ method. The phase II SORAYA trial enrolled patients with PR-ROC with high FRα tumor expression, defined as at least 75% of viable tumor cells exhibiting at least 2$^+$ membrane staining intensity (Matulonis et al. 2023a). Patients with platinum-refractory disease, defined as disease progression during or within 3 months of first-line platinum therapy, and patients who had received more than three prior lines of chemotherapy were excluded; prior bevacizumab was required. Of 105 patients evaluable for efficacy, 51% had received three prior lines of therapy and 48% had received prior PARPi. The study found an ORR of 32.4% with a median duration of response of 6.9 months. Based on these results, mirvetuximab received FDA accelerated approval for the treatment of patients FRα-positive PROC who have received one to three prior lines of therapy.

The confirmatory MIRASOL trial was a randomized phase III trial comparing mirvetuximab soravtansine to the investigator's choice of chemotherapy (PLD, paclitaxel, or topotecan) in patients with one to three prior lines of therapy and high FRα expression, again assessed using the PS2 method with a cutoff of 75%. The study reported substantial clinical benefit to mirvetuximab over chemotherapy, with investigator-assessed median PFS of 5.6 months in the mirvetuximab group versus 4.0 months in the chemotherapy group ($P < 0.001$) and median OS of 16.5 versus 12.75 months, respectively (HR 0.67, 95% CI 0.50–0.89; $P = 0.005$). The ORR was 42.3% for mirvetuximab versus 15.9% for investigator's choice chemotherapy (Moore et al. 2023). Additionally, grade 3 and higher adverse events were less common with mirvetuximab. These results led to the full FDA approval of mirvetuximab soravtansine for the treatment of FRα-high, PR-ROC patients who have received one to three prior systemic treatment regimens along with the VENTANA FOLR1 RxDx Assay as a companion diagnostic. This approval marked the first ADC with proven efficacy and survival benefit in ovarian cancer and first biomarker-driven therapy approval in ovarian cancer.

Bevacizumab

In addition, bevacizumab in combination with chemotherapy has been approved for PR-ROC based on the results of the phase II AURELIA trial (Pujade-Lauraine et al. 2014). In this study, patients with PR-ROC were randomized to chemotherapy (weekly paclitaxel, PLD, or topotecan) with or without bevacizumab. The primary end point was PFS, and crossover to single-agent bevacizumab at the time of progression was allowed. ORR was significantly increased in the bevacizumab cohort (31% vs. 13%), and the mPFS was nearly doubled at 6.7 versus 3.4 months (HR 0.48, 95% CI 0.38–0.60; $P < 0.001$); however, there was no significant difference in OS. The greatest PFS benefit was seen in patients treated with weekly paclitaxel (ORR 53.3%, mPFS 10.4 mo, 95% CI 7.9–11.9 mo) on subgroup analysis (Poveda et al. 2015), which is an improvement over the known ORR of ~10% for single-agent non-platinum agents in this setting. Importantly, patients also reported improvement in abdominal and gastrointestinal symptoms with bevacizumab, and patients with ascites at baseline required fewer paracenteses in the bevacizumab group compared with chemotherapy alone. Bevacizumab has also demonstrated single-agent activity in ROC with response rates ranging from 16% to 21% (Burger et al. 2007) and therefore remains an acceptable treatment regimen in patients who are not candidates for further chemotherapy.

PARPi

As described above, while PARPi were preliminarily FDA approved for treatment of ROC, including PR disease, these approvals were withdrawn after final OS analyses showed no significant improvement.

Radiation

While ovarian cancer is frequently radiosensitive, radiation has limited utility in the up-front treatment of ovarian cancer given the need to cover a large volume at risk of recurrence in the abdomen and pelvis. In the modern era, more targeted forms of radiation may be indicated in specific clinical scenarios. The use of advanced radiotherapy techniques such as adjuvant whole abdominal intensity-modulated radiotherapy (IMRT) following primary surgery and chemotherapy for advanced ovarian cancer and stereotactic body radiotherapy (SBRT) for treatment of oligometastatic recurrent disease have been reviewed elsewhere (Fields et al. 2017; Kowalchuk et al. 2020; Corrigan et al. 2022), and prospective clinical research on this topic remains active (Macchia et al. 2022). Advanced interventional radiology techniques for oligometastatic disease such as radiofrequency, microwave, or cryogenic ablation can also be effective (Yuan et al. 2021).

INVESTIGATIONAL STRATEGIES FOR RECURRENT OVARIAN CANCER

ADCs and Combinations

As discussed above, mirvetuximab is FDA approved for the treatment of FRα-high PROC after receipt of one to three prior lines of therapy. Efforts are now focusing on evaluating mirvetuximab in earlier lines of therapy and in combination. The phase 2 PICCOLO trial tested the efficacy and safety of mirvetuximab monotherapy for patients with FRα-high ROC who are platinum-ineligible and have received at least two prior lines of therapy (Secord et al. 2024). Of 79 patients enrolled, the ORR was 51.9% (95% CI 40.4, 63.3) with mDOR of 8.3 months (95% CI 5.5, 10.8) and mPFS of 6.9 months (95% CI 5.9, 9.6) (Secord et al. 2024). Additionally, preclinical data demonstrate that mirvetuximab can potentiate the activity of other chemotherapeutic agents (Ponte et al. 2016); thus, mirvetuximab is being tested in combination with other therapies in both PS-ROC and PR-ROC with an aim to extend the benefit of mirvetuximab to tumors with lower FRα expression levels. Several combinations have been investigated as part of the FORWARD II trial (NCT02606305), including with bevacizumab (O'Malley et al. 2020; Gilbert et al. 2023), carboplatin (Moore et al. 2018b), pembrolizumab (Matulonis et al. 2018), and the triplet combination of mirvetuximab, carboplatin, and bevacizumab (Richardson et al. 2024). The combination of mirvetuximab with bevacizumab demonstrated a tolerable safety profile and an ORR of 44% (95% CI 33, 54) in patients with

FRα-expressing PROC, which included tumors with FRα PS2$^+$ IHC ≥25%, demonstrating a benefit in lower FRα-expressing tumors (Gilbert et al. 2023). This combination has been included in the NCCN guidelines for patients with PROC with FRα ≥25%. Based on these results, the phase III GLORIOSA trial (NCT05445778) (O'Malley et al. 2023) is investigating the combination of mirvetuximab and bevacizumab versus bevacizumab alone as maintenance therapy in PS-ROC. Beyond mirvetuximab, there are many other ADCs in development for the treatment of EOC (for review, see Karpel et al. 2023) including other FRα-targeting ADCs (e.g., MORAb-202/farletuzumab ecteribulin, STRO-002/luveltamab tazevibulin, rinatabart sesutecan, LY4170156, IMGN151) as well as ADCs targeting other tumor antigens such as HER2, Trop2, and CDH6, among others (Table 2).

Notably, trastuzumab deruxtecan (T-DXd) is a humanized anti-HER2 monoclonal antibody linked to a potent topoisomerase I inhibitor payload (Ogitani et al. 2016) that demonstrated excellent activity in the phase II DESTINY PanTumor02 (DPT02) trial in patients with recurrent advanced or metastatic HER2-expressing solid tumors including EOC. In EOC patients with 2^+ or 3^+ HER2 expression, the ORR was 45% and median DOR was 11.3 months, with four CRs (Meric-Bernstam et al. 2024). Based on the results of this trial, T-DXd has received tumor agnostic approval for all tumors with HER2 3^+ expression by IHC and is included in NCCN guidelines (National Comprehensive Cancer Network 2024) for HER2-positive disease (2^+ or 3^+ by IHC). DTP02 is ongoing and continues to evaluate ovarian cancer patients with HER2 1^+ expression. GOG-3086/REFRaME-01 is an ongoing phase 2/3 two-part study designed to evaluate the efficacy and safety of the FRα-targeting ADC, luveltamab tazevibulin, versus investigator's choice chemotherapy in patients with recurrent FRα-expressing PROC (NCT05870748) (Naumann et al. 2023). Similarly, the phase 2/3 REJOICE-Ovarian01 trial is assessing the optimal dosing, efficacy, and safety of the CHD6-targeting ADC, raludotatug deruxtecan, compared to the investigator's choice of chemotherapy (NCT06161025) (Ray-Coquard et al. 2024).

Ongoing active areas of investigation related to ADCs in EOC include identification of novel tumor-specific targets, mechanisms of primary and acquired ADC resistance, the optimal sequencing of ADCs, and ADCs in combination therapy, including with standard chemotherapy, antiangiogenic agents, and ICI.

VEGFi with PARPi

Preclinical data demonstrate that DNA repair is dysregulated in hypoxic tumor microenvironments (Bindra et al. 2007), suggesting that VEGFi-induced hypoxia could render tumors more susceptible to death from DNA damage. In support of this hypothesis, the combination of cediranib, an anti-VEGF tyrosine kinase inhibitor, and olaparib initially showed impressive improvement in PFS (HR 0.42, 95% CI 0.23–0.76; $P = 0.005$) in patients with PS-ROC, with the benefit strongest in *BRCAwt* patients (Liu et al. 2014). These results led to the phase III NRG GY004 study comparing olaparib versus olaparib/cediranib versus platinum-doublet chemotherapy in PS-ROC, which found no improvement in PFS with the olaparib/cediranib combination compared to chemotherapy and worse patient-reported outcomes (Liu et al. 2022). However, both olaparib and olaparib/cediranib had substantial clinical activity in the subset of patients with g*BRCAm*, which excluded patients with first-line PARPi exposure. ICON9 is an ongoing phase III trial evaluating maintenance therapy with olaparib/cediranib compared with olaparib alone following platinum-based chemotherapy in PS-ROC (NCT03 278717) (Elyashiv et al. 2021).

The combination of VEGFi and PARPi may also have activity in the PR-ROC population. The phase II OCTOVA trial randomized patients who relapsed within 12 months of platinum-based chemotherapy to olaparib alone (300 mg twice daily), weekly paclitaxel (80 mg/m^2), or olaparib (300 mg twice daily) plus cediranib (20 mg daily). In this heavily pretreated population, including 22% with prior PARPi exposure and 34% with prior antiangiogenic exposure, the combination of olaparib and cediranib showed promising activity, with an extended PFS of 5.4 versus 3.7 months with olaparib alone (HR 0.73; 60% CI 0.59, 0.89; $P = 0.1$), with no difference between weekly paclitaxel and olaparib alone (Nicum et al. 2024). The phase II BAROCCO trial randomized patients with PR-ROC to weekly paclitaxel (80 mg/m^2) or olaparib (300 mg twice daily) with cediranib (20 mg daily or 20 mg 5 d/wk) (Colombo et al. 2022). Again, patients were heavily pretreated, with 60% having three or more prior lines of chemotherapy. No difference in PFS was seen among groups, although the investigators argued that the oral doublet could be an attractive alternative to IV chemotherapy in this challenging population. The phase III GY005 study (NCT02502266) is investigating the combination of olaparib and cediranib in patients with non-*gBRCAm* PR-ROC. Initial results presented at the SGO 2024 Annual Meeting showed no improvement in PFS or OS with olaparib and cediranib versus SOC therapy (Lee et al. 2022, 2024).

Immunotherapy Combinations

As in the first-line setting, single-agent ICIs have shown minimal activity in the vast majority of patients with recurrent EOC. The phase III NINJA trial evaluated nivolumab monotherapy compared with chemotherapy in women with PROC (Hamanishi et al. 2021) and reported significantly worse PFS and nonsignificantly lower ORR (7.6% vs. 13.2%; $P = 0.191$) for nivolumab compared to nonplatinum chemotherapy, further underscoring the lack of efficacy of ICI as monotherapy in PROC. This has been largely attributed to tumor heterogeneity and an immunosuppressive tumor microenvironment (Kumar et al. 2024), leading to a focus on combination approaches. Dual immune checkpoint blockade with the combination of nivolumab and ipilimumab yielded superior ORR compared to nivolumab alone (31.4% vs. 12.2%) in the GY-003 trial, although PFS was only minimally extended at 3.9 months in the ipilimumab plus nivolumab group (Zamarin et al. 2020). The F_c-enhanced anti-CTLA-4 antibody, botensilimab, is also being tested in combination with balstilimab, an anti-PD-1 agent, in a phase I study of advanced solid tumors (NCT03860272). In the PROC cohort, there was promising activity with an ORR of 33% (95% CI 15.6%–55.3%) (Bockorny et al. 2023). Multiple anti-TIGIT monoclonal antibodies are also under investigation in combination with anti-PD-1/PD-L1 agents, chemotherapy, and other drugs (summarized in Moufarrij and O'Cearbhaill 2024).

ICIs have also been tested in combination with chemotherapy with modest results. The phase III ATALANTE/ENGOT-ov29 study of atezolizumab added to chemotherapy and bevacizumab in patients with PS-ROC did not show significant improvement in outcomes (Kurtz et al. 2023). Similarly, in the phase II/III NRG-GY009 trial, atezolizumab added to PLD with or without bevacizumab did not extend median PFS or OS in patients with PROC (NCT02839707) (O'Cearbhaill et al. 2023). Atezolizumab also did not add benefit to nonplatinum chemotherapy with bevacizumab in patients with recurrent EOC who are not candidates for platinum-based chemotherapy in the phase III AGO-OVAR 2.29/ENGOT-ov34 trial (NCT03343831) (Marmé et al. 2024). However, a small phase II trial of the combination of pembrolizumab, oral cyclophosphamide, and bevacizumab in patients with recurrent EOC, the majority of which were PR, reported an ORR of 47.5%, clinical benefit rate of 95.0%, and median PFS of 10.0 months (90% CI 6.5–17.4) (Zsiros et al. 2021); based on these results, this combination is now included on the NCCN guidelines.

The combination of PARPi with ICI has also been evaluated in recurrent EOC, given preclinical evidence discussed previously (Jiao et al. 2017; Césaire et al. 2018). The phase I/II TOPACIO/KEYNOTE-162 trial (NCT02657889) tested the combination of pembrolizumab and niraparib in patients with PR-ROC or with triple negative breast cancer and reported an ORR of 18% in the ovarian cohort, including three complete responses (Konstantinopoulos et al. 2019). However, the phase II MOONSTONE study assessed the efficacy of niraparib and dostarlimab in *BRCAwt* recurrent PR-ROC and was terminated prematurely due to futility (Randall et al.

2023). The triplet combination of PARPi, VEGFi, and ICI was evaluated in the phase II OPAL-A trial and exhibited a 17.1% response rate in PR-ROC that was largely *BRCAwt*- and HRD-negative (Liu et al. 2024). Collectively, these studies have consistently demonstrated that a small (~10%) population of EOC derives benefit from ICI alone, yet the ability to prospectively identify these patients has remained elusive. The addition of other agents in combination can modestly improve response rates, but with increased toxicity. An improved understanding of biomarkers of response and toxicity risk will be necessary for bringing immunotherapies into standard practice for patients with EOC.

Beyond ICI, additional immunotherapy approaches under active investigation include bispecific antibodies that simultaneously target an ovarian cancer-specific antigen and an immune cell receptor (e.g., ubamatamab/REGN4018) (Van Nieuwenhuysen et al. 2022), cytokine therapies (e.g., the engineered IL-2 variant, nemvaleukin) (Winer et al. 2022), cancer vaccines (Sellars et al. 2022), and oncolytic viruses (e.g., Olvi-Vec) (Holloway et al. 2023). In addition, adoptive cell therapy (ACT) approaches are actively being investigated as monotherapy and in combination with ICI in ovarian cancer (recently reviewed in Gitto et al. 2024). ACTs can use endogenous tumor-reactive T cells, known as tumor-infiltrating lymphocytes, or peripheral blood-sourced T cells, which are then engineered ex vivo to express a tumor antigen-specific T-cell receptor or chimeric antigen receptor to promote their activity against tumor cells (Son et al. 2022). Although T-cell-based therapies are the furthest along in development, more recent strategies include natural killer cell- and macrophage-based ACT, which also have the potential to modify the tumor microenvironment (Klichinsky et al. 2020; Rodriguez-Garcia et al. 2021). While promising, ACT approaches require further refinement before being incorporated into standard treatment for EOC patients, including evaluation earlier in a patient's treatment course, developing methods to decrease production time and reduce cost and refining strategies to mitigate toxicities.

TARGETED THERAPIES FOR SPECIFIC HISTOLOGICAL EPITHELIAL OVARIAN CANCER SUBTYPES

Investigational approaches are increasingly being tailored to specific histologic subtypes of EOC and their associated molecular and genetic features. Given the relative rarity of non-high-grade serous subtypes, these efforts have required national and international collaboration but are yielding promising advances in both treatment de-escalation and novel therapeutics with some notable examples discussed below.

Low-Grade Serous Ovarian Cancer

The predominant cancer driver mutations in LGSOC include KRAS, BRAF, ERBB2, NRAS, NF1, and PIK3CA, highlighting the dominant role of the mitogen-activated protein kinase (MAPK) pathway (also known as the Ras-Raf-MEK-ERK pathway) in this disease (Table 5). Thus, MEK inhibitors have been a focus of clinical interest for recurrent disease. The selective MEK1/2 inhibitor, trametinib (2 mg once daily), demonstrated favorable activity compared to the investigator's choice of standard therapy in the phase II/III GOG-281 trial with mPFS of 13.0 months with trametinib versus 7.2 months (HR 0.48, 95% CI 0.36–0.64; $P < 0.0001$) for the standard therapy group (Gershenson et al. 2022). The MILO/ENGOT-ov11 was a similar trial in recurrent LGSOC investigating the MEK1/2 inhibitor binimetinib (45 mg twice daily) and did not meet its primary end point of PFS when compared to chemotherapy. However, a post hoc analysis found improved response rates and longer PFS in patients with tumors harboring MAPK pathway mutations, suggesting this could be another option for recurrent LGSOC (Monk et al. 2020). Activation of focal adhesion kinase (FAK) has been found to be a common resistance mechanism to RAF/MEK inhibition; therefore, the combination of the RAF/MEK clamp, avutometinib, with the FAK inhibitor, defactinib, is being investigated, with preliminary results from the phase II ENGOT-ov60/GOG-3052/RAMP 201 trial demonstrating an ORR of 31% for the combination

Table 5. Clinical trials in low-grade serous ovarian cancer

Study name	Study drug(s)	Patient population	Study arms
NCT04095364 GY-019	Letrozole	Stage II–IV LGSOC after up-front cytoreductive surgery	Carboplatin + paclitaxel followed by letrozole maintenance
			Letrozole
NCT05601700 LEPRE	Letrozole	Stage III and IV LGSOC after up-front cytoreductive surgery	Carboplatin + paclitaxel
			Letrozole
NCT06394804 CHAMELEON	Avutometinib Defactinib	Newly diagnosed unresectable LGSOC or residual disease after primary cytoreductive surgery	Avutometinib + defactinib + letrozole
NCT06072781 RAMP 301 GOG-3097 ENGOT-ov81	Avutometinib Defactinib	Recurrent LGSOC after progression on platinum-based chemotherapy	Avutometinib + defactinib
			Physician's choice chemotherapy
NCT05113368	Regorafenib	Recurrent LGSOC	Regorafenib + fulvestrant

(LGSOC) Low-grade serous ovarian cancer.

(44% in KRAS-mutant, 17% in KRAS-wild-type), with a disease control rate of 61% at 6 months (Banerjee et al. 2023; Grisham et al. 2024). The phase III RAMP-301 trial (NCT06072781) comparing the avutometinib/defactinib combination versus the investigator's choice of chemotherapy is ongoing. Thus, at present, regimens for recurrent LGSOC recommended by the NCCN include trametinib, binimetinib, and dabrafenib + trametinib (for BRAF V600E-positive tumors), as well as hormonal therapy, chemotherapy, or observation.

Clear Cell Ovarian Cancer

Clear cell ovarian cancer has relatively poor chemotherapy responsiveness compared with HGSOC. Although ICI have shown poor activity in pooled trials of EOCs, subset analyses have suggested that clear cell carcinomas may be more likely to respond to immunotherapy (Sia et al. 2022). Mutations in the SWI/SNF chromatin remodeling subunit ARID1A and in PIK3CA also occur in ~50% of clear cell ovarian cancers. Thus, ongoing phase II trials are re-exploring the efficacy of immunotherapy specifically in clear cell ovarian cancers, for example, with the combination of kinase inhibitor lenvatinib with pembrolizumab (NCT05296512) or with dostarlimab and the PP2A inhibitor LB-100 (NCT06065462). A phase II trial including 44 patients with recurrent clear cell carcinomas of gynecologic origin (36 patients with ovarian primary) found a 14% ORR with nivolumab alone and 33% with ipilimumab + nivolumab, including four complete responses with the immunotherapy combination (Dizon et al. 2024).

Mucinous Ovarian Cancer

Growing knowledge about the distinct molecular features of mucinous ovarian tumors may help guide future treatment selection, as these tumors rarely harbor *BRCA1/2* mutations or HRD deficiency but more commonly feature *ERBB2* amplification, *KRAS* mutations, MMR amplification as well as deficiency, and ER positivity, raising the possibility of treatment with targeted agents, hormonal therapy, or immunotherapy (Gorringe et al. 2020). Additionally, given the histological similarity of mucinous ovarian cancers to gastrointestinal malignancies, there has been interest in treating these with gastrointestinal cancer chemotherapy regimens. GOG0241 randomized patients with mucinous ovarian cancer to carboplatin/paclitaxel or oxaliplatin/capecitabine, with or without bevacizumab (Gore et al. 2015, 2019). Ultimately, the trial was terminated early due to poor recruitment, finding no differences in survival among the treatment groups. The authors cited difficulties with confirming the diagnosis of mucinous ovarian cancer on central pathology review, difficulty with obtaining study drugs, and overall rarity of the histological subtype as major challenges. Nevertheless, interest persists in improving the treatment of mucinous EOCs specifically, and an ongoing clinical trial called HIMOC is focusing on use of HIPEC preferentially for this ovarian cancer subtype (NCT05123807).

CONCLUDING REMARKS AND CURRENT AREAS OF FOCUS

An improved understanding of the molecular biology of specific EOC subsets, as well as the tumor microenvironment, has accelerated drug development and interest in clinical trial development both in the newly diagnosed setting as well as in ROC. In newly diagnosed ovarian cancer, PARPi efficacy has been demonstrated beyond *BRCA*-related cancers, especially in HRD^+ cancers. For recurrent disease, the approval of the first ADC for ovarian cancer, mirvetuximab, has paved the way for testing additional ADCs with various targets and payloads, as well as in combination with other agents. Continued active investigations into new chemotherapy drug classes, combinatorial immunotherapy approaches, and innovative surgical techniques such as HIPEC and novel radiation modalities, together with novel diagnostic tools to allow for individualized therapy, offer hope for further improved outcomes for patients with advanced ovarian cancer. Challenges ahead include increasing the cure rate of newly diagnosed advanced ovarian cancer, strategies to sensitize ovarian cancers to immunotherapy, and novel approaches and drug development for the treatment of platinum-resistant ROC.

REFERENCES

Aghajanian C, Blank SV, Goff BA, Judson PL, Teneriello MG, Husain A, Sovak MA, Yi J, Nycum LR. 2012. OCEANS: a randomized, double-blind, placebo-controlled phase III trial of chemotherapy with or without bevacizumab in patients with platinum-sensitive recurrent epithelial ovarian, primary peritoneal, or fallopian tube cancer. *J Clin Oncol* **30:** 2039–2045. doi:10.1200/JCO.2012.42.0505

Aghajanian C, Goff B, Nycum LR, Wang YV, Husain A, Blank SV. 2015. Final overall survival and safety analysis of OCEANS, a phase 3 trial of chemotherapy with or without bevacizumab in patients with platinum-sensitive recurrent ovarian cancer. *Gynecol Oncol* **139:** 10–16. doi:10.1016/j.ygyno.2015.08.004

Armstrong DK, Bundy B, Wenzel L, Huang HQ, Baergen R, Lele S, Copeland LJ, Walker JL, Burger RA; Gynecologic Oncology Group. 2006. Intraperitoneal cisplatin and paclitaxel in ovarian cancer. *N Engl J Med* **354:** 34–43. doi:10.1056/NEJMoa052985

Aronson SL, Lopez-Yurda M, Koole SN, Schagen van Leeuwen JH, Schreuder HWR, Hermans RHM, de Hingh IHJT, van Gent MDJM, Arts HJG, van Ham MAPC, et al. 2023. Cytoreductive surgery with or without hyperthermic intraperitoneal chemotherapy in patients with advanced ovarian cancer (OVHIPEC-1): final survival analysis of a randomised, controlled, phase 3 trial. *Lancet Oncol* **24:** 1109–1118. doi:10.1016/S1470-2045(23)00396-0

Banerjee SN, Lassen Ring K, Van Nieuwenhuysen E, Fabbro M, Aghajanian C, Oaknin A, Colombo N, Santin A, Clamp AR, Moore KN, et al. 2023. Initial efficacy and safety results from ENGOT-ov60/GOG-3052/RAMP 201: a phase 2 study of avutometinib (VS-6766) ± defactinib in recurrent low-grade serous ovarian cancer (LGSOC). *J Clin Oncol* **41**(Suppl 16): 5515. doi:10.1200/JCO.2023.41.16_suppl.5515

Bartels HC, Rogers AC, McSharry V, McVey R, Walsh T, O'Brien D, Boyd WD, Brennan DJ. 2019. A meta-analysis of morbidity and mortality in primary cytoreductive surgery compared to neoadjuvant chemotherapy in advanced ovarian malignancy. *Gynecol Oncol* **154:** 622–630. doi:10.1016/j.ygyno.2019.07.011

Bartoletti M, Pelizzari G, Gerratana L, Bortot L, Lombardi D, Nicoloso M, Scalone S, Giorda G, Baldassarre G, Sorio R, et al. 2020. Bevacizumab or PARP-inhibitors maintenance therapy for platinum-sensitive recurrent ovarian cancer: a network meta-analysis. *Int J Mol Sci* **21:** 3805. doi:10.3390/ijms21113805

Bax HJ, Chauhan J, Stavraka C, Santaolalla A, Osborn G, Khiabany A, Grandits M, López-Abente J, Palhares LCGF, Chan Wah Hak C, et al. 2023. Folate receptor α in ovarian cancer tissue and patient serum is associated with disease burden and treatment outcomes. *Br J Cancer* **128:** 342–353. doi:10.1038/s41416-022-02031-x

Bell J, Brady MF, Young RC, Lage J, Walker JL, Look KY, Rose GS, Spirtos NM; Gynecologic Oncology Group. 2006. Randomized phase III trial of three versus six cycles of adjuvant carboplatin and paclitaxel in early stage epithelial ovarian carcinoma: a Gynecologic Oncology Group study. *Gynecol Oncol* **102:** 432–439. doi:10.1016/j.ygyno.2006.06.013

Belotte J, Felicetti B, Baines AJ, YoussefAgha A, Rojas-Espaillat L, Ortiz AG, Provencher D, Vázquez RM, Cortijo LG, Zeng X. 2024. Comparing niraparib versus platinum-taxane doublet chemotherapy as neoadjuvant treatment in patients with newly diagnosed homologous recombination-deficient stage III/IV ovarian cancer: study protocol for cohort C of the open-label, phase 2, randomized controlled multicenter OPAL trial. *Trials* **25:** 301. doi:10.1186/s13063-024-08142-5

Bindra RS, Crosby ME, Glazer PM. 2007. Regulation of DNA repair in hypoxic cancer cells. *Cancer Metastasis Rev* **26:** 249–260. doi:10.1007/s10555-007-9061-3

Binju M, Padilla MA, Singomat T, Kaur P, Suryo Rahmanto Y, Cohen PA, Yu Y. 2019. Mechanisms underlying acquired platinum resistance in high grade serous ovarian cancer—a mini review. *Biochim Biophys Acta Gen Subj* **1863:** 371–378. doi:10.1016/j.bbagen.2018.11.005

Bockorny B, Matulonis U, O'Day S, Margolin K, El-Khoueiry A, Wilky B, Sanborn R, Balmanoukian A, Bullock A, Wulf G, et al. 2023. Botensilimab, a novel innate/adaptive immune activator, plus balstilimab (anti-PD-1) in patients with recurrent platinum refractory/resistant ovarian cancer (041). *Gynecol Oncol* **176:** S35–S36. doi:10.1016/j.ygyno.2023.06.514

Bogani G, Ditto A, Lopez S, Bertolina F, Murgia F, Pinelli C, Chiappa V, Raspagliesi F. 2020. Adjuvant chemotherapy vs. observation in stage I clear cell ovarian carcinoma: a systematic review and meta-analysis. *Gynecol Oncol* **157:** 293–298. doi:10.1016/j.ygyno.2019.12.045

Bookman MA, Brady MF, McGuire WP, Harper PG, Alberts DS, Friedlander M, Colombo N, Fowler JM, Argenta PA, De Geest K, et al. 2009. Evaluation of new platinum-based treatment regimens in advanced-stage ovarian cancer: a phase III trial of the Gynecologic Cancer Intergroup. *J Clin Oncol* **27:** 1419–1425. doi:10.1200/JCO.2008.19.1684

Bristow RE, Eisenhauer EL, Santillan A, Chi DS. 2007. Delaying the primary surgical effort for advanced ovarian cancer: a systematic review of neoadjuvant chemotherapy and interval cytoreduction. *Gynecol Oncol* **104:** 480–490. doi:10.1016/j.ygyno.2006.11.002

Burger RA, Sill MW, Monk BJ, Greer BE, Sorosky JI. 2007. Phase II trial of bevacizumab in persistent or recurrent epithelial ovarian cancer or primary peritoneal cancer: a Gynecologic Oncology Group study. *J Clin Oncol* **25:** 5165–5171. doi:10.1200/JCO.2007.11.5345

Burger RA, Brady MF, Bookman MA, Fleming GF, Monk BJ, Huang H, Mannel RS, Homesley HD, Fowler J, Greer BE, et al. 2011. Incorporation of bevacizumab in the primary treatment of ovarian cancer. *N Engl J Med* **365:** 2473–2483. doi:10.1056/NEJMoa1104390

Cadoo KA, Simpkins F, Mathews CA, Kabil N, Bennett J, Aghajanian C. 2020. Olaparib treatment in patients (pts) with platinum-sensitive relapsed (PSR) ovarian cancer (OC) by *BRCA* mutation (*BRCAm*) and homologous recombination deficiency (HRD) status: phase II LIGHT study. *J Clin Oncol* **38**(15 Suppl)**:** 6013. doi:10.1200/JCO.2020.38.15_suppl.6013

Cancer Genome Atlas Research Network. 2011. Integrated genomic analyses of ovarian carcinoma. *Nature* **474:** 609–615. doi:10.1038/nature10166

Césaire M, Thariat J, Candéias SM, Stefan D, Saintigny Y, Chevalier F. 2018. Combining PARP inhibition, radiation, and immunotherapy: a possible strategy to improve the treatment of cancer? *Int J Mol Sci* **19:** 3793. doi:10.3390/ijms19123793

Chan JK, Brady MF, Penson RT, Huang H, Birrer MJ, Walker JL, DiSilvestro PA, Rubin SC, Martin LP, Davidson SA, et al. 2016. Weekly vs. every-3-week paclitaxel and carboplatin for ovarian cancer. *N Engl J Med* **374:** 738–748. doi:10.1056/NEJMoa1505067

Chang SJ, Hodeib M, Chang J, Bristow RE. 2013. Survival impact of complete cytoreduction to no gross residual disease for advanced-stage ovarian cancer: a meta-analysis. *Gynecol Oncol* **130:** 493–498. doi:10.1016/j.ygyno.2013.05.040

Chi DS, Eisenhauer EL, Lang J, Huh J, Haddad L, Abu-Rustum NR, Sonoda Y, Levine DA, Hensley M, Barakat RR. 2006. What is the optimal goal of primary cytoreductive surgery for bulky stage IIIC epithelial ovarian carcinoma (EOC)? *Gynecol Oncol* **103:** 559–564. doi:10.1016/j.ygyno.2006.03.051

Clamp AR, James EC, McNeish IA, Dean A, Kim JW, O'Donnell DM, Gallardo-Rincon D, Blagden S, Brenton J, Perren TJ, et al. 2019. Weekly dose-dense chemotherapy in first-line epithelial ovarian, fallopian tube, or primary peritoneal carcinoma treatment (ICON8): primary progression free survival analysis results from a GCIG phase 3 randomised controlled trial. *Lancet* **394:** 2084–2095. doi:10.1016/S0140-6736(19)32259-7

Clamp AR, James EC, McNeish IA, Dean A, Kim JW, O'Donnell DM, Gallardo-Rincon D, Blagden S, Brenton J, Perren TJ, et al. 2022. Weekly dose-dense chemotherapy in first-line epithelial ovarian, fallopian tube, or primary peritoneal cancer treatment (ICON8): overall survival results from an open-label, randomised, controlled, phase 3 trial. *Lancet Oncol* **23:** 919–930. doi:10.1016/S1470-2045(22)00283-2

Classe JM, Meeus P, Leblanc E, Wernert R, Quenet F, Marchal F, Houvenaeghel G, Bats AS, Ferron G, Brigand C, et al. 2023. Hyperthermic intraperitoneal chemotherapy in platinum-sensitive relapsed epithelial ovarian cancer: the CHIPOR randomized phase III trial. *J Clin Oncol* **41:** 5510. doi:10.1200/JCO.2023.41.16_suppl.5510

Classe JM, Meeus P, Hudry D, Wernert R, Quenet F, Marchal F, Houvenaeghel G, Bas AS, Lecuru F, Ferron G, et al. 2024. Hyperthermic intraperitoneal chemotherapy for recurrent ovarian cancer (CHIPOR): a randomised, open-label, phase 3 trial. *Lancet Oncol* **25:** 1551–1562. doi:10.1016/S1470-2045(24)00531-X

Cobb LP, Davis J, Hull S, Vining DJ, Fellman BM, Yuan Y, Westin SN, Taylor JS, Bevers MW, Shafer A, et al. 2022. A pilot phase II study of neoadjuvant fulvestrant plus abemaciclib in women with advanced low-grade serous carcinoma. *J Clin Oncol* **40:** 5522. doi:10.1200/JCO.2022.40.16_suppl.5522

Coleman RL, Oza AM, Lorusso D, Aghajanian C, Oaknin A, Dean A, Colombo N, Weberpals JI, Clamp A, Scambia G, et al. 2017a. Rucaparib maintenance treatment for recurrent ovarian carcinoma after response to platinum therapy (ARIEL3): a randomised, double-blind, placebo-controlled, phase 3 trial. *Lancet* **390:** 1949–1961. doi:10.1016/S0140-6736(17)32440-6

Coleman RL, Brady MF, Herzog TJ, Sabbatini P, Armstrong DK, Walker JL, Kim BG, Fujiwara K, Tewari KS, O'Malley DM, et al. 2017b. Bevacizumab and paclitaxel-carboplatin chemotherapy and secondary cytoreduction in recurrent, platinum-sensitive ovarian cancer (NRG Oncology/Gynecologic Oncology Group study GOG-0213): a multicentre, open-label, randomised, phase 3 trial. *Lancet Oncol* **18:** 779–791. doi:10.1016/S1470-2045(17)30279-6

Coleman RL, Spirtos NM, Enserro D, Herzog TJ, Sabbatini P, Armstrong DK, Kim JW, Park SY, Kim BG, Nam JH, et al. 2019. Secondary surgical cytoreduction for recurrent ovarian cancer. *N Engl J Med* **381:** 1929–1939. doi:10.1056/NEJMoa1902626

Coleman RL, Oza A, Lorusso D, Aghajanian C, Oaknin A, Dean A, Colombo N, Weberpals J, Clamp AR, Scambia G, et al. 2022. Overall survival results from ArieL3: a phase 3 randomized, double-blind study of rucaparib vs placebo following response to platinum-based chemotherapy for recurrent ovarian carcinoma. *Int J Gynecol Cancer* **32:** A3–A5.

Collinson F, Qian W, Fossati R, Lissoni A, Williams C, Parmar M, Ledermann J, Colombo N, Swart A; ICON1 Collaborators. 2014. Optimal treatment of early-stage ovarian cancer. *Ann Oncol* **25:** 1165–1171. doi:10.1093/annonc/mdu116

Colombo N, Tomao F, Benedetti Panici P, Nicoletto MO, Tognon G, Bologna A, Lissoni AA, DeCensi A, Lapresa M, Mancari R, et al. 2022. Randomized phase II trial of weekly paclitaxel vs. cediranib-olaparib (continuous or intermittent schedule) in platinum-resistant high-grade epithelial ovarian cancer. *Gynecol Oncol* **164:** 505–513. doi:10.1016/j.ygyno.2022.01.015

Copeland LJ, Brady MF, Burger RA, Rodgers WH, Huang HQ, Cella D, O'Malley DM, Street DG, Tewari KS, Bender DP, et al. 2022. Phase III randomized trial of maintenance taxanes versus surveillance in women with advanced ovarian/tubal/peritoneal cancer: a Gynecologic Oncology Group 0212: NRG Oncology study. *J Clin Oncol* **40:** 4119–4128. doi:10.1200/JCO.22.00146

Corrigan KL, Yoder A, De B, Lin L, Jhingran A, Joyner MM, Eifel PJ, Colbert LE, Lu KH, Klopp AH. 2022. Long-term survival following definitive radiation therapy for recurrence or oligometastases in gynecological malignancies: a landmark analysis. *Gynecol Oncol* **164:** 550–557. doi:10.1016/j.ygyno.2021.12.022

da Costa AA, Valadares CV, Baiocchi G, Mantoan H, Saito A, Sanches S, Guimarães AP, Achatz MI. 2015. Neoadjuvant chemotherapy followed by interval debulking surgery and the risk of platinum resistance in epithelial ovarian cancer. *Ann Surg Oncol* **22:** 971–978. doi:10.1245/s10434-015-4623-z

D'Andrea AD. 2018. Mechanisms of PARP inhibitor sensitivity and resistance. *DNA Repair (Amst)* **71:** 172–176. doi:10.1016/j.dnarep.2018.08.021

Della Corte L, Conte C, Palumbo M, Guerra S, Colacurci D, Riemma G, De Franciscis P, Giampaolino P, Fagotti A, Bifulco G, et al. 2023. Hyperthermic intraperitoneal chemotherapy (HIPEC): new approaches and controversies on the treatment of advanced epithelial ovarian cancer—systematic review and meta-analysis. *J Clin Med* **12:** 7012. doi:10.3390/jcm12227012

Dellinger TH, Han ES. 2021. State of the science: the role of HIPEC in the treatment of ovarian cancer. *Gynecol Oncol* **160:** 364–368. doi:10.1016/j.ygyno.2020.12.029

De Placido S, Scambia G, Di Vagno G, Naglieri E, Lombardi AV, Biamonte R, Marinaccio M, Cartenì G, Manzione L, Febbraro A, et al. 2004. Topotecan compared with no therapy after response to surgery and carboplatin/paclitaxel in patients with ovarian cancer: multicenter Italian Trials in Ovarian Cancer (MITO-1) randomized study. *J Clin Oncol* **22:** 2635–2642. doi:10.1200/JCO.2004.09.088

DiSilvestro P, Banerjee S, Colombo N, Scambia G, Kim BG, Oaknin A, Friedlander M, Lisyanskaya A, Floquet A, Leary A, et al. 2023. Overall survival with maintenance olaparib at a 7-year follow-up in patients with newly diagnosed advanced ovarian cancer and a *BRCA* mutation: the SOLO1/GOG 3004 trial. *J Clin Oncol* **41:** 609–617. doi:10.1200/JCO.22.01549

Disis ML, Taylor MH, Kelly K, Beck JT, Gordon M, Moore KM, Patel MR, Chaves J, Park H, Mita AC, et al. 2019. Efficacy and safety of avelumab for patients with recurrent or refractory ovarian cancer: phase 1b results from the JAVELIN solid tumor trial. *JAMA Oncol* **5:** 393–401. doi:10.1001/jamaoncol.2018.6258

Dizon DS, Mathews CA, MacLaughlan David S, Machan JT, Hadfield MJ, Marks EI, Bansal R, McGinn C, Hassinger F, et al. 2024. Final results of BrUOG 354: a randomized phase II trial of nivolumab alone or in combination with ipilimumab for people with ovarian and other extra-renal clear cell carcinomas. *J Clin Oncol* **42:** LBA5500. doi:10.1200/JCO.2024.42.17_suppl.LBA5500

du Bois A, Kristensen G, Ray-Coquard I, Reuss A, Pignata S, Colombo N, Denison U, Vergote I, Del Campo JM, Ottevanger P, et al. 2016. Standard first-line chemotherapy with or without nintedanib for advanced ovarian cancer (AGO-OVAR 12): a randomised, double-blind, placebo-controlled phase 3 trial. *Lancet Oncol* **17:** 78–89. doi:10.1016/S1470-2045(15)00366-6

El Hajj H, Vanseymortier M, Hudry D, Bogart E, Abdeddaim C, Leblanc E, Le Deley MC, Narducci F. 2021. Rationale and study design of the CHIPPI-1808 trial: a phase III randomized clinical trial evaluating hyperthermic intraperitoneal chemotherapy (HIPEC) for stage III ovarian cancer patients treated with primary or interval cytoreductive surgery. *ESMO Open* **6:** 100098. doi:10.1016/j.esmoop.2021.100098

Elyashiv O, Ledermann J, Parmar G, Farrelly L, Counsell N, Feeney A, El-Khouly F, Macdonald I, Neto A, Arthur-Darkwa E, et al. 2021. ICON 9—an international phase III randomized study to evaluate the efficacy of maintenance therapy with olaparib and cediranib or olaparib alone in patients with relapsed platinum-sensitive ovarian cancer following a response to platinum-based chemotherapy. *Int J Gynecol Cancer* **31:** 134–138. doi:10.1136/ijgc-2020-002073

Essel KG, Behbakht K, Lai T, Hand L, Evans E, Dvorak J, Ding K, Konecny G, Moore KN. 2021. PARPi after PARPi in epithelial ovarian cancer. *Gynecol Oncol Rep* **35:** 100699. doi:10.1016/j.gore.2021.100699

Everett EN, French AE, Stone RL, Pastore LM, Jazaeri AA, Andersen WA, Taylor PT Jr. 2006. Initial chemotherapy followed by surgical cytoreduction for the treatment of stage III/IV epithelial ovarian cancer. *Am J Obstet Gynecol* **195:** 568–574. doi:10.1016/j.ajog.2006.03.075

Fagotti A, Ferrandina G, Fanfani F, Ercoli A, Lorusso D, Rossi M, Scambia G. 2006. A laparoscopy-based score to predict surgical outcome in patients with advanced ovarian carcinoma: a pilot study. *Ann Surg Oncol* **13:** 1156–1161. doi:10.1245/ASO.2006.08.021

Fagotti A, Ferrandina G, Fanfani F, Garganese G, Vizzielli G, Carone V, Salerno MG, Scambia G. 2008. Prospective validation of a laparoscopic predictive model for optimal cytoreduction in advanced ovarian carcinoma. *Am J Obstet Gynecol* **199:** 642.e1–642.e6. doi:10.1016/j.ajog.2008.06.052

Fagotti A, Ferrandina MG, Vizzielli G, Pasciuto T, Fanfani F, Gallotta V, Margariti PA, Chiantera V, Costantini B, Gueli Alletti S, et al. 2020. Randomized trial of primary debulking surgery versus neoadjuvant chemotherapy for advanced epithelial ovarian cancer (SCORPION-NCT01461850). *Int J Gynecol Cancer* **30:** 1657–1664. doi:10.1136/ijgc-2020-001640

Fagotti A, Costantini B, Fanfani F, Giannarelli D, De Iaco P, Chiantera V, Mandato V, Giorda G, Aletti G, Greggi S, et al. 2025. Hyperthermic intraperitoneal chemotherapy in platinum-sensitive recurrent ovarian cancer: a randomized trial on survival evaluation (HORSE; MITO-18). *J Clin Oncol* **43:** 852–860. doi:10.1200/JCO.24.00686

Farmer H, McCabe N, Lord CJ, Tutt AN, Johnson DA, Richardson TB, Santarosa M, Dillon KJ, Hickson I, Knights C, et al. 2005. Targeting the DNA repair defect in *BRCA* mutant cells as a therapeutic strategy. *Nature* **434:** 917–921. doi:10.1038/nature03445

Ferrandina G, Ludovisi M, Lorusso D, Pignata S, Breda E, Savarese A, Del Medico P, Scaltriti L, Katsaros D, Priolo D, et al. 2008. Phase III trial of gemcitabine compared with pegylated liposomal doxorubicin in progressive or recurrent ovarian cancer. *J Clin Oncol* **26:** 890–896. doi:10.1200/JCO.2007.13.6606

Fields EC, McGuire WP, Lin L, Temkin SM. 2017. Radiation treatment in women with ovarian cancer: past, present, and future. *Front Oncol* **7:** 177. doi:10.3389/fonc.2017.00177

Finn RS, Dering J, Conklin D, Kalous O, Cohen DJ, Desai AJ, Ginther C, Atefi M, Chen I, Fowst C, et al. 2009. PD 0332991, a selective cyclin D kinase 4/6 inhibitor, preferentially inhibits proliferation of luminal estrogen receptor-positive human breast cancer cell lines in vitro. *Breast Cancer Res* **11:** 1–13.

Fotopoulou C, Zang R, Gultekin M, Cibula D, Ayhan A, Liu D, Richter R, Braicu I, Mahner S, Harter P, et al. 2013. Value of tertiary cytoreductive surgery in epithelial ovarian cancer: an international multicenter evaluation. *Ann Surg Oncol* **20:** 1348–1354. doi:10.1245/s10434-012-2673-z

Frenel JS, Kim JW, Aryal N, Asher R, Berton D, Vidal L, Pautier P, Ledermann JA, Penson RT, Oza AM, et al. 2022. Efficacy of subsequent chemotherapy for patients with *BRCA1/2*-mutated recurrent epithelial ovarian cancer progressing on olaparib versus placebo maintenance: post-hoc analyses of the SOLO2/ENGOT Ov-21 trial. *Ann Oncol* **33:** 1021–1028. doi:10.1016/j.annonc.2022.06.011

Fujiwara K, Vergote IB, Sehouli J, Salutari V, Zola P, Madry R, Wenham RM, Korach J, Pautier P, Cibula D, et al. 2019. ENGOT-OV43/KEYLYNK-001: a phase III trial of pembrolizumab plus chemotherapy with olaparib maintenance for first-line treatment of *BRCA*-nonmutated advanced epithelial ovarian cancer. *Ann Oncol* **30:** ix89.

Gadducci A, Multinu F, Cosio S, Carinelli S, Ghioni M, Aletti GD. 2021. Clear cell carcinoma of the ovary: epidemiology, pathological and biological features, treatment options and clinical outcomes. *Gynecol Oncol* **162:** 741–750. doi:10.1016/j.ygyno.2021.06.033

Garcia Garcia Y, de Juan Ferré A, Mendiola C, Barretina-Ginesta MP, Gaba Garcia L, Santaballa Bertrán A, Bover Barcelo I, Gil-Martin M, Manzano A, Rubio Pérez MJ, et al. 2019. Efficacy and safety results from GEICO 1205, a randomized phase II trial of neoadjuvant chemotherapy with or without bevacizumab for advanced epithelial ovarian cancer. *Int J Gynecol Cancer* **29:** 1050–1056. doi:10.1136/ijgc-2019-000256

Gershenson DM, Bodurka DC, Lu KH, Nathan LC, Milojevic L, Wong KK, Malpica A, Sun CC. 2015. Impact of age and primary disease site on outcome in women with low-grade serous carcinoma of the ovary or peritoneum: results of a large single-institution registry of a rare tumor. *J Clin Oncol* **33:** 2675–2682. doi:10.1200/JCO.2015.61.0873

Gershenson DM, Bodurka DC, Coleman RL, Lu KH, Malpica A, Sun CC. 2017. Hormonal maintenance therapy for women with low-grade serous cancer of the ovary or peritoneum. *J Clin Oncol* **35:** 1103–1111. doi:10.1200/JCO.2016.71.0632

Gershenson DM, Miller A, Brady WE, Paul J, Carty K, Rodgers W, Millan D, Coleman RL, Moore KN, Banerjee S, et al. 2022. Trametinib versus standard of care in patients with recurrent low-grade serous ovarian cancer (GOG 281/LOGS): an international, randomised, open-label, multicentre, phase 2/3 trial. *Lancet* **399:** 541–553. doi:10.1016/S0140-6736(21)02175-9

Gilbert L, Oaknin A, Matulonis UA, Mantia-Smaldone GM, Lim PC, Castro CM, Provencher D, Memarzadeh S, Method M, Wang J, et al. 2023. Safety and efficacy of mirvetuximab soravtansine, a folate receptor α (FRα)-targeting antibody-drug conjugate (ADC), in combination with bevacizumab in patients with platinum-resistant ovarian cancer. *Gynecol Oncol* **170:** 241–247. doi:10.1016/j.ygyno.2023.01.020

Gillen J, Miller A, Bell-McGuinn KM, Schilder RJ, Walker JL, Mathews CA, Duska LR, Guntupalli SR, O'Cearbhaill R, Hays J, et al. 2021. Post hoc analyses of GOG 9923: does *BRCA* status affect toxicities?: an NRG oncology study. *Gynecol Oncol* **161:** 512–515. doi:10.1016/j.ygyno.2021.01.037

Gitto SB, Ihewulezi CJN, Powell DJ. 2024. Adoptive T cell therapy for ovarian cancer. *Gynecol Oncol* **186:** 77–84. 10.1016/j.ygyno.2024.04.001

González-Martín A, Pothuri B, Vergote I, DePont Christensen R, Graybill W, Mirza MR, McCormick C, Lorusso D, Hoskins P, Freyer G, et al. 2019. Niraparib in patients with newly diagnosed advanced ovarian cancer. *N Engl J Med* **381:** 2391–2402. doi:10.1056/NEJMoa1910962

Gordon AN, Fleagle JT, Guthrie D, Parkin DE, Gore ME, Lacave AJ. 2001. Recurrent epithelial ovarian carcinoma: a randomized phase III study of pegylated liposomal doxorubicin versus topotecan. *J Clin Oncol* **19:** 3312–3322. doi:10.1200/JCO.2001.19.14.3312

Gore ME, Hackshaw A, Brady WE, Penson RT, Zaino RJ, McCluggagge WG, Ganesan R, Wilkinson N, Perren T, Montes A, et al. 2015. Multicentre trial of carboplatin/paclitaxel versus oxaliplatin/capecitabine, each with/without bevacizumab, as first line chemotherapy for patients with mucinous epithelial ovarian cancer (mEOC). *J Clin Oncol* **33**(15_Suppl)**:** 5528. doi:10.1200/jco.2015.33.15_suppl.5528

Gore M, Hackshaw A, Brady WE, Penson RT, Zaino R, McCluggage WG, Ganesan R, Wilkinson N, Perren T, Montes A, et al. 2019. An international, phase III randomized trial in patients with mucinous epithelial ovarian cancer (mEOC/GOG 0241) with long-term follow-up: and experience of conducting a clinical trial in a rare gynecological tumor. *Gynecol Oncol* **153:** 541–548. doi:10.1016/j.ygyno.2019.03.256

Gorringe KL, Cheasley D, Wakefield MJ, Ryland GL, Allan PE, Alsop K, Amarasinghe KC, Ananda S, Bowtell DDL, Christie M, et al. 2020. Therapeutic options for mucinous ovarian carcinoma. *Gynecol Oncol* **156:** 552–560. doi:10.1016/j.ygyno.2019.12.015

Grisham RN, Aghajanian C, Van Nieuwenhuysen E, Rodrigues M, Ring KL, Santin AD, Colombo N, Prendergast EN, Thaker PH, Moore KN, et al. 2024. Efficacy and safety of avutometinib ± defactinib in recurrent low-grade serous ovarian cancer: primary analysis of ENGOT-OV60/GOG-3052/RAMP 201. In *International Gynecologic Cancer Society Annual Meeting*, Dublin.

Hamanishi J, Takeshima N, Katsumata N, Ushijima K, Kimura T, Takeuchi S, Matsumoto K, Ito K, Mandai M, Nakai H, et al. 2021. Nivolumab versus gemcitabine or pegylated liposomal doxorubicin for patients with platinum-resistant ovarian cancer: open-label, randomized trial in Japan (NINJA). *J Clin Oncol* **39:** 3671–3681. doi:10.1200/JCO.21.00334

Hanahan D, Weinberg RA. 2011. Hallmarks of cancer: the next generation. *Cell* **144:** 646–674. doi:10.1016/j.cell.2011.02.013

Hardy-Bessard AC, Moore KN, Mirza MR, Asselain B, Redondo A, Pfisterer J, Pignata S, Provencher DM, Cibula D, Reyners AKL, et al. 2019. ENGOT-OV44/FIRST study: a randomized, double-blind, adaptive, phase III study of platinum-based therapy with dostarlimab (TSR-042) + niraparib versus standard-of-care (SOC) platinum-based therapy as first-line treatment of stage 3/4 non-mucinous epithelial ovarian cancer (OC). *J Clin Oncol* **37:** TPS5600. doi:10.1200/JCO.2019.37.15_suppl.TPS5600

Harrison R, Zighelboim I, Cloven NG, Marcus JZ, Coleman RL, Karam A. 2021. Secondary cytoreductive surgery for recurrent ovarian cancer: an SGO clinical practice statement. *Gynecol Oncol* **163:** 448–452. doi:10.1016/j.ygyno.2021.10.008

Harter P, du Bois A, Hahmann M, Hasenburg A, Burges A, Loibl S, Gropp M, Huober J, Fink D, Schröder W, et al. 2006. Surgery in recurrent ovarian cancer: the Arbeitsgemeinschaft Gynaekologische Onkologie (AGO) DESKTOP OVAR trial. *Ann Surg Oncol* **13:** 1702–1710. doi:10.1245/s10434-006-9058-0

Harter P, Sehouli J, Vergote I, Ferron G, Reuss A, Meier W, Greggi S, Mosgaard BJ, Selle F, Guyon F, et al. 2021. Randomized trial of cytoreductive surgery for relapsed ovarian cancer. *N Engl J Med* **385:** 2123–2131. doi:10.1056/NEJMoa2103294

Harter P, Mouret-Reynier MA, Lorusso D, Cropet C, Guerra EM, Wolfrum-Ristau P, Matsumoto T, Vergote I, Colombo N, Unelma Mainpaa J, et al. 2023a. Efficacy of subsequent therapies in patients (pts) with advanced ovarian cancer (AOC) in the phase III PAOLA-1/ENGOT-ov25 trial according to whether disease progression occurred during or after the end of olaparib (ola) maintenance. *J Clin Oncol* **41**(16_suppl): 5550–5550. doi:10.1200/JCO.2023.41.16_suppl.5550

Harter P, Trillsch F, Okamoto A, Reuss A, Kim JW, Rubio-Pérex MJ, Vardar MA, Scambia G, Tredan O, Nyvang GB, et al. 2023b. Durvalumab with paclitaxel/carboplatin (PC) and bevacizumab (bev), followed by maintenance durvalumab, bev, and olaparib in patients (pts) with newly diagnosed advanced ovarian cancer (AOC) without a tumor *BRCA1/2* mutation (non-*tBRCAm*): results from the randomized, placebo (pbo)-controlled phase III DUO-O trial. *J Clin Oncol* **41:** LBA5506. doi:10.1200/JCO.2023.41.17_suppl.LBA5506

Heinzelmann-Schwarz VA, Kurzeder C, Schmid S, Gabriel N, Mueller A, Fehr MK, Marth C, Du Bois A, Klar M. 2021. ENGOT-ov54/Swiss-GO-2/MATAO including LOGOS (Low-Grade Ovarian Cancer Sub-Study): MAintenance Therapy with Aromatase inhibitor in epithelial Ovarian cancer—a randomized, double-blinded, placebo-controlled, multicenter phase III trial. *J Clin Oncol* **39:** TPS5598. doi:10.1200/JCO.2021.39.15_suppl.TPS5598

Heitz F, Marth C, Henry S, Reuss A, Cibula D, Gaba Garcia L, Colombo N, Schmalfeld B, de Gregorio N, Wimberger P, et al. 2023. AGO-OVAR 28/ENGOT-ov57. Niraparib alone versus niraparib in combination with bevacizumab in patients with carboplatin-taxane-based chemotherapy in advanced ovarian cancer: a multicenter randomized phase III trial. *Int J Gynecol Cancer* **33:** 1966–1969. doi:10.1136/ijgc-2023-004944

Herzog TJ, Hays JL, Barlin JN, Buscema J, Cloen NG, Kong LR, Tyagi NK, Lanneau G, Long BJ, Marsh RL, et al. 2023. ARTISTRY-7: a phase 3, multicenter study of nemvaleukin alfa in combination with pembrolizumab versus chemotherapy in patients with platinum-resistant epithelial ovarian, fallopian tube, or primary peritoneal cancer (GOG-3063; ENGOT-OV68). *J Clin Oncol* **41:** TPS5612. doi:10.1200/JCO.2023.41.16_suppl.TPS5612

Holloway R, Thaker P, Mendivil A, Ahmad S, Bell M, Chambers S, Chan JK, Coleman RL, Crafton S, Crane E, et al. 2022. TP026/#1435 phase 3 study of efficacy & safety of Olvi-Vec and platinum-doublet + bevacizumab compared to platinum-doublet + bevacizumab in platinum-resistant/refractory ovarian cancer (ONPRIME; GOG-3076)[NCT05281471]. *Int J Gynecol Cancer* **32:** A236.

Holloway RW, Mendivil AA, Kendrick JE, Abaid LN, Brown JV, LeBlanc J, McKenzie ND, Mori KM, Ahmad S. 2023. Clinical activity of olvimulogene nanivacirepvec-primed immunochemotherapy in heavily pretreated patients with platinum-resistant or platinum-refractory ovarian cancer: the nonrandomized phase 2 VIRO-15 clinical trial. *JAMA Oncol* **9:** 903–908. doi:10.1001/jamaoncol.2023.1007

Horowitz NS, Miller A, Rungruang B, Richard SD, Rodriguez N, Bookman MA, Hamilton CA, Krivak TC, Maxwell GL. 2015. Does aggressive surgery improve outcomes? Interaction between preoperative disease burden and complex surgery in patients with advanced-stage ovarian cancer: an analysis of GOG 182. *J Clin Oncol* **33:** 937–943. doi:10.1200/JCO.2014.56.3106

Hou JY, Chapman JS, Kalashnikova E, Pierson W, Smith-McCune K, Pineda G, Vattakalam RM, Ross A, Mills M, Suarez CJ, et al. 2022. Circulating tumor DNA monitoring for early recurrence detection in epithelial ovarian cancer. *Gynecol Oncol* **167:** 334–341. doi:10.1016/j.ygyno.2022.09.004

Hwang WT, Adams SF, Tahirovic E, Hagemann IS, Coukos G. 2012. Prognostic significance of tumor-infiltrating T cells in ovarian cancer: a meta-analysis. *Gynecol Oncol* **124:** 192–198. doi:10.1016/j.ygyno.2011.09.039

Jiang R, Feng Y, Chen Y, Cheng X, Shi T, Gao W, Jia H, Jiang S, Guo Y, Huang X, et al. 2024. Surgery versus no surgery in platinum-sensitive relapsed ovarian cancer: final overall survival analysis of the SOC-1 randomized phase 3 trial. *Nat Med* **2024:** 1–8.

Jiao S, Xia W, Yamaguchi H, Wei Y, Chen MK, Hsu JM, Hsu JL, Yu WH, Du Y, Lee HH, et al. 2017. PARP inhibitor upregulates PD-L1 expression and enhances cancer-associated immunosuppression. *Clin Cancer Res* **23:** 3711–3720. doi:10.1158/1078-0432.CCR-16-3215

Kalli KR, Oberg AL, Keeney GL, Christianson TJ, Low PS, Knutson KL, Hartmann LC. 2008. Folate receptor α as a tumor target in epithelial ovarian cancer. *Gynecol Oncol* **108:** 619–626. doi:10.1016/j.ygyno.2007.11.020

Karpel HC, Powell SS, Pothuri B. 2023. Antibody-drug conjugates in gynecologic cancer. *Am Soc Clin Oncol Educ Book* **43:** e390772. doi:10.1200/EDBK_390772

Katsumata N, Yasuda M, Isonishi S, Takahashi F, Michimae H, Kimura E, Aoki D, Jobo T, Kodama S, Terauchi F, et al. 2013. Long-term results of dose-dense paclitaxel and carboplatin versus conventional paclitaxel and carboplatin for treatment of advanced epithelial ovarian, fallopian tube, or primary peritoneal cancer (JGOG 3016): a randomised, controlled, open-label trial. *Lancet Oncol* **14:** 1020–1026. doi:10.1016/S1470-2045(13)70363-2

Kaufman B, Shapira-Frommer R, Schmutzler RK, Audeh MW, Friedlander M, Balmaña J, Mitchell G, Fried G, Stemmer SM, Hubert A, et al. 2015. Olaparib monotherapy in patients with advanced cancer and a germline *BRCA1/2* mutation. *J Clin Oncol* **33:** 244–250. doi:10.1200/JCO.2014.56.2728

Kayikcioglu F, Köse MF, Boran N, Calişkan E, Tulunay G. 2001. Neoadjuvant chemotherapy or primary surgery in advanced epithelial ovarian carcinoma. *Int J Gynecol Cancer* **11:** 466–470. doi:10.1046/j.1525-1438.2001.01064.x

Kehoe S, Hook J, Nankivell M, Jayson GC, Kitchener H, Lopes T, Luesley D, Perren T, Bannoo S, Mascarenhas M, et al. 2015. Primary chemotherapy versus primary surgery for newly diagnosed advanced ovarian cancer (CHORUS): an open-label, randomised, controlled, non-inferiority trial. *Lancet* **386:** 249–257. doi:10.1016/S0140-6736(14)62223-6

Kim H, Xu H, George E, Hallberg D, Kumar S, Jagannathan V, Medvedev S, Kinose Y, Devins K, Verma P, et al. 2020. Combining PARP with ATR inhibition overcomes PARP inhibitor and platinum resistance in ovarian cancer models. *Nat Commun* **11:** 3726. doi:10.1038/s41467-020-17127-2

Klichinsky M, Ruella M, Shestova O, Lu XM, Best A, Zeeman M, Schmierer M, Gabrusiewicz K, Anderson NR, Petty NE, et al. 2020. Human chimeric antigen receptor macrophages for cancer immunotherapy. *Nat Biotechnol* **38:** 947–953. doi:10.1038/s41587-020-0462-y

Konstantinopoulos PA, Ceccaldi R, Shapiro GI, D'Andrea AD. 2015. Homologous recombination deficiency: exploiting the fundamental vulnerability of ovarian cancer. *Cancer Discov* **5:** 1137–1154. doi:10.1158/2159-8290.CD-15-0714

Konstantinopoulos PA, Waggoner S, Vidal GA, Mita M, Moroney JW, Holloway R, Van Le L, Sachdev JC, Chapman-Davis E, Colon-Otero G, et al. 2019. Single-arm phases 1 and 2 trial of niraparib in combination with pembrolizumab in patients with recurrent platinum-resistant ovarian carcinoma. *JAMA Oncol* **5:** 1141–1149. doi:10.1001/jamaoncol.2019.1048

Konstantinopoulos PA, Norquist B, Lacchetti C, Armstrong D, Grisham RN, Goodfellow PJ, Kohn EC, Levine DA, Liu JF, Lu KH, et al. 2020. Germline and somatic tumor testing in epithelial ovarian cancer: ASCO guideline. *J Clin Oncol* **38:** 1222–1245. doi:10.1200/JCO.19.02960

Koole S, van Stein R, Sikorska K, Barton D, Perrin L, Brennan D, Zivanovic O, Mosgaard BJ, Fagotti A, Colombo PE, et al. 2020. Primary cytoreductive surgery with or without hyperthermic intraperitoneal chemotherapy (HIPEC) for FIGO stage III epithelial ovarian cancer: OVHIPEC-2, a phase III randomized clinical trial. *Int J Gynecol Cancer* **30:** 888–892. doi:10.1136/ijgc-2020-001231

Koole SN, Schouten PC, Hauke J, Kluin RJC, Nederlof P, Richters LK, Krebsbach G, Sikorska K, Alkemade M, Opdam M, et al. 2022. Effect of HIPEC according to HRD/*BRCAwt* genomic profile in stage III ovarian cancer: results from the phase III OVHIPEC trial. *Int J Cancer* **151:** 1394–1404. doi:10.1002/ijc.34124

Kowalchuk RO, Waters MR, Richardson KM, Spencer K, Larner JM, Irvin WP, Kersh CR. 2020. Stereotactic body radiation therapy in the treatment of ovarian cancer. *Radiat Oncol* **15:** 108. doi:10.1186/s13014-020-01564-w

Kristeleit R, Lisyanskaya A, Fedenko A, Dvorkin M, de Melo AC, Shparyk Y, Rakhmatullina I, Bondarenko I, Colombo N, Svintsitskiy V, et al. 2022. Rucaparib versus standard-of-care chemotherapy in patients with relapsed ovarian cancer and a deleterious *BRCA1* or *BRCA2* mutation (ARIEL4): an international, open-label, randomised, phase 3 trial. *Lancet Oncol* **23:** 465–478. doi:10.1016/S1470-2045(22)00122-X

Kristeleit R, O'Malley D, Lim MC, McNeish I, Herzog TJ, Wilson M, Fehm TN, Coleman RL, Van Gorp T, Oza AM, et al. 2024a. 49MO updated progression-free survival (PFS) in patients (pts) with newly diagnosed advanced ovarian cancer (OC) treated with rucaparib (RUC) in ATHENA-MONO. *ESMO Open* **9**(Suppl 5): 103556. doi:10.1016/j.esmoop.2024.103556

Kristeleit R, O'Malley D, Lim MC, Miller R, Herzog T, Wilson M, De Vivo R, Coleman R, Oaknin A, Oza A, et al. 2024b. Interim post-progression data and updated survival in patients with newly diagnosed advanced ovarian cancer in ATHENA-MONO. *Gynecol Oncol* **190:** S10–S11. doi:10.1016/j.ygyno.2024.07.022

Kumar S, Acharya S, Karthikeyan M, Biswas P, Kumari S. 2024. Limitations and potential of immunotherapy in ovarian cancer. *Front Immunol* **14:** 1292166. doi:10.3389/fimmu.2023.1292166

Kurtz JE, Pujade-Lauraine E, Oaknin A, Belin L, Leitner K, Cibula D, Denys H, Rosengarten O, Rodrigues M, de Gregorio N, et al. 2023. Atezolizumab combined with bevacizumab and platinum-based therapy for platinum-sensitive ovarian cancer: placebo-controlled randomized phase III ATALANTE/ENGOT-ov29 trial. *J Clin Oncol* **41:** 4768–4778. doi:10.1200/JCO.23.00529

Leath C, Scambia G, Valencia RV, Colombo N, Cibula D, Bidzinski M, Kim JW, Nam JH, Madry R, Hernancez C. 2022. Overall survival by number of prior lines of chemotherapy in patients with *BRCA*-mutated platinum-sensitive relapsed ovarian cancer receiving olaparib treatment or non-platinum chemotherapy in SOLO3. In *IGCS 2022 Annual Global Meeting*, New York.

Ledermann J, Harter P, Gourley C, Friedlander M, Vergote I, Rustin G, Scott C, Meier W, Shapira-Frommer R, Safra T, et al. 2012. Olaparib maintenance therapy in platinum-sensitive relapsed ovarian cancer. *N Engl J Med* **366:** 1382–1392. doi:10.1056/NEJMoa1105535

Ledermann JA, Harter P, Gourley C, Friedlander M, Vergote I, Rustin G, Scott C, Meier W, Shapira-Frommer R, Safra T, et al. 2016. Overall survival in patients with platinum-sensitive recurrent serous ovarian cancer receiving olaparib maintenance monotherapy: an updated analysis from a randomised, placebo-controlled, double-blind, phase 2 trial. *Lancet Oncol* **17:** 1579–1589. doi:10.1016/S1470-2045(16)30376-X

Lee EK, Liu JF. 2019. Antibody-drug conjugates in gynecologic malignancies. *Gynecol Oncol* **153:** 694–702. doi:10.1016/j.ygyno.2019.03.245

Lee JM, Moore RG, Ghamande S, Park MS, Diaz JP, Chapman J, Kendrick J, Slomovitz BM, Tewari KS, Lowe ES, et al. 2022. Cediranib in combination with olaparib in patients without a germline *BRCA1/2* mutation and with recurrent platinum-resistant ovarian cancer: phase IIb CONCERTO trial. *Clin Cancer Res* **28:** 4186–4193. doi:10.1158/1078-0432.CCR-21-1733

Lee JM, Brady MF, Miller A, Moore RG, MacKay H, McNally L, Lea J, Street D, Lheureux S, McDonald ME, et al. 2024. Cediranib and olaparib combination compared with cediranib or olaparib alone, or chemotherapy in platinum-resistant or primary platinum-refractory ovarian cancer: NRG-GY005. *J Clin Oncol* **42:** 4305–4316. doi:10.1200/JCO.24.00683

Li Q, Cohn D, Waller A, Backes F, Copeland L, Fowler J, Salani R, O'Malley D. 2014. Outpatient rapid 4-step desensitization for gynecologic oncology patients with mild to low-risk, moderate hypersensitivity reactions to carboplatin/cisplatin. *Gynecol Oncol* **135:** 90–94. doi:10.1016/j.ygyno.2014.07.104

Lim MC, Chang SJ, Park B, Yoo HJ, Yoo CW, Nam BH, Park SY, HIPEC for Ovarian Cancer Collaborators. 2022. Survival after hyperthermic intraperitoneal chemotherapy and primary or interval cytoreductive surgery in ovarian cancer: a randomized clinical trial. *JAMA Surg* **157:** 374–383. doi:10.1001/jamasurg.2022.0143

Lim MC, Kim JH, Park B, Lee JY, Chang SJ, Lee YY, Choi CH, Park JY, Kim DY, Hong DG, et al. 2024. Rationale and study design of the KOV-HIPEC-04: a phase III randomized controlled trial in primary stage III and IV ovarian cancer after interval cytoreductive surgery (FOCUS). *J Clin Oncol* **42:** TPS5636. doi:10.1200/JCO.2024.42.16_suppl.TPS5636

Liu JF, Barry WT, Birrer M, Lee JM, Buckanovich RJ, Fleming GF, Rimel B, Buss MK, Nattam S, Hurteau J, et al. 2014. Combination cediranib and olaparib versus olaparib alone for women with recurrent platinum-sensitive ovarian cancer: a randomised phase 2 study. *Lancet Oncol* **15:** 1207–1214. doi:10.1016/S1470-2045(14)70391-2

Liu JF, Brady MF, Matulonis UA, Miller A, Kohn EC, Swisher EM, Cella D, Tew WP, Cloven NG, Muller CY, et al. 2022. Olaparib with or without cediranib versus platinum-based chemotherapy in recurrent platinum-sensitive ovarian cancer (NRG-GY004): a randomized, open-label, phase III trial. *J Clin Oncol* **40:** 2138–2147. doi:10.1200/JCO.21.02011

Liu JF, Gaillard S, Wahner Hendrickson AE, Yeku O, Diver E, Gunderson Jackson C, Arend R, Ratner E, Samnotra V, et al. 2024. Niraparib, dostarlimab, and bevacizumab as combination therapy in pretreated, advanced platinum-resistant ovarian cancer: findings from cohort A of the OPAL phase II trial. *JCO Precis Oncol* **8:** e2300693.

Macchia G, Jereczek-Fossa BA, Lazzari R, Cerrotta A, Deodato F, Ippolito E, Aristei C, Gambacorta MA, Scambia G, Valentini V, et al. 2022. Efficacy and safety of stereotactic body radiotherapy (SBRT) in oligometastatic/persistent/recurrent ovarian cancer: a prospective, multicenter phase II study (MITO-RT3/RAD). *Int J Gynecol Cancer* **32:** 939–943. doi:10.1136/ijgc-2021-002709

Mahdi H, Moslemi-Kebria M, Levinson KL, Gojayev A, Lockhart D, Ali-Fehmi R, Munkarah AR. 2013. Prevalence and prognostic impact of lymphadenectomy and lymph node metastasis in clinically early-stage ovarian clear cell carcinoma. *Int J Gynecol Cancer* **23:** 1226–1230. doi:10.1097/IGC.0b013e3182856736

Manning-Geist BL, Chi DS, Long Roche K, Zivanovic O, Sonoda Y, Gardner GJ, O'Cearbhaill RE, Abu-Rustum NR, Leitao MM Jr. 2021. Tertiary cytoreduction for recurrent ovarian carcinoma: an updated and expanded analysis. *Gynecol Oncol* **162:** 345–352. doi:10.1016/j.ygyno.2021.05.015

Manning-Geist B, Gordhandas S, Hodgson A, Zhou QC, Iasonos A, Chi DS, Ellenson L, Aghajanian CA, Abu-Rustum NR, Leitao M, et al. 2022. Management of patients with early-stage ovarian clear cell carcinoma: risk stratification and fertility conservation. *Int J Gynecol Cancer* **32:** 1576–1582. doi:10.1136/ijgc-2022-003935

Markman M. 2015. Maintenance chemotherapy in the management of epithelial ovarian cancer. *Cancer Metastasis Rev* **34:** 11–17. doi:10.1007/s10555-014-9537-x

Markman M, Walker JL. 2006. Intraperitoneal chemotherapy of ovarian cancer: a review, with a focus on practical aspects of treatment. *J Clin Oncol* **24:** 988–994. doi:10.1200/JCO.2005.05.2456

Markman M, Hall J, Spitz D, Weiner S, Carson L, Van Le L, Baker M. 2002. Phase II trial of weekly single-agent paclitaxel in platinum/paclitaxel-refractory ovarian cancer. *J Clin Oncol* **20:** 2365–2369. doi:10.1200/JCO.2002.09.130

Markman M, Liu PY, Wilczynski S, Monk B, Copeland LJ, Alvarez RD, Jiang C, Alberts D, Southwest Oncology Group; Gynecologic Oncology Group. 2003. Phase III randomized trial of 12 versus 3 months of maintenance paclitaxel in patients with advanced ovarian cancer after complete response to platinum and paclitaxel-based chemotherapy: a Southwest Oncology Group and Gynecologic Oncology Group trial. *J Clin Oncol* **21:** 2460–2465. doi:10.1200/JCO.2003.07.013

Markman M, Markman J, Webster K, Zanotti K, Kulp B, Peterson G, Belinson J. 2004. Duration of response to second-line, platinum-based chemotherapy for ovarian cancer: implications for patient management and clinical trial design. *J Clin Oncol* **22:** 3120–3125. doi:10.1200/JCO.2004.05.195

Markman M, Liu PY, Moon J, Monk BJ, Copeland L, Wilczynski S, Alberts D. 2009. Impact on survival of 12 versus 3 monthly cycles of paclitaxel (175 mg/m^2) administered to patients with advanced ovarian cancer who attained a complete response to primary platinum-paclitaxel: follow-up of a Southwest Oncology Group and Gynecologic Oncology Group phase 3 trial. *Gynecol Oncol* **114:** 195–198. doi:10.1016/j.ygyno.2009.04.012

Marmé F, Harter P, Redondo A, Reuss A, Ray-Coquard IL, Lindemann K, Kurzeder C, Van Nieuwenhuysen E, Bellier C, Pietzner K, et al. 2024. Atezolizumab versus placebo in combination with bevacizumab and non-platinum-based chemotherapy in recurrent ovarian cancer: final overall and progression-free survival results from the AGO-OVAR 2.29/ENGOT-ov34 study. *Gynecol Cancer* **42:** LBA5501. doi:10.1200/JCO.2024.42.17_suppl.LBA5501

Matulonis UA, Moore KN, Martin LP, Vergote IB, Castro C, Gilbert L, Male K, Birrer MJ, O'Malley DM. 2018. Mirvetuximab soravtansine, a folate receptor α (FRα)-targeting antibody-drug conjugate (ADC), with pembrolizumab in platinum-resistant ovarian cancer (PROC): initial results of an expansion cohort from FORWARD II, a phase Ib study. *Ann Oncol* **29:** viii339. doi:10.1093/annonc/mdy285.157

Matulonis UA, Shapira-Frommer R, Santin AD, Lisyanskaya AS, Pignata S, Vergote I, Raspagliesi F, Sonke GS, Birrer M, Provencher DM, et al. 2019. Antitumor activity and safety of pembrolizumab in patients with advanced recurrent ovarian cancer: results from the phase II KEYNOTE-100 study. *Ann Oncol* **30:** 1080–1087. doi:10.1093/annonc/mdz135

Matulonis UA, Lorusso D, Oaknin A, Pignata S, Dean A, Denys H, Colombo N, Van Gorp T, Konner JA, Marin MR, et al. 2023a. Efficacy and safety of mirvetuximab soravtansine in patients with platinum-resistant ovarian cancer with high folate receptor α expression: results from the SORAYA study. *J Clin Oncol* **41:** 2436–2445. doi:10.1200/JCO.22.01900

Matulonis U, Herrstedt J, Oza A, Mahner S, Redondo A, Berton D, Berek J, Haslund C, Marmé F, González-Martin A, et al. 2023b. Final overall survival and long-term safety in the ENGOT-OV16/NOVA phase III trial of niraparib in patients with recurrent ovarian cancer (LBA 6). *Gynecol Oncol* **176:** S31–S32. doi:10.1016/j.ygyno.2023.06.508

McGuire WP, Hoskins WJ, Brady MF, Kucera PR, Partridge EE, Look KY, Clarke-Pearson DL, Davidson M. 1996. Cyclophosphamide and cisplatin compared with paclitaxel and cisplatin in patients with stage III and stage IV ovarian cancer. *N Engl J Med* **334:** 1–6. doi:10.1056/NEJM199601043340101

McLaughlin PMJ, Klar M, Zwimpfer TA, Dutilh G, Vetter M, Marth C, du Bois A, Schade-Brittinger C, Reuss A, Bommer C, et al. 2022. Maintenance Therapy with Aromatase Inhibitor in epithelial Ovarian Cancer (MATAO): study protocol of a randomized double-blinded placebo-controlled multi-center phase III trial. *BMC Cancer* **22:** 508. doi:10.1186/s12885-022-09555-8

Mehta DA, Hay JW. 2014. Cost-effectiveness of adding bevacizumab to first line therapy for patients with advanced ovarian cancer. *Gynecol Oncol* **132:** 677–683. doi:10.1016/j.ygyno.2014.01.021

Meric-Bernstam F, Makker V, Oaknin A, Oh DY, Banerjee S, González-Martín A, Jung KH, Ługowska I, Manso L, Manzano A, et al. 2024. Efficacy and safety of trastuzumab deruxtecan in patients with HER2-expressing solid tumors: primary results from the DESTINY-PanTumor02 phase II trial. *J Clin Oncol* **42:** 47–58. doi:10.1200/JCO.23.02005

Miller DS, Blessing JA, Krasner CN, Mannel RS, Hanjani P, Pearl ML, Waggoner SE, Boardman CH. 2009. Phase II evaluation of pemetrexed in the treatment of recurrent or persistent platinum-resistant ovarian or primary peritoneal carcinoma: a study of the Gynecologic Oncology Group. *J Clin Oncol* **27:** 2686–2691. doi:10.1200/JCO.2008.19.2963

Mirza MR, Monk BJ, Herrstedt J, Oza AM, Mahner S, Redondo A, Fabbro M, Ledermann JA, Lorusso D, Vergote I, et al. 2016. Niraparib maintenance therapy in platinum-sensitive, recurrent ovarian cancer. *N Engl J Med* **375:** 2154–2164. doi:10.1056/NEJMoa1611310

Mitchell SK, Crson LF, Judson P, Downs LS Jr. 2005. Efficacy and tolerability of lower-dose topotecan in recurrent ovarian cancer: a retrospective case review. *Int J Gynecol Cancer* **15:** 793–798. doi:10.1136/ijgc-00009577-200509000-00013

Monberg MJ, Hall JP, Moon R, Higson O, McLaurin K, Dalvi T. 2019. Real-world bevacizumab utilization and outcomes in first-line ovarian cancer. *J Clin Oncol* **37:** 5578–5578. doi:10.1200/JCO.2019.37.15_suppl.5578

Monk BJ, Grisham RN, Banerjee S, Kalbacher E, Mirza MR, Romero I, Vuylsteke P, Coleman RL, Hilpert F, Oza AM, et al. 2020. MILO/ENGOT-ov11: binimetinib versus physician's choice chemotherapy in recurrent or persistent low-grade serous carcinomas of the ovary, fallopian tube, or primary peritoneum. *J Clin Oncol* **38:** 3753–3762. doi:10.1200/JCO.20.01164

Monk BJ, Colombo N, Oza AM, Fujiwara K, Birrer MJ, Randall L, Poddubskaya EV, Scambia G, Shparyk YV, Lim MC, et al. 2021a. Chemotherapy with or without avelumab followed by avelumab maintenance versus chemotherapy alone in patients with previously untreated epithelial ovarian cancer (JAVELIN Ovarian 100): an open-label, randomised, phase 3 trial. *Lancet Oncol* **22:** 1275–1289. doi:10.1016/S1470-2045(21)00342-9

Monk BJ, Coleman RL, Fujiwara K, Wilson MK, Oza AM, Oaknin A, O'Malley DM, Lorusso D, Westin SN, Safra T, et al. 2021b. ATHENA (GOG-3020/ENGOT-ov45): a randomized, phase III trial to evaluate rucaparib as monotherapy (ATHENA-MONO) and rucaparib in combination with nivolumab (ATHENA-COMBO) as maintenance treatment following frontline platinum-based chemotherapy in ovarian cancer. *Int J Gynecol Cancer* **31:** 1589–1594.

Monk BJ, Parkinson C, Lim MC, O'Malley DM, Oaknin A, Wilson MK, Coleman RL, Lorusso D, Bessette P, Ghamande S, et al. 2022. A randomized, phase III trial to evaluate rucaparib monotherapy as maintenance treatment in patients with newly diagnosed ovarian cancer (ATHENA–MONO/GOG-3020/ENGOT-ov45). *J Clin Oncol* **40:** 3952–3964. doi:10.1200/JCO.22.01003

Monk BJ, González-Martin A, Buckley L, Matulonis UA, Rimel BJ, Wu X, Moore KN, Mirza MR. 2023. Safety and management of niraparib monotherapy in ovarian cancer clinical trials. *Int J Gynecol Cancer* **33:** 971–981. doi:10.1136/ijgc-2022-004079

Monk BJ, Oaknin A, O'Malley DM, Wilson M, Lorusso D, Westin S, Oza AM, Zagouri F, Herzog TJ, Mikheeva O, et al. 2024a. LBA30 ATHENA-COMBO, a phase III, randomized trial comparing rucaparib (RUCA) + nivolumab (NIVO) combination therapy vs RUCA monotherapy as maintenance treatment in patients (pts) with newly diagnosed ovarian cancer (OC). *Ann Oncol* **35:** S1223–S1224. doi:10.1016/j.annonc.2024.08.2269

Monk BJ, Barretina-Ginesta MP, Pothuri B, Vergote I, Graybill W, Mirza MR, McCormick CC, Lorusso D, Moore RG, Freyer G, et al. 2024b. Niraparib first-line maintenance therapy in patients with newly diagnosed advanced ovarian cancer: final overall survival results from the PRIMA/ENGOT-OV26/GOG-3012 trial. *Ann Oncol* **35:** 981–992. doi:10.1016/j.annonc.2024.08.2241

Moore KN, Ponte J, LoRusso P, Birrer MJ, Bauer TM, Borghaei H, O'Malley DM, Ruiz-Soto R, Lutz R, Malik L. 2014. Relationship of pharmacokinetics (PK), toxicity, and initial evidence of clinical activity with IMGN853, a folate receptor α (FRα) targeting antibody drug conjugate in patients (Pts) with epithelial ovarian cancer (EOC) and other FRα-positive solid tumors. *J Clin Oncol* **32:** 5571. doi:10.1200/jco.2014.32.15_suppl.5571

Moore KN, Borghaei H, O'Malley DM, Jeong W, Seward SM, Bauer TM, Perez RP, Matulonis UA, Running KL, Zhang X, et al. 2017a. Phase 1 dose-escalation study of mirvetuximab soravtansine (IMGN853), a folate receptor α-targeting antibody-drug conjugate, in patients with solid tumors. *Cancer* **123:** 3080–3087. doi:10.1002/cncr.30736

Moore KN, Martin LP, O'Malley DM, Matulonis UA, Konner JA, Perez RP, Bauer TM, Ruiz-Soto R, Birrer MJ. 2017b. Safety and activity of mirvetuximab soravtansine (IMGN853), a folate receptor α–targeting antibody–drug conjugate, in platinum-resistant ovarian, fallopian tube, or primary peritoneal cancer: a phase I expansion study. *J Clin Oncol* **35:** 1112–1118. doi:10.1200/JCO.2016.69.9538

Moore KN, Colombo N, Scambia G, Kim BG, Oaknin A, Friedlander M, Lisyanskaya A, Floquet A, Leary A, Sanke GS, et al. 2018a. Maintenance olaparib following platinum-based chemotherapy in newly diagnosed patients (pts) with advanced ovarian cancer (OC) and a *BRCA1/2* mutation (*BRCAm*): phase III SOLO1 trial. *Ann Oncol* **29:** viii727. doi:10.1093/annonc/mdy424.041

Moore KN, O'Malley DM, Vergote I, Martin LP, Gonzalez-Martin A, Malek K, Birrer MJ. 2018b. Safety and activity findings from a phase 1b escalation study of mirvetuximab soravtansine, a folate receptor α (FRα)-targeting antibody-drug conjugate (ADC), in combination with carboplatin in patients with platinum-sensitive ovarian cancer. *Gynecol Oncol* **151:** 46–52. doi:10.1016/j.ygyno.2018.07.017

Moore KN, Secord AA, Geller MA, Miller DS, Cloven N, Fleming GF, Wahner Hendrickson AE, Azodi M, DiSilvestro P, et al. 2019. Niraparib monotherapy for late-line treatment of ovarian cancer (QUADRA): a multicentre, open-label, single-arm, phase 2 trial. *Lancet Oncol* **20:** 636–648. doi:10.1016/S1470-2045(19)30029-4

Moore KN, Oza AM, Colombo N, Oaknin A, Scambia G, Lorusso D, Konecny GE, Banerjee S, Murphy CG, Tanyi JL, et al. 2021. Phase III, randomized trial of mirvetuximab soravtansine versus chemotherapy in patients with platinum-resistant ovarian cancer: primary analysis of FORWARD I. *Ann Oncol* **32:** 757–765. doi:10.1016/j.annonc.2021.02.017

Moore KN, Angelergues A, Konecny GE, García Y, Banerjee S, Lorusso D, Lee JY, Moroney JW, Colombo N, Roszak A, et al. 2023. Mirvetuximab soravtansine in FRα-positive, platinum-resistant ovarian cancer. *N Engl J Med* **389:** 2162–2174. doi:10.1056/NEJMoa2309169

Morice P, Gouy S, Leary A. 2019. Mucinous ovarian carcinoma. *N Engl J Med* **380:** 1256–1266. doi:10.1056/NEJMra1813254

Morice PM, Leary A, Dolladille C, Chrétien B, Poulain L, González-Martín A, Moore K, O'Reilly EM, Ray-Coquard I, Alexandre J. 2021. Myelodysplastic syndrome and acute myeloid leukaemia in patients treated with PARP inhibitors: a safety meta-analysis of randomised controlled trials and a retrospective study of the WHO pharmacovigilance database. *Lancet Haematol* **8:** e122–e134. doi:10.1016/S2352-3026(20)30360-4

Morris R, Alvarez RD, Andrews S, Malone J, Bryant C, Heilbrun LK, Smith D, Schimp V, Munkarah A. 2008. Topotecan weekly bolus chemotherapy for relapsed platinum-sensitive ovarian and peritoneal cancers. *Gynecol Oncol* **109:** 346–352. doi:10.1016/j.ygyno.2008.02.028

Moubarak M, Harter P, Ataseven B, Traut A, Welz J, Baert T, Heitz F. 2022. Re-treatment with PARPi in patients with recurrent epithelial ovarian cancer: a single institutional experience. *Gynecol Oncol Rep* **40:** 100939. doi:10.1016/j.gore.2022.100939

Moufarrij S, O'Cearbhaill RE. 2024. Novel therapeutics in ovarian cancer: expanding the toolbox. *Curr Oncol* **31:** 97–114. doi:10.3390/curroncol31010007

Musacchio L, Salutari V, Pignata S, Braicu E, Cibula D, Colombo N, Frenel JS, Zagouri F, Carbone V, Ghizzoni V, et al. 2021. Randomized phase III trial on niraparib-TSR-042 (dostarlimab) versus physician's choice chemotherapy in recurrent ovarian, fallopian tube, or primary peritoneal cancer patients not candidate for platinum retreatment: NItCHE trial (MITO 33). *Int J Gynecol Cancer* **31:** 1369–1373. doi:10.1136/ijgc-2021-002593

Mutch DG, Prat J. 2014. 2014 FIGO staging for ovarian, fallopian tube and peritoneal cancer. *Gynecol Oncol* **133:** 401–404. doi:10.1016/j.ygyno.2014.04.013

Mutch DG, Orlando M, Goss T, Teneriello MG, Gordon AN, McMeekin SD, Wang Y, Scribner DR Jr, Marciniack M, Naumann RW, et al. 2007. Randomized phase III trial of gemcitabine compared with pegylated liposomal doxorubicin in patients with platinum-resistant ovarian cancer. *J Clin Oncol* **25:** 2811–2818. doi:10.1200/JCO.2006.09.6735

Nagao S, Fujiwara K, Yamamoto K, Tanabe H, Okamoto A, Takehara K, Saito M, Fujiwara H, Tan DSP, Yamaguchi S, et al. 2023. Intraperitoneal carboplatin for ovarian cancer—a phase 2/3 trial. *NEJM Evid* **2:** EVIDoa2200225. doi:10.1056/EVIDoa2200225

National Comprehensive Cancer Network. 2024. Ovarian cancer including fallopian tube cancer and primary peritoneal cancer (Version 3.2024). https://www.nccn.org/professionals/physician_gls/pdf/ovarian.pdf

Naumann R, Gonzalez Martin A, Herzog TJ, Coleman RL, Ray-Coquard IL, Miller R, Lu L, Dokainish H, Berman C, Oaknin A, et al. 2023. 818TiP REFRaME-O1/ENGOT-OV79/GOG-3086: a phase II/III open-label study evaluating the efficacy and safety of luveltamab tazevibulin versus investigator's choice of chemotherapy in women with relapsed platinum-resistant epithelial ovarian cancer expressing folate receptor α (FolRα). *Ann Oncol* **34:** S540–S541. doi:10.1016/j.annonc.2023.09.1993

Neijt JP, Engelholm SA, Tuxen MK, Sørensen PG, Hansen M, Sessa C, de Swart CA, Hirsch FR, Lund B, van Houwelingen HC. 2000. Exploratory phase III study of paclitaxel and cisplatin versus paclitaxel and carboplatin in advanced ovarian cancer. *J Clin Oncol* **18:** 3084–3092. doi:10.1200/JCO.2000.18.17.3084

Nickles Fader A, Java J, Ueda S, Bristow RE, Armstrong DK, Bookman MA, Gershenson DM; Gynecologic Oncology Group (GOG). 2013. Survival in women with grade 1 serous ovarian carcinoma. *Obstet Gynecol* **122:** 225–232. doi:10.1097/AOG.0b013e31829ce7ec

Nicum S, McGregor N, Austin R, Collins L, Dutton S, McNeish I, Glasspool R, Hall M, Roux R, Michael A, et al. 2024. Results of a randomised phase II trial of olaparib, chemotherapy or olaparib and cediranib in patients with platinum-resistant ovarian cancer. *Br J Cancer* **130:** 941–950. doi:10.1038/s41416-023-02567-6

O'Cearbhaill R, Sill M, Duong H, Waggoner S, Grisham R, Backes F, Mannel R, Tanyi J, Powell M, Mahews C, et al. 2023. PO005LBA/#1579 a randomized, phase II/III study of pegylated-liposomal-doxorubicin and atezolizumab (IND# 134427) versus pegylated-liposomal-doxorubicin, bevacizumab and atezolizumab versus pegylated-liposomal-doxorubicin and bevacizumab in platinum-resistant ovarian cancer (NRG-GY009). *Int J Gynecol Cancer* **33:** 4.

Ogitani Y, Aida T, Hagihara K, Yamaguchi J, Ishii C, Harada N, Soma M, Okamoto H, Oitate M, Arakawa S, et al. 2016. DS-8201a, a novel HER2-targeting ADC with a novel DNA topoisomerase I inhibitor, demonstrates a promising antitumor efficacy with differentiation from T-DM1. *Clin Cancer Res* **22:** 5097–5108. doi:10.1158/1078-0432.CCR-15-2822

O'Malley DM, Matulonis UA, Birrer MJ, Castro CM, Gilbert L, Vergote I, Martin LP, Mantia-Smaldone GM, Martin AG, Bratos R, et al. 2020. Phase Ib study of mirvetuximab soravtansine, a folate receptor α (FRα)-targeting antibody-drug conjugate (ADC), in combination with bevacizumab in patients with platinum-resistant ovarian cancer. *Gynecol Oncol* **157:** 379–385. doi:10.1016/j.ygyno.2020.01.037

O'Malley DM, Nyers TKN, Zamagni C, Diver E, Lorusso D. 2023. GLORIOSA: a randomized, open-label, phase 3 study of mirvetuximab soravtansine with bevacizumab vs. bevacizumab as maintenance in platinum-sensitive ovarian, fallopian tube, or primary peritoneal cancer. *J Clin Oncol* **41**(16_suppl): TPS5622. doi:10.1200/JCO.2023.41.16_suppl.TPS5622

Onda T, Satoh T, Ogawa G, Saito T, Kasamatsu T, Nakanishi T, Mizutani T, Takehara K, Okamoto A, Ushijima K, et al. 2020. Comparison of survival between primary debulking surgery and neoadjuvant chemotherapy for stage III/IV ovarian, tubal and peritoneal cancers in phase III randomised trial. *Eur J Cancer* **130:** 114–125. doi:10.1016/j.ejca.2020.02.020

O'Shannessy DJ, Somers EB, Smale R, Fu YS. 2013. Expression of folate receptor-α (FRA) in gynecologic malignancies and its relationship to the tumor type. *Int J Gynecol Pathol* **32:** 258–268. doi:10.1097/PGP.0b013e3182774562

Oza AM, Cook AD, Pfisterer J, Embleton A, Ledermann JA, Pujade-Lauraine E, Kristensen G, Carey MS, Beale P, Cervantes A, et al. 2015. Standard chemotherapy with or without bevacizumab for women with newly diagnosed ovarian cancer (ICON7): overall survival results of a phase 3 randomised trial. *Lancet Oncol* **16:** 928–936. doi:10.1016/S1470-2045(15)00086-8

Ozols RF, Bundy BN, Greer BE, Fowler JM, Clarke-Pearson D, Burger RA, Mannel RS, DeGeest K, Hartenbach EM, Baergen R, et al. 2003. Phase III trial of carboplatin and paclitaxel compared with cisplatin and paclitaxel in patients with optimally resected stage III ovarian cancer: a Gynecologic Oncology Group study. *J Clin Oncol* **21:** 3194–3200. doi:10.1200/JCO.2003.02.153

Parmar MK, Ledermann JA, Colombo N, du Bois A, Delaloye JF, Kristensen GB, Wheeler S, Swart AM, Qian W, Torri V, et al. 2003. Paclitaxel plus platinum-based chemotherapy versus conventional platinum-based chemotherapy in women with relapsed ovarian cancer: the ICON4/AGO-OVAR-2.2 trial. *Lancet* **361:** 2099–2106. doi:10.1016/S0140-6736(03)13718-X

Pavlidis N, Rassy E, Vermorken JB, Assi T, Kattan J, Boussios S, Smith-Gagen J. 2021. The outcome of patients with serous papillary peritoneal cancer, fallopian tube cancer, and epithelial ovarian cancer by treatment eras: 27 years data from the SEER registry. *Cancer Epidemiol* **75:** 102045. doi:10.1016/j.canep.2021.102045

Perren TJ, Swart AM, Pfisterer J, Ledermann JA, Pujade-Lauraine E, Kristensen G, Carey MS, Beale P, Cervantes A, Kurzeder C, et al. 2011. A phase 3 trial of bevacizumab in ovarian cancer. *N Engl J Med* **365:** 2484–2496. doi:10.1056/NEJMoa1103799

Petrillo M, Paris I, Vizzielli G, Amadio G, Cosentino F, Salutari V, Scambia G, Fagotti A. 2015. Neoadjuvant chemotherapy followed by maintenance therapy with or without bevacizumab in unresectable high-grade serous ovarian cancer: a case-control study. *Ann Surg Oncol* **22:** 952–958. doi:10.1245/s10434-015-4651-8

Pfisterer J, Plante M, Vergote I, du Bois A, Hirte H, Lacave AJ, Wagner U, Stähle A, Stuart G, Kimmig R, et al. 2006a. Gemcitabine plus carboplatin compared with carboplatin in patients with platinum-sensitive recurrent ovarian cancer: an intergroup trial of the AGO-OVAR, the NCIC CTG, and the EORTC GCG. *J Clin Oncol* **24:** 4699–4707. doi:10.1200/JCO.2006.06.0913

Pfisterer J, Weber B, Reuss A, Kimmig R, du Bois A, Wagner U, Bourgeois H, Meier W, Costa S, Blohmer JU, et al. 2006b. Randomized phase III trial of topotecan following carboplatin and paclitaxel in first-line treatment of advanced ovarian cancer: a gynecologic cancer intergroup trial of the AGO-OVAR and GINECO. *J Natl Cancer Inst* **98:** 1036–1045. doi:10.1093/jnci/djj296

Pfisterer J, Joly F, Kristensen G, Rau J, Mahner S, Pautier P, El-Balat A, Kurtz JE, Canzler U, Sehouli J, et al. 2023. Optimal treatment duration of bevacizumab as front-line therapy for advanced ovarian cancer: AGO-OVAR

17 BOOST/GINECO OV118/ENGOT Ov-15 Open-Label Randomized Phase III Trial. *J Clin Oncol* **41:** 893–902. doi:10.1200/JCO.22.01010

Pierson WE, Peters PN, Chang MT, Chen LM, Quigley DA, Ashworth A, Chapman JS. 2020. An integrated molecular profile of endometrioid ovarian cancer. *Gynecol Oncol* **157:** 55–61. doi:10.1016/j.ygyno.2020.02.011

Pignata S, Scambia G, Ferrandina G, Savarese A, Sorio R, Breda E, Gebbia V, Musso P, Frigerio L, Del Medico P, et al. 2011. Carboplatin plus paclitaxel versus carboplatin plus pegylated liposomal doxorubicin as first-line treatment for patients with ovarian cancer: the MITO-2 randomized phase III trial. *J Clin Oncol* **29:** 3628–3635. doi:10.1200/JCO.2010.33.8566

Pignata S, Scambia G, Katsaros D, Gallo C, Pujade-Lauraine E, De Placido S, Bologna A, Weber B, Raspagliesi F, Panici PB, et al. 2014. Carboplatin plus paclitaxel once a week versus every 3 weeks in patients with advanced ovarian cancer (MITO-7): a randomised, multicentre, open-label, phase 3 trial. *Lancet Oncol* **15:** 396–405. doi:10.1016/S1470-2045(14)70049-X

Pignata S, Scambia G, Bologna A, Signoriello S, Vergote IB, Wagner U, Lorusso D, Murgia V, Sorio R, Ferrandina G, et al. 2017. Randomized controlled trial testing the efficacy of platinum-free interval prolongation in advanced ovarian cancer: the MITO-8, MaNGO, BGOG-Ov1, AGO-Ovar2.16, ENGOT-Ov1, GCIG study. *J Clin Oncol* **35:** 3347–3353. doi:10.1200/JCO.2017.73.4293

Pignata S, Lorusso D, Joly F, Gallo C, Colombo N, Sessa C, Bamias A, Salutari V, Selle F, Frezzini S, et al. 2021. Carboplatin-based doublet plus bevacizumab beyond progression versus carboplatin-based doublet alone in patients with platinum-sensitive ovarian cancer: a randomised, phase 3 trial. *Lancet Oncol* **22:** 267–276. doi:10.1016/S1470-2045(20)30637-9

Ponte JF, Ab O, Lanieri L, Lee J, Coccia J, Bartle LM, Themeles M, Zhou Y, Pinkas J, Ruiz-Soto R. 2016. Mirvetuximab soravtansine (IMGN853), a folate receptor α–targeting antibody-drug conjugate, potentiates the activity of standard of care therapeutics in ovarian cancer models. *Neoplasia* **18:** 775–784. doi:10.1016/j.neo.2016.11.002

Postow MA, Callahan MK, Wolchok JD. 2015. Immune checkpoint blockade in cancer therapy. *J Clin Oncol* **33:** 1974–1982. doi:10.1200/JCO.2014.59.4358

Poveda AM, Selle F, Hilpert F, Reuss A, Savarese A, Vergote I, Witteveen P, Bamias A, Scotto N, Mitchell L, et al. 2015. Bevacizumab combined with weekly paclitaxel, pegylated liposomal doxorubicin, or topotecan in platinum-resistant recurrent ovarian cancer: analysis by chemotherapy cohort of the randomized phase III AURELIA trial. *J Clin Oncol* **33:** 3836–3838. doi:10.1200/JCO.2015.63.1408

Pujade-Lauraine E, Wagner U, Aavall-Lundqvist E, Gebski V, Heywood M, Vasey PA, Volgger B, Vergote I, Pignata S, Ferrero A, et al. 2010. Pegylated liposomal doxorubicin and carboplatin compared with paclitaxel and carboplatin for patients with platinum-sensitive ovarian cancer in late relapse. *J Clin Oncol* **28:** 3323–3329. doi:10.1200/JCO.2009.25.7519

Pujade-Lauraine E, Hilpert F, Weber B, Reuss A, Poveda A, Kristensen G, Sorio R, Vergote I, Witteveen P, Bamias A, et al. 2014. Bevacizumab combined with chemotherapy for platinum-resistant recurrent ovarian cancer: the AURELIA open-label randomized phase III trial. *J Clin Oncol* **32:** 1302–1308. doi:10.1200/JCO.2013.51.4489

Pujade-Lauraine E, Ledermann JA, Selle F, Gebski V, Penson RT, Oza AM, Korach J, Huzarski T, Poveda A, Pignata S, et al. 2017. Olaparib tablets as maintenance therapy in patients with platinum-sensitive, relapsed ovarian cancer and a *BRCA1/2* mutation (SOLO2/ENGOT-Ov21): a double-blind, randomised, placebo-controlled, phase 3 trial. *Lancet Oncol* **18:** 1274–1284. doi:10.1016/S1470-2045(17)30469-2

Pujade-Lauraine E, Selle F, Scambia G, Asselain B, Marmé F, Lindemann K, Colombo N, Mądry R, Glasspool R, Vergote I, et al. 2023. Maintenance olaparib rechallenge in patients with platinum-sensitive relapsed ovarian cancer previously treated with a PARP inhibitor (OReO/ENGOT-ov38): a phase IIIb trial. *Ann Oncol* **34:** 1152–1164. doi:10.1016/j.annonc.2023.09.3110

Randall LM, O'Malley DM, Monk BJ, Coleman RL, Gaillard S, Adams S, Duska LR, Dalton H, Holloway RW, Huang M, et al. 2023. Niraparib and dostarlimab for the treatment of recurrent platinum-resistant ovarian cancer: results of a phase II study (MOONSTONE/GOG-3032). *Gynecol Oncol* **178:** 161–169. doi:10.1016/j.ygyno.2023.10.005

Rauh-Hain JA, Nitschmann CC, Worley MJ Jr, Bradford LS, Berkowitz RS, Schorge JO, Campos SM, del Carmen MG, Horowitz NS. 2013. Platinum resistance after neoadjuvant chemotherapy compared to primary surgery in patients with advanced epithelial ovarian carcinoma. *Gynecol Oncol* **129:** 63–68. doi:10.1016/j.ygyno.2013.01.009

Rauh-Hain JA, Melamed A, Wright A, Gockley A, Clemmer JT, Schorge JO, Del Carmen MG, Keating NL. 2017. Overall survival following neoadjuvant chemotherapy vs primary cytoreductive surgery in women with epithelial ovarian cancer: analysis of the National Cancer Database. *JAMA Oncol* **3:** 76–82. doi:10.1001/jamaoncol.2016.4411

Ray-Coquard I, Pautier P, Pignata S, Pérol D, González-Martín A, Berger R, Fujiwara K, Vergote I, Colombo N, Mäenpää J, et al. 2019. Olaparib plus bevacizumab as first-line maintenance in ovarian cancer. *N Engl J Med* **381:** 2416–2428. doi:10.1056/NEJMoa1911361

Ray-Coquard I, Richardson DL, Hasegawa K, Mailley C, Re S, Gopal Kundu M, Lin J, Moore KN. 2024. REJOICE-Ovarian01: a phase 2/3 study of raludotatug deruxtecan (R-DXd) in patients with platinum-resistant ovarian cancer. *J Clin Oncol* **42:** TPS5625. doi:10.1200/JCO.2024.42.16_suppl.TPS5625

Richardson DL, Moore KN, Vergote I, Gilbert L, Martin LP, Mantia-Smaldone GM, Castro CM, Provencher D, Matulonis UA, Stec J, et al. 2024. Phase 1b study of mirvetuximab soravtansine, a folate receptor α (FRα)-targeting antibody-drug conjugate, in combination with carboplatin and bevacizumab in patients with platinum-sensitive ovarian cancer. *Gynecol Oncol* **185:** 186–193. doi:10.1016/j.ygyno.2024.01.045

Rodriguez-Garcia A, Lynn RC, Poussin M, Eiva MA, Shaw LC, O'Connor RS, Minutolo NG, Casado-Medrano V, Lopez G, Matsuyama T, et al. 2021. CAR-T cell-mediated depletion of immunosuppressive tumor-associated macrophages promotes endogenous antitumor immunity and augments adoptive immunotherapy. *Nat Commun* **12:** 877. doi:10.1038/s41467-021-20893-2

Rose PG, Blessing JA, Mayer AR, Homesley HD. 1998. Prolonged oral etoposide as second-line therapy for platinum-resistant and platinum-sensitive ovarian carcinoma: a Gynecologic Oncology Group study. *J Clin Oncol* **16:** 405–410. doi:10.1200/JCO.1998.16.2.405

Rouzier R, Gouy S, Selle F, Lambaudie E, Floquet A, Fourchotte V, Pomel C, Colombo PE, Kalbacher E, Martin-Francoise S, et al. 2017. Efficacy and safety of bevacizumab-containing neoadjuvant therapy followed by interval debulking surgery in advanced ovarian cancer: results from the ANTHALYA trial. *Eur J Cancer* **70:** 133–142. doi:10.1016/j.ejca.2016.09.036

Rustin G, Van Der Burg M. 2009. A randomized trial in ovarian cancer (OC) of early treatment of relapse based on CA125 level alone versus delayed treatment based on conventional clinical indicators (MRC OV05/EORTC 55955 trials). *J Clin Oncol* **27**(18 Suppl): 1. doi:10.1200/jco.2009.27.18_suppl.1

Safra T, Menczer J, Bernstein R, Shpigel S, Inbar MJ, Grisaru D, Golan A, Levy T. 2007. Efficacy and toxicity of weekly topotecan in recurrent epithelial ovarian and primary peritoneal cancer. *Gynecol Oncol* **105:** 205–210. doi:10.1016/j.ygyno.2006.11.017

Salani R, Khanna N, Frimer M, Bristow RE, Chen LM. 2017. An update on post-treatment surveillance and diagnosis of recurrence in women with gynecologic malignancies: Society of Gynecologic Oncology (SGO) recommendations. *Gynecol Oncol* **146:** 3–10. doi:10.1016/j.ygyno.2017.03.022

Salutari V, Marchetti C, Ghizzoni V, Giudice E, Giannarelli D, Tudisco R, Carbone MV, Costantini B, Naldini A, Ricci C, et al. 2023. # 881 The NUVOLA TRIAL: neoadjuvant chemoteraphy in unresectable ovarian cancer with olaparib and weekly carboplatin plus paclitaxel. A phase II open-label multi-centre study. *Int J Gynecol Cancer* **33:** A430–A431.

Sato E, Olson SH, Ahn J, Bundy B, Nishikawa H, Qian F, Jungbluth AA, Frosina D, Gnjatic S, Ambrosone C, et al. 2005. Intraepithelial $CD8^+$ tumor-infiltrating lymphocytes and a high $CD8^+$/regulatory T cell ratio are associated with favorable prognosis in ovarian cancer. *Proc Natl Acad Sci* **102:** 18538–18543. doi:10.1073/pnas.0509182102

Schettino C, Musacchio L, Bartoletti M, Chiodini P, Arenare L, Baldassarre G, Califano D, Capoluongo E, Costi MP, D'Incalci M, et al. 2022. Olaparib beyond progression compared with platinum chemotherapy after secondary cytoreductive surgery in patients with recurrent ovarian cancer: phase III randomized, open-label MITO 35b study, a project of the MITO-MANGO groups. *Int J Gynecol Cancer* **32:** 799–803. doi:10.1136/ijgc-2022-003435

Schwartz PE, Rutherford TJ, Chambers JT, Kohorn EI, Thiel RP. 1999. Neoadjuvant chemotherapy for advanced ovarian cancer: long-term survival. *Gynecol Oncol* **72:** 93–99. doi:10.1006/gyno.1998.5236

Secord AA, Carr BR, Lewin S, Diver E, Ayuk SM, Wang Y, Murphy C, Salutari V, Barquin Gardia A, Galvez Montosa F, et al. 2024. 718MO mirvetuximab soravtansine (MIRV) in recurrent platinum-sensitive ovarian cancer (PSOC) with high folate receptor-α (FRα) expression: results from the PICCOLO trial. *Ann Oncol* **35:** S549–S550. doi:10.1016/j.annonc.2024.08.780

Sellars MC, Wu CJ, Fritsch EF. 2022. Cancer vaccines: building a bridge over troubled waters. *Cell* **185:** 2770–2788. doi:10.1016/j.cell.2022.06.035

Shi T, Zhu J, Feng Y, Tu D, Zhang Y, Zhang P, Jia H, Huang X, Cai Y, Yin S, et al. 2021. Secondary cytoreduction followed by chemotherapy versus chemotherapy alone in platinum-sensitive relapsed ovarian cancer (SOC-1): a multicentre, open-label, randomised, phase 3 trial. *Lancet Oncol* **22:** 439–449. doi:10.1016/S1470-2045(21)00006-1

Shih KK, Chi DS, Barakat RR, Leitao MM Jr. 2010. Tertiary cytoreduction in patients with recurrent epithelial ovarian, fallopian tube, or primary peritoneal cancer: an updated series. *Gynecol Oncol* **117:** 330–335. doi:10.1016/j.ygyno.2010.01.046

Shuqing L, Zhiling Z. 2023. Patients with stage IA ovarian clear cell carcinoma do not require chemotherapy following surgery. *Cancer Med* **12:** 6668–6674. doi:10.1002/cam4.5453

Sia TY, Manning-Geist B, Gordhandas S, Murali R, Marra A, Liu YL, Friedman CF, Hollmann TJ, Zivanovic O, Chi DS, et al. 2022. Treatment of ovarian clear cell carcinoma with immune checkpoint blockade: a case series. *Int J Gynecol Cancer* **32:** 1017–1024. doi:10.1136/ijgc-2022-003430

Son J, George GC, Nardo M, Krause KJ, Jazaeri AA, Biter AB, Hong DS. 2022. Adoptive cell therapy in gynecologic cancers: a systematic review and meta-analysis. *Gynecol Oncol* **165:** 664–670. doi:10.1016/j.ygyno.2022.03.013

Spiliotis J, Halkia E, Lianos E, Kalantzi N, Grivas A, Efstathiou E, Giassas S. 2015. Cytoreductive surgery and HIPEC in recurrent epithelial ovarian cancer: a prospective randomized phase III study. *Ann Surg Oncol* **22:** 1570–1575. doi:10.1245/s10434-014-4157-9

Sugiyama T, Kamura T, Kigawa J, Terakawa N, Kikuchi Y, Kita T, Suzuki M, Sato I, Taguchi K. 2000. Clinical characteristics of clear cell carcinoma of the ovary: a distinct histologic type with poor prognosis and resistance to platinum-based chemotherapy. *Cancer* **88:** 2584–2589. doi:10.1002/1097-0142(20000601)88:11<2584::AID-CNCR22>3.0.CO;2-5

Swisher EM, Lin KK, Oza AM, Scott CL, Giordano H, Sun J, Konecny GE, Coleman RL, Tinker AV, O'Malley DM, et al. 2017. Rucaparib in relapsed, platinum-sensitive high-grade ovarian carcinoma (ARIEL2 part 1): an international, multicentre, open-label, phase 2 trial. *Lancet Oncol* **18:** 75–87. doi:10.1016/S1470-2045(16)30559-9

Tan DS, Kaye S. 2007. Ovarian clear cell adenocarcinoma: a continuing enigma. *J Clin Pathol* **60:** 355–360. doi:10.1136/jcp.2006.040030

Teneriello MG, Tseng PC, Crozier M, Encarnacion C, Hancock K, Messing MJ, Boehm KA, Williams A, Asmar L. 2009. Phase II evaluation of nanoparticle albumin-bound paclitaxel in platinum-sensitive patients with recurrent ovarian, peritoneal, or fallopian tube cancer. *J Clin Oncol* **27:** 1426–1431. doi:10.1200/JCO.2008.18.9548

Tewari D, Java JJ, Salani R, Armstrong DK, Markman M, Herzog T, Monk BJ, Chan JK. 2015. Long-term survival advantage and prognostic factors associated with intraperitoneal chemotherapy treatment in advanced ovarian cancer: a gynecologic oncology group study. *J Clin Oncol* **33:** 1460–1466. doi:10.1200/JCO.2014.55.9898

Tewari KS, Burger RA, Enserro D, Norquist BM, Swisher EM, Brady MF, Bookman MA, Fleming GF, Huang H, Homesley HD, et al. 2019. Final overall survival of a randomized trial of bevacizumab for primary treatment of ovarian cancer. *J Clin Oncol* **37:** 2317–2328. doi:10.1200/JCO.19.01009

Travis LB, Holowaty EJ, Bergfeldt K, Lynch CF, Kohler BA, Wiklund T, Curtis RE, Hall P, Andersson M, Pukkala E, et al. 1999. Risk of leukemia after platinum-based chemotherapy for ovarian cancer. *N Engl J Med* **340:** 351–357. doi:10.1056/NEJM199902043400504

Trimbos JB, Parmar M, Vergote I, Guthrie D, Bolis G, Colombo N, Vermorken JB, Torri V, Mangioni C, Pecorelli S, et al. 2003. International Collaborative Ovarian Neoplasm trial 1 and Adjuvant ChemoTherapy in Ovarian Neoplasm trial: two parallel randomized phase III trials of adjuvant chemotherapy in patients with early-stage ovarian carcinoma. *J Natl Cancer Inst* **95:** 105–112. doi:10.1093/jnci/95.2.105

Tseng JH, Cowan RA, Zhou Q, Iasonos A, Byrne M, Polcino T, Polen-De C, Gardner GJ, Sonoda Y, Zivanovic O, et al. 2018. Continuous improvement in primary debulking surgery for advanced ovarian cancer: do increased complete gross resection rates independently lead to increased progression-free and overall survival? *Gynecol Oncol* **151:** 24–31. doi:10.1016/j.ygyno.2018.08.014

Tyulyandina A, Rumyantsev A, Pokataev I, Nechushkina V, Morhkov K, Sergeev Y, Mochalnikova V, Bulanov A, Stenina M, Tjulandin S. 2019. Phase II study: letrozole maintenance therapy after first-line chemotherapy in patients with advanced serous and endometrioid ovarian cancer. *Ann Oncol* **30:** v418. doi:10.1093/annonc/mdz250.032

van Driel WJ, Koole SN, Sikorska K, Schagen van Leeuwen JH, Schreuder HWR, Hermans RHM, de Hingh IHJT, van der Velden J, Arts HJ, Massuger LFAG, et al. 2018. Hyperthermic intraperitoneal chemotherapy in ovarian cancer. *N Engl J Med* **378:** 230–240. doi:10.1056/NEJMoa1708618

van Meurs HS, Tajik P, Hof MH, Vergote I, Kenter GG, Mol BW, Buist MR, Bossuyt PM. 2013. Which patients benefit most from primary surgery or neoadjuvant chemotherapy in stage IIIC or IV ovarian cancer? An exploratory analysis of the European Organisation for Research and Treatment of Cancer 55971 randomised trial. *Eur J Cancer* **49:** 3191–3201. doi:10.1016/j.ejca.2013.06.013

Van Nieuwenhuysen E, O'Malley D, O'Cearbhaill RE, Moore KN, Hamilton EP, Yeku O, Bouberhan S, Hou JY, Yoo SY, Brouwer-Visser J, et al. 2022. 523MO ubamatamab (REGN4018, MUC16xCD3 bispecific antibody) monotherapy in patients with recurrent ovarian cancer (OC): phase I dose-escalation analysis. *Ann Oncol* **33:** S784. doi:10.1016/j.annonc.2022.07.651

Varga A, Piha-Paul S, Ott PA, Mehnert JM, Berton-Rigaud D, Morosky A, Yang P, Ruman J, Matei D. 2019. Pembrolizumab in patients with programmed death ligand 1-positive advanced ovarian cancer: analysis of KEYNOTE-028. *Gynecol Oncol* **152:** 243–250. doi:10.1016/j.ygyno.2018.11.017

Vasey PA, Jayson GC, Gordon A, Gabra H, Coleman R, Atkinson R, Parkin D, Paul J, Hay A, Kaye SB, et al. 2004. Phase III randomized trial of docetaxel–carboplatin versus paclitaxel–carboplatin as first-line chemotherapy for ovarian carcinoma. *J Natl Cancer Inst* **96:** 1682–1691. doi:10.1093/jnci/djh323

Vergote I, De Wever I, Tjalma W, Van Gramberen M, Decloedt J, van Dam P. 1998. Neoadjuvant chemotherapy or primary debulking surgery in advanced ovarian carcinoma: a retrospective analysis of 285 patients. *Gynecol Oncol* **71:** 431–436. doi:10.1006/gyno.1998.5213

Vergote I, Tropé CG, Amant F, Kristensen GB, Ehlen T, Johnson N, Verheijen RH, van der Burg ME, Lacave AJ, Panici PB, et al. 2010. Neoadjuvant chemotherapy or primary surgery in stage IIIC or IV ovarian cancer. *N Engl J Med* **363:** 943–953. doi:10.1056/NEJMoa0908806

Vergote I, Scambia G, O'Malley DM, Van Calster B, Park SY, Del Campo JM, Meier W, Bamias A, Colombo N, Wenham RM, et al. 2019. Trebananib or placebo plus carboplatin and paclitaxel as first-line treatment for advanced ovarian cancer (TRINOVA-3/ENGOT-ov2/GOG-3001): a randomised, double-blind, phase 3 trial. *Lancet Oncol* **20:** 862–876. doi:10.1016/S1470-2045(19)30178-0

Vizzielli G, Giudice MT, Nardelli F, Costantini B, Salutari V, Inzani FS, Zannoni GF, Chiantera V, Di Giorgio A, Pacelli F, et al. 2024. Pressurized intraperitoneal aerosol chemotherapy (PIPAC) applied to platinum-resistant recurrence of ovarian tumor: a single-institution experience (ID: PARROT trial). *Ann Surg Oncol* **31:** 1207–1216. doi:10.1245/s10434-023-14648-0

Walker JL, Brady MF, Wenzel L, Fleming GF, Huang HQ, DiSilvestro PA, Fujiwara K, Alberts DS, Zheng W, Tewari KS, et al. 2019. Randomized trial of intravenous versus intraperitoneal chemotherapy plus bevacizumab in advanced ovarian carcinoma: an NRG oncology/gynecologic oncology group study. *J Clin Oncol* **37:** 1380–1390. doi:10.1200/JCO.18.01568

Westin S, Michael V, Fellman B, Meyer L, Taylor T, Alvarado T, Grinsfelder M, Fleming N, Shafer A, Cobb L, et al. 2023. Now: neoadjuvant olaparib window trial in patients with newly diagnosed *BRCA* mutant ovarian cancer (LBA 1). *Gynecol Oncol* **176:** S2–S3. doi:10.1016/j.ygyno.2023.06.467

Wethington SL, Shah PD, Martin L, Tanyi JL, Latif N, Morgan M, Torigian DA, Rodriguez D, Smith SA, Dean E, et al. 2023. Combination ATR (ceralasertib) and PARP (olaparib) I nhibitor (CAPRI) trial in acquired PARP inhibitor–resistant homologous recombination–deficient ovarian cancer. *Clin Cancer Res* **29:** 2800–2807. doi:10.1158/1078-0432.CCR-22-2444

Wilson MK, Pujade-Lauraine E, Aoki D, Mirza MR, Lorusso D, Oza AM, du Bois A, Vergote I, Reuss A, Bacon M, et al. 2017. Fifth ovarian cancer consensus conference of the gynecologic cancer intergroup: recurrent disease. *Ann Oncol* **28:** 727–732. doi:10.1093/annonc/mdw663

Winer I, Valshampayan U, Gilbert L, Rosen S, Gandhi S, Wang Y, Du Y, Sun L, Dalal R, Desai M, et al. 2022. Clinical outcomes of ovarian cancer patients treated with the novel engineered cytokine nemvaleukin alfa in combination with the PD-1 inhibitor pembrolizumab: recent data from ARTISTRY-1 (077). *Gynecol Oncol* **166:** S49. doi:10.1016/S0090-8258(22)01295-1

Wong C, Wellman TL, Lounsbury KM. 2003. VEGF and HIF-1α expression are increased in advanced stages of epithelial ovarian cancer. *Gynecol Oncol* **91:** 513–517. doi:10.1016/j.ygyno.2003.08.022

Wright AA, Bohlke K, Armstrong DK, Bookman MA, Cliby WA, Coleman RL, Dizon DS, Kash JJ, Meyer LA, Moore KN, et al. 2016. Neoadjuvant chemotherapy for newly diagnosed, advanced ovarian cancer: Society of Gynecologic Oncology and American Society of Clinical Oncology clinical practice guideline. *J Clin Oncol* **34:** 3460–3473. doi:10.1200/JCO.2016.68.6907

Young RC, Walton LA, Ellenberg SS, Homesley HD, Wilbanks GD, Decker DG, Miller A, Park R, Major F Jr. 1990. Adjuvant therapy in stage I and stage II epithelial ovarian cancer: results of two prospective randomized trials. *N Engl J Med* **322:** 1021–1027. doi:10.1056/NEJM199004123221501

Yuan F, Wei SH, Konecny GE, Memarzadeh S, Suh RD, Sayre J, Lu DS, Raman SS. 2021. Image-guided percutaneous thermal ablation of oligometastatic ovarian and non-ovarian gynecologic tumors. *J Vasc Interv Radiol* **32:** 729–738. doi:10.1016/j.jvir.2021.01.270

Zamarin D, Burger RA, Sill MW, Powell DJ Jr, Lankes HA, Feldman MD, Zivanovic O, Gunderson C, Ko E, Mathews C, et al. 2020. Randomized phase II trial of nivolumab versus nivolumab and ipilimumab for recurrent or persistent ovarian cancer: an NRG oncology study [erratum in *J Clin Oncol* **38:** 2702. doi:10.1200/JCO.20.01943]. *J Clin Oncol* **38:** 1814–1823. doi:10.1200/JCO.19.02059

Zhang L, Conejo-Garcia JR, Katsaros D, Gimotty PA, Massobrio M, Regnani G, Makrigiannakis A, Gray H, Schlienger K, Liebman MN, et al. 2003. Intratumoral T cells, recurrence, and survival in epithelial ovarian cancer. *N Engl J Med* **348:** 203–213. doi:10.1056/NEJMoa020177

Zhu JW, Wong F, Szymiczek A, Ene GEV, Zhang S, May T, Narod SA, Kotsopoulos J, Akbari MR. 2023. Evaluating the utility of ctDNA in detecting residual cancer and predicting recurrence in patients with serous ovarian cancer. *Int J Mol Sci* **24:** 14388. doi:10.3390/ijms241814388

Zimmermann M, Bernier C, Kaiser B, Fournier S, Li L, Desjardins J, Skeldon A, Rimkunas V, Veloso A, Young JTF, et al. 2022. Guiding ATR and PARP inhibitor combinations with chemogenomic screens. *Cell Rep* **40:** 111081. doi:10.1016/j.celrep.2022.111081

Zivanovic O, Chi DS, Zhou Q, Iasonos A, Konner JA, Makker V, Grisham RN, Brown AK, Nerenstone S, Diaz JP, et al. 2021. Secondary cytoreduction and carboplatin hyperthermic intraperitoneal chemotherapy for platinum-sensitive recurrent ovarian cancer: an MSK team ovary phase II study. *J Clin Oncol* **39:** 2594–2604. doi:10.1200/JCO.21.00605

Zsiros E, Lynam S, Attwood KM, Wang C, Chilakapati S, Gomez EC, Liu S, Akers S, Lele S, Frederick PJ, et al. 2021. Efficacy and safety of pembrolizumab in combination with bevacizumab and oral metronomic cyclophosphamide in the treatment of recurrent ovarian cancer: a phase 2 nonrandomized clinical trial. *JAMA Oncol* **7:** 78–85. doi:10.1001/jamaoncol.2020.5945

Harnessing Antitumor Immunity in Ovarian Cancer

Katherine C. Kurnit[1] and Kunle Odunsi[1,2]

[1]Department of Obstetrics and Gynecology, University of Chicago, Chicago, Illinois 60637, USA
[2]University of Chicago Medicine Comprehensive Cancer Center, Chicago, Illinois 60637, USA
Correspondence: odunsia@bsd.uchicago.edu

Despite progress in other tumor types, immunotherapy is not yet part of the standard of care treatment for high-grade serous ovarian cancer patients. Although tumor infiltration by T cells is frequently observed in patients with ovarian cancer, clinical responses to immunotherapy remain low. Mechanisms for immune resistance in ovarian cancer have been explored and may provide insight into future approaches to improve response to immunotherapy agents. In this review, we discuss what is known about the immune landscape in ovarian cancer, review the available data for immunotherapy-based strategies in these patients, and provide possible future directions.

Despite multiple approvals of new therapeutic agents in the past 10 years, high-grade serous ovarian cancer remains a leading cause of gynecologic cancer deaths (Siegel et al. 2022). New agents targeting DNA damage repair and angiogenesis have led to improvements in progression-free survival, but only small changes to overall survival have occurred in the recent past (Wu et al. 2018). Immunotherapy has changed the treatment landscape for many solid tumors, including melanoma (Larkin et al. 2019), lung cancer (Reck et al. 2016), and endometrial cancer (Makker et al. 2020), but thus far no immunotherapy agents have been approved specifically for ovarian cancer patients.

In this review, we will discuss the current immune landscape in ovarian cancer with a focus on high-grade serous carcinomas, as these are the most prevalent epithelial ovarian cancer (EOC) subtype and 5-yr survival outcomes remain poor (Peres et al. 2019; Siegel et al. 2022). We will review the literature to date evaluating immunotherapy-based strategies in patients with ovarian cancer, and end with a discussion of future directions that may help guide the development of newer immunotherapy approaches going forward.

TUMOR IMMUNE LANDSCAPE AND RATIONALE FOR IMMUNOTHERAPY

Immunologic destruction of tumors is a multistep, coordinated process that can be modulated or targeted at several critical points to elicit tumor rejection. Immune rejection of ovarian cancer has been demonstrated in many preclinical animal models. Correlative human studies in patients with ovarian cancer also strongly support the

Cite this article as *Cold Spring Harb Perspect Med* doi: 10.1101/cshperspect.a041336

role for immune system involvement in patient outcomes. Several studies by our group and others demonstrate that tumor infiltration by $CD8^+$ T cells (TIL) improves outcomes of EOC patients (Zhang et al. 2003; Curiel et al. 2004; Sato et al. 2005), suggesting that these tumors are immunogenic. A confirmatory large study of more than 5500 EOC patients by the Ovarian Tumor Tissue Analysis (OTTA) consortium (2017) also showed that $CD8^+$ TIL was significantly associated with longer overall survival (2.8, 3.0, 3.8, and 5.1 yr for patients with no, low, moderate, or high levels of $CD8^+$ TIL, respectively). Some translational studies suggest that TIL density may be influenced by genomic subtypes. For example, data show that TIL may be increased in tumors with homologous recombination deficiency and/or *BRCA* alterations (Strickland et al. 2016; Morse et al. 2019; van Wagensveld et al. 2022) and may be lower in tumors with Cyclin E1 amplification (Guo et al. 2019; Lederman 2019; van Wagensveld et al. 2022). Whether these differences in immune microenvironment between these genomic subgroups of ovarian cancer account for differences in survival between genomic subgroups remains yet to be determined (Nakayama et al. 2010; van Wagensveld et al. 2022).

Unfortunately, despite the known tumor infiltration of lymphocytes, efforts to harness the immune system in ovarian cancer have met with limited success. To harness the antitumor immune response, all of the steps in the cancer-immunity cycle must be optimal and include (Chen and Mellman 2013; Odunsi 2017; Kandalaft et al. 2019) (1) generation of sufficient numbers of effector T cells with high avidity recognition of tumor-associated antigens (TAAs), (2) trafficking and infiltration into the tumor, (3) overcoming inhibitory networks in the tumor microenvironment (TME), (4) direct recognition of TAA and generation of an effector antitumor response, and (5) persistence of the antitumor T cells.

B cells have been investigated to a lesser degree, but some studies have similarly demonstrated better outcomes in patients whose tumors demonstrate a greater infiltration of intratumoral or peritumoral B $CD20^+$ B cells (Milne et al. 2009; Nielsen et al. 2012; Gupta et al. 2019). These B cells are often organized into tertiary lymphoid structures (TLSs), which have been proposed to establish a localized immune response. B cells can promote antitumor immunity via several mechanisms. First, they produce isotype-switched antibodies that in some cases recognize extracellular domains on the tumor cell surface, thus redirecting the cytotoxic activity of natural killer (NK) and myeloid cells against tumor cells. Second, they produce cytokines that could create a microenvironment that allows for effector T-cell survival. Third, they are capable of cross-presenting antigens to T cells and, finally, they can provide tonic signals to T lymphocytes, for example, through ICOS ligand, CD80, or CD86. However, other studies have shown a worse prognosis associated with infiltration of $CD19^+$ B cells (Dong et al. 2006; Yang et al. 2013), suggesting a nuanced role of these populations as well. Mirroring our expanding knowledge of T cells, a newer cell population of regulatory B cells (Bregs) has been described (Wei et al. 2016). Defining a specific surface protein for Breg identification has been difficult (Gupta et al. 2019), but some proposed markers include $CD1d^+$, $CD5^+$, or $CD24^{hi}$/$CD38^{hi}$ (Mizoguchi et al. 2002; Garaud et al. 2018; Mohd Jaya et al. 2021). Regardless of the markers present, though, their presence from a functional standpoint is clear, as a subset of B cells has been found to produce several immune-suppressive cytokines, including IL-10 (Mizoguchi et al. 2002; Garaud et al. 2018), consistent with a Breg phenotype. Additionally, Bregs have been shown to convert $CD4^+$ T cells into regulatory T cells (Tregs) in breast cancer (Olkhanud et al. 2011) and lead to an immune-suppressed tumor environment through this mechanism as well. It is clear from these studies that information regarding subpopulations of T cells and B cells is critical to understanding tumor biology and potentially to guiding prognostic discussions and treatment choices. However, finding efficient and clinically relevant methods for characterizing these populations in the clinical setting remains elusive, and these types of analyses currently are limited to the research setting.

An array of studies have also reviewed the role of tumor-associated macrophages. Macrophages make up one, if not the largest, subgroup

 Cite this article as *Cold Spring Harb Perspect Med* doi: 10.1101/cshperspect.a041336

of tumor-infiltrating cells (El-Arabey et al. 2020; Liu et al. 2020). Similar to other tumor types, subpopulations of macrophages with proinflammatory and anti-inflammatory characteristics have been described in ovarian cancer. A meta-analysis of nine studies evaluating the presence of macrophages in ovarian tumors looked at these so-called M1 (proinflammatory) and M2 (anti-inflammatory) populations (Yuan et al. 2017). Patients whose tumors demonstrated a high M1:M2 ratio had improved overall survival. Building on this work more recently, ubiquitin-protein ligase E3 component n-recognin 5 (UBR5) was found to help regulate overall tumor-associated macrophage infiltration in ovarian tumors (Song et al. 2020). This protein is known to be overexpressed in many ovarian cancers and has been associated with poorer prognosis (O'Brien et al. 2008; Bradley et al. 2014). With the loss of UBR5, there was an increased M1 phenotype among tumor-associated macrophages and, ultimately, an improved response to therapy suggesting a relationship between these macrophage populations and treatment response. In general, however, these designations of M1 and M2 macrophage subpopulations are likely oversimplified, and definitions among the studies thus far have varied to some degree. Recent single-cell RNA-seq data in breast cancer showed that it was much more likely that macrophages are present with varying degrees of proinflammatory and anti-inflammatory characteristics, rather than as discrete populations of M1 and M2 macrophages (Azizi et al. 2018). This coexpression of varying pro- and anti-inflammatory markers in macrophages was also supported by data in gliomas (Müller et al. 2017). Nonetheless, these studies of macrophages in ovarian cancer have shown a similar general trend in the relationship between an improved prognosis and a proinflammatory macrophage phenotype that is suggestive of a possible positive prognostic role of these proinflammatory macrophages in ovarian carcinomas (Yuan et al. 2017).

Myeloid-derived suppressor cells (MDSCs) are another well-known immune cell population understood to be associated with immune suppression (Groth et al. 2019) that have been described in ovarian carcinomas (Mabuchi et al. 2021). Local environmental factors such as chronic low-grade inflammation likely contribute to the formation of MDSCs from myeloid progenitor cells (Ostrand-Rosenberg et al. 2020) as well as tumor cells (Ouzounova et al. 2017). While myelocytic and granulocytic MDSCs (m-MDSC and g-MDSC) have protumor functions, the mechanisms by which they promote tumor growth and invasion are not overlapping. Similar to other immune-suppressive immune cells, MDSCs have been associated with poorer prognoses in patients with ovarian cancer (Wu et al. 2017). While data about the specific role of the MDSC subpopulations is more limited in ovarian cancer, data from ovarian cancer patients have shown MDSCs to be present both in ascites (Obermajer et al. 2011) as well as tumor cells (Cui et al. 2013), suggesting that their roles may be relevant in this tumor type as well and further work is needed.

Based primarily on mouse data, tumor-associated neutrophils have been divided into N1 (antitumorigenic) and N2 (immunosuppressive and protumorigenic) populations with distinct transcriptional profiles (Shaul et al. 2016). Normal neutrophils can acquire a suppressor phenotype within ovarian cancer ascites fluid and these were defined as "suppressor neutrophils" (Singel et al. 2019a) to indicate their complete distinctiveness from PMN-MDSC and N2 neutrophils. The acquisition of this suppressor phenotype requires complement signaling, and it can be induced not only by ovarian cancer ascites fluid, but also by malignant effusions from patients with different metastatic cancers, showing the generalizability of the findings (Singel et al. 2019a). Neutrophils may also impact the metastatic potential of premalignant lesions by forming neutrophil extracellular traps (Lee et al. 2019; Singel et al. 2019b). High levels of tumor-associated neutrophils have been associated with a worse prognosis and have been associated with dysfunctional cytotoxicity in CD8 cells and immune evasion (Yang et al. 2020). However, other studies show no prognostic impact (Henriksen et al. 2020). Making this discussion more complicated are the technical considerations of evaluating the presence of neutrophils in tumors. Frozen tumor samples, or even fresh tumors that are not used immediately, may have a loss of neutrophil populations (Price and Dale 1977; Restivo et al. 2022), highlighting the technical error that can impair our ability to objectively evaluate this question.

The roles of other immune cells have also been described. Dendritic cells are important mediators of adaptive and innate immune responses (Ning et al. 2021) and can also be immunogenic (antitumor) or tolerogenic (protumor) (Mabuchi et al. 2021). Dendritic cells are antigen-presenting cells for proinflammatory T cells, but also can invoke immune-suppressive signaling impacting T-cell populations (Ning et al. 2021). In one study, high proportions of lysosomal-associated membrane protein 3 (LAMP3) dendritic cells relative to B-cell infiltration were associated with improved overall survival (Truxova et al. 2018). Survival was increased further when tumors had high proportions of $CD8^+$ T cells as well. NK cells are another population present in many ovarian carcinomas. One study showed that, after $CD8^+$ T cells, $CD56^+$ (NK) cells were the second largest subset of $CD103^+$ tumor-infiltrating immune cells (Webb et al. 2014). However, data are mixed about the prognostic impact of NK cells, and their presence in intrastromal versus intratumoral compartments may have a differing impact on prognosis (Hoogstad-van Evert et al. 2018; Truxova et al. 2018; Nersesian et al. 2021). A recent study showed that a certain subpopulation of NK cells, called decidual NK cells, appears to expand in patients with ovarian cancer, and may aid in the tumor's ability to avoid targeting by the immune system (Gonzalez et al. 2021).

In general, a wide range of immune cells are present within many ovarian tumors. The ratios of certain populations vary between patients and may also vary between metastatic sites. Understanding the unique makeup and interactions of each individual's tumor may help guide a more personalized discussion of prognosis and treatment options in the future, and translational work in this area is ongoing. Trial designs that include biopsies before and on-treatment for a variety of treatment approaches may not only provide insight into the diversity of interpatient tumor immune environments but may also further delineate the impact of different treatment strategies on tumor-immune interactions. Investigations should move beyond traditional immunohistochemistry evaluations of tumors and incorporate more quantitative strategies such as flow cytometry and spatial transcriptomics that allow for more granular comparisons.

IMMUNOTHERAPY

Given the obvious interaction between the host immune system and high-grade serous ovarian cancers, many trials have evaluated the role of various immunotherapy agents in patients with ovarian cancer. The largest class of therapeutics that have been investigated are the immune checkpoint inhibitors, and a summary of select phase 2 and phase 3 data is listed in Table 1. Unfortunately, results from many of these studies have been disappointing. Single-agent immune checkpoint inhibitors have not been investigated in the primary setting but have been investigated in the recurrent setting. Response rates to single-agent anti-PD-(L)1 treatment have largely been below 15% (Disis et al. 2019; Matulonis et al. 2019; Zamarin et al. 2020; Hamanishi et al. 2021). It is notable, however, that some of those patients who did respond to treatment experienced durable responses, akin to many other tumor types. Dual checkpoint inhibitor therapy was slightly more successful in one recent study showing a response rate closer to 30% (Zamarin et al. 2020), although this was not replicated in a second study (Hinchcliff et al. 2021). Of note, the response rates seen with many historical platinum-resistant regimens that are currently considered to be standard of care are very low (Markman et al. 2003; Pujade-Lauraine et al. 2014), so longer durations of response with tolerable toxicity may make immunotherapy regimens reasonable options despite disappointing response rates.

More recently, immune checkpoint inhibitor trials in ovarian cancer have looked at combinations with other agents, frequently cytotoxic regimens. In the primary treatment setting, both avelumab and atezolizumab have been evaluated in phase III clinical trials. These immune checkpoint inhibitors were studied in combination with standard therapy backbones that included carboplatin and paclitaxel (Monk et al. 2021;

Table 1. Select list of completed phase 2 or 3 clinical trials of immune checkpoint inhibitors in patients with epithelial ovarian cancer[a]

References	Design	Arms	Population	Results
Immune checkpoint inhibitor alone				
Ouzounova et al. 2017; Zamarin et al. 2020	Phase 2 Randomized	Nivolumab versus Nivolumab + ipilimumab for four doses followed by nivolumab	Measurable 1–3 prior lines PFI < 12 mo *N* = 100 total	ORR within 6 mo: Nivolumab: 12.2%; combo: 31.4% (combination) with response in 6 mo Odds ratio = 3.28, 85% CI 1.54 not reached Median PFS: 2 versus 3.9 mo; stratified HR 0.53 (95% CI 0.34–0.82)
Obermajer et al. 2011; Matulonis et al. 2019	Phase 2 Single arm	Pembrolizumab	Cohort A: 1–2 prior lines PFI 3–12 mo Cohort B: 4–6 prior lines PFI ≥ 3 mo Cohort A: *n* = 285 Cohort B: *n* = 91	ORR: Cohort A: 7.4% Cohort B: 9.9% Cohort A: PD-L1 ≥ 10: 16.7% Cohort B: PD-L1 ≥ 10: 18.2% Cohort A: PFS: 2.1 mo (2.1–2.2) Cohort B: FPS: 2.1 (2.1–2.6)
Cui et al. 2013; Hamanishi et al. 2021	Phase 3 Randomized	Nivolumab versus Gemcitabine or pegylated liposomal doxorubicin	Platinum-resistant 0–1 lines after becoming platinum-resistant	Median OS: Nivo: 10.1 mo (95% CI 8.3–14.1) versus Chemo: 12.1 mo (9.3–15.3) HR 1.0 (0.8–1.3) Median PFS: Nivo: 2.0 mo (1.9–2.2) versus Chemo: 3.8 mo (3.6–4.2) HR 1.5 (1.2–1.9)
Shaul et al. 2016; Hinchcliff et al. 2021 (Abstract)	Phase 2 Randomized	Tremelimumab for four doses followed by durvalumab (sequential arm) versus Tremelimumab + durvalumab for four doses followed by durvalumab (combination arm)	Platinum-resistant or refractory High-grade serous Unlimited prior lines *N* = 61	Median PFS: Sequential: 1.84 mo (95% CI 1.77–2.17) Combination: 1.87 mo (95% CI 1.77–2.43)

Continued

Table 1. *Continued*

References	Design	Arms	Population	Results
Immune checkpoint inhibitor in combination				
Singel et al. 2019b; Monk et al. 2021	Phase 3 Randomized	Carboplatin + paclitaxel followed by avelumab maintenance versus Carboplatin + paclitaxel + avelumab followed by avelumab maintenance versus Carboplatin + paclitaxel	Newly diagnosed stage III or IV epithelial ovarian cancer Neoadjuvant or primary debulking *N* = 998	Median PFS (IQR): Avelumab maintenance: 16.8 mo (13.5–not reached) Avelumab throughout: 18.1 mo (14.8–not reached) Chemo alone: not reached (18.2–not reached) Stratified HR relative to chemo alone: Avelumab maintenance: 1.43 (95% CI 1.05–1.95) Avelumab throughout: 1.14 (0.83–1.56)
Yang et al. 2020; Moore et al. 2021	Phase 3 Randomized Placebo-controlled	Carboplatin + paclitaxel + bevacizumab + atezolizumab versus Carboplatin + paclitaxel + bevacizumab + placebo	Newly diagnosed stage III or IV ovarian cancer Primary debulking with macroscopic residual disease or plan for neoadjuvant chemotherapy *N* = 1031	Median PFS: Atezolizumab: 19.5 mo Placebo: 18.4 mo HR 0.92 (95% CI 0.79–1.07)
Henriksen et al. 2020; Pujade-Lauraine et al. 2021	Phase 3 Randomized	Avelumab versus Pegylated liposomal doxorubicin + avelumab versus Pegylated liposomal doxorubicin	Platinum-resistant or platinum-refractory disease Up to three prior lines in platinum-sensitive setting; no prior lines in platinum-resistant setting *N* = 566	PFS (95% CI): Combo: 3.7 mo (3.3–5.1) PLD: 3.5 mo (2.1–4.0) Avelumab: 1.9 mo (1.8–1.9) Stratified HR (93.1% CI): Combo: HR 0.78 (0.59–1.24) Avelumab: HR 1.68 (1.32–2.60)
Price and Dale 1977; Liu et al. 2019	Phase 2 Single arm	Nivolumab + bevacizumab	Recurrent EOC 1–3 prior lines within 12 mo from last platinum therapy *N* = 38	ORR: 28.9% (95% CI 15.4–45.9) ORR: 40.0% (95% CI 19.1–64.0) in platinum-sensitive ORR: 16.7% (95% CI 3.6–41.4) in platinum-resistant

Cite this article as *Cold Spring Harb Perspect Med* doi: 10.1101/cshperspect.a041336

Table 1. *Continued*

References	Design	Arms	Population	Results
Ning et al. 2021; Zsiros et al. 2021	Phase 2 Single arm	Pembrolizumab + bevacizumab + oral cyclophosphamide	Recurrent EOC Platinum-resistant or platinum-sensitive with unable to have more platinum $N = 40$	ORR: 47.5% Median PFS: 10.0 mo (90% CI 6.5–17.4)
Truxova et al. 2018; Konstantinopoulos et al. 2019	Pooled phase 1 and phase 2 Single arm	Niraparib + pembrolizumab	Platinum-resistant or unable to have more platinum Up to five prior lines $N = 62$	ORR 18% (90% CI 11–29)

(PLD) Pegylated liposomal doxorubicin, (ORR) objective response rate, (PFS) progression-free survival, (IQR) interquartile range, (HR) hazard ratio, (CI) confidence interval.

[a]"Ovarian cancer" refers to ovarian, fallopian tube, or primary peritoneal cancers.

Moore et al. 2021), with GOG 3015 also including bevacizumab (anti-VEGFR). Unfortunately, neither study found a progression-free survival benefit with the addition of immune checkpoint inhibitor therapy. In the recurrent treatment setting, immune checkpoint blockade has similarly been combined with standard of care cytotoxic chemotherapy. Results of one such study also failed to show a benefit over the standard of care regimens (Pujade-Lauraine et al. 2021). Studies evaluating the addition of newer, targeted therapies to immune checkpoint inhibitors in the recurrent ovarian cancer setting have been somewhat more successful. A phase II trial of bevacizumab with nivolumab showed some success, with a response rate of 40% in patients with platinum-sensitive disease (Liu et al. 2019). However, only 17% of patients with platinum-resistant disease had an objective response rate (Liu et al. 2019), similar to results from the phase Ib study of atezolizumab and bevacizumab (Moroney et al. 2020). Another phase II trial studied the combination of metronomic oral cyclophosphamide, pembrolizumab, and bevacizumab. Low dose of cyclophosphamide was used for its immunomodulatory effects, particularly to selectively target Tregs, as shown in other studies (André et al. 2014). This study demonstrated a response rate of 47.5% with durable responses (Zsiros et al. 2021), findings that are certainly worthy of further investigation. Other studies have combined immune checkpoint inhibitors with novel targeted therapies such as PARP inhibitors or other antiangiogenic drugs (Konstantinopoulos et al. 2019; Zimmer et al. 2019) with only marginally better success. However, many other studies of immune checkpoint inhibitor therapy combinations are ongoing in both the frontline (e.g., NCT03740165, NCT04417192, NCT03522246) and recurrent settings (e.g., NCT05116189, NCT03660826).

In addition to the immune checkpoint inhibitors, newer immunotherapy classes are also under investigation. Multiple studies of a variety of ovarian cancer vaccines have been published (Chow et al. 2020). One phase I/II trial of a peptide-based dendritic cell vaccine for consolidation therapy in patients with recurrent ovarian cancer who were HLA-A2 positive showed promising results (Chu et al. 2012). Dendritic cells were loaded with peptides for human telomerase reverse transcriptase and HER2/NEU, which are found in high proportions of recurrent ovarian cancers, and pan-DR epitope, which binds to the majority of the most common HLA-DRs. Unfortunately, only 11 patients were enrolled and the study was closed early due to issues with the supply of the vaccine. Another pilot study evaluated the use of dendritic cells pulsed with whole-tumor cell lysate in recurrent ovarian cancer patients either alone, with bevacizumab, or with low-dose cyclophosphamide and bevacizumab combined (Tanyi et al. 2018). Although there were only two partial responses, 13 of the 25 patients had stable disease for a median of 14 mo. Vaccines targeting cancer tumor antigens have perhaps been the most successful. Multiple cancer tumor antigen vaccine trials have targeted NY-ESO-1 (Odunsi et al. 2007, 2014; Diefenbach et al. 2008; Sabbatini et al. 2012), with some recurrent ovarian cancer patients showing durable responses. Successes with oncolytic viruses have been modest, with best responses largely restricted to prolonged disease stability (Vasey et al. 2002; Galanis et al. 2010; Kim et al. 2013; Hoare et al. 2018).

More recently, the use of cell therapy in ovarian cancer patients has been explored (Sarivalasis et al. 2021), both through intravenous and intraperitoneal approaches. Given the improved prognosis associated with higher numbers of tumor-infiltrating lymphocytes discussed above, the first studies focused primarily on the use of tumor-infiltrating lymphocytes that are harvested and then reinfused following lymphodepletion. Unfortunately, response rates were fairly limited (Sarivalasis et al. 2021), even after cotreatment with other immune checkpoint inhibitors (Kverneland et al. 2020). More recently, studies have begun investigating engineered T cells, such as engineered T-cell receptor (TCR) or chimeric antigen receptor T (CAR-T) cell therapy. These therapies have largely targeted TAAs. Such antigens include cancer–testis antigens (NY-ESO-1, MAGE-A4), folate receptor α, MUC-1, and HER2. Two cell therapy trials that included patients with ovarian cancer were presented at the European Society for Medical Oncology in 2022.

 Cite this article as *Cold Spring Harb Perspect Med* doi: 10.1101/cshperspect.a041336

The first reported updated data from the SURPASS trial, which evaluated a TCR therapy targeting MAGE-A4 and included multiple ovarian cancer patients. Across all patients included, the objective response rate was 28%, and the disease control rate was 81% (Hong et al. 2022). The second trial was a CAR-T-cell therapy targeting CLAUDIN 6 and a CLAUDIN 6-encoding CAR-T-cell-amplifying RNA vaccine in patients with CLAUDIN 6-positive tumors. Four ovarian cancer patients were included. Among the entire cohort, the objective response rate was 33% and the disease control rate was 67% (Mackensen et al. 2022). Many other studies are ongoing and results in ovarian cancer patients are still limited. A selection of ongoing T-cell therapy clinical trials is listed in Table 2.

POTENTIAL MECHANISMS OF IMMUNE RESISTANCE

The clinical data summarized in the preceding section underscore the amount of information yet to be learned about the role of the immune system in ovarian cancer. Recently, many studies have focused on identifying potential mechanisms for immune resistance in the clinical setting (Macpherson et al. 2020). One of the broadest issues with these analyses is the heterogeneity of ovarian cancer from a molecular standpoint. Based on the Cancer Genome Atlas Research Network (2011) and other large-scale molecular analyses, we now know that even high-grade serous ovarian cancer has diversity from a genomic and transcriptomic standpoint and is not a single, homogenous entity. These diverse molecular subtypes are likely to have differences in immune environments, such as those highlighted above, with tumors that are homologous recombination deficient or Cyclin E1 amplified (Strickland et al. 2016; Guo et al. 2019; Lederman 2019; Morse et al. 2019; van Wagensveld et al. 2022). Setting aside the heterogeneity of ovarian cancer, though, a major barrier to the successful deployment of cancer immunotherapy for ovarian cancer patients is the immunosuppressive TME. Even if large numbers of tumor-specific T cells are generated in patients by an immunotherapy, these T cells might not readily destroy tumor targets in vivo. Some of the dominant immune resistance mechanisms in ovarian cancer include: extrinsic suppression of $CD8^+$ effector cells by Tregs (Curiel et al. 2004; Barnett et al. 2010), metabolic deregulation via tryptophan catabolism by the immunoregulatory enzyme indoleamine-2,3-dioxygenase (IDO) (Okamoto et al. 2005; Inaba et al. 2009; Qian et al. 2009; Godin-Ethier et al. 2011; Hornyák et al. 2018), IL-6 (Kolomeyevskaya et al. 2015), IL-10 (Mustea et al. 2006; Rabinovich et al. 2010), prostaglandin E_2 (PGE_2) (Rask et al. 2006; Qiu et al. 2014; Bronger et al. 2016), and vascular endothelial growth factor (VEGF) (Zhang et al. 2003; Duncan et al. 2008). Additionally, engagement of T-cell inhibitory receptors such as PD-1 (programmed cell death-1), CTLA-4 (cytotoxic T lymphocyte-associated protein-4), LAG-3 (lymphocyte activation gene-3), TIM-3 (T-cell immunoglobulin and mucin protein-3), and others (reviewed elsewhere, Nirschl and Drake 2013) also can contribute to resistance. Many of these mechanisms also correlate with tumor progression and poor prognosis (Rodriguez et al. 2018). Collectively, this redundant immunosuppressive network facilitates tumor progression by restraining endogenous antitumor immunity and serves as an important obstacle that must be overcome to implement efficacious immunotherapeutic strategies.

Classical checkpoints such as PD-L1 and CTLA-4/B7, as well as other cell surface proteins, including CD40/L, OX40/L, GITR/L, and CD70/CD27, have been shown to be relevant in ovarian cancer (Hamanishi et al. 2007; Ryan et al. 2010; Guo et al. 2014; Lu et al. 2014; Webb et al. 2015, 2016; Tu et al. 2020; Cai et al. 2021). Even when T-cell stimulation and efficient checkpoint blockade are successful, however, the mixed results of immunotherapy studies including cell therapy trials suggest that there may be an element of T-cell exhaustion. Up-regulation of other checkpoints secondary to ongoing stimulation of the TILs may also occur. In preclinical work evaluating $CD8^+$ T cells expressing the cancer–testis antigen NY-ESO-1, up-regulation of the inhibitory molecules PD-1 and LAG3 was associated with decreased T-cell function as measured by levels of IFN-γ and TNF-α production (Matsuzaki et al. 2010).

Table 2. Selection of ongoing CAR-T or TCR-cell therapy trials for ovarian cancer[a] patients in the United States

NCT #	Title	Phase	T-cell therapy	Ovarian cancer population
NCT03318900	T-cell infusion, aldesleukin, and utomilumab in treating patients with recurrent ovarian cancer	1/1b	Leukapheresis, followed by cyclophosphamide, $CD8^+$ T-cell infusion, then utomilumab (monoclonal antibody agonist for the T-cell costimulatory receptor 4-1BB/CD137)	Recurrent high-grade epithelial ovarian cancer; at least one prior line; platinum-resistant; tumor expression of PRAME or COL6A3; specific HLA
NCT03691376	Genetically engineered cells (NY-ESO-1 TCR-engineered T cells and HSCs) after melphalan conditioning regimen in treating patients with recurrent or refractory ovarian, fallopian tube, or primary peritoneal cancer	1	Autologous NY-ESO-1 engineered CD4-TCR CD34 HSC, then autologous NY-ESO-1 CD8 T cells; melphalan	Recurrent epithelial ovarian cancer; tumor positive for NY-ESO-1; specific HLA
NCT03907527	Modified immune cells (autologous CAR-T cells) in treating patients with advanced, recurrent platinum-resistant ovarian, fallopian tube or primary peritoneal cancer	1/1b	PRGN-3005 autologous CAR-T cells	Recurrent ovarian cancer; platinum-resistant
NCT05225363	Modified immune cells (TAG72-CAR-T cells) for the treatment of patients with platinum-resistant epithelial ovarian cancer	1	TAG72 CAR-T cells; fludarabine and cyclophosphamide	Recurrent epithelial ovarian cancer; platinum-resistant; tumor is positive for TAG72
NCT05617755	AB-1015, an integrated circuit T (ICT)-cell therapy in patients with platinum-resistant epithelial ovarian cancer	1	AB-1015 (integrated circuit T cells); fludarabine and cyclophosphamide	Platinum-resistant high-grade serous ovarian[a] cancer; no more than three prior lines
NCT05316129	Infusion of autologous T cells engineered to target FSH receptor in recurrent ovarian cancer	1	Autologous T cells are genetically modified to express a chimeric endocrine receptor targeting the follicle-stimulating hormone receptor (FSHCER T cells)	Recurrent high-grade ovarian cancer; tumor is positive for FSH receptor; at least two prior lines and up to six prior lines
NCT04670068	Phase I study of autologous CAR-T cells targeting the B7-H3 antigen in recurrent epithelial ovarian	1	B7-H3 CAR-T cells; fludarabine and cyclophosphamide	Recurrent ovarian cancer; platinum-resistant or refractory; up to four prior lines
NCT03585764	MOv19-BBz CAR-T cells in aFR expressing recurrent high-grade serous ovarian, fallopian tube, or primary peritoneal cancer	1	Lentiviral transduced MOv19-BBz CAR-T cells; with or without fludarabine and cyclophosphamide	Recurrent high-grade serous epithelial ovarian cancer; at least two prior lines; tumor positive for folate receptor α

Continued

Table 2. *Continued*

NCT #	Title	Phase	T-cell therapy	Ovarian cancer population
NCT03054298	CAR-T cells in mesothelin-expressing cancers	1	Lentiviral transduced huCART-meso cells; with or without cyclophosphamide	Persistent or recurrent serous epithelial ovarian cancer
NCT03017131	Genetically modified T cells and decitabine in treating patients with recurrent or refractory ovarian, primary peritoneal, or fallopian tube cancer	1	NY-ESO-1-specific T cells; decitabine and cyclophosphamide	Recurrent ovarian cancer; platinum-resistant or refractory, or if platinum-sensitive at least two lines of therapy; HLA specific
NCT03907852	Phase 1/2 trial of Gavo-cel (TC-210) in patients with advanced mesothelin-expressing cancer	1/2	TC-210 (Gavocabtagene autoleucel, engineered T cells expressing a single-domain antibody that recognizes human mesothelin, fused to the CD3-epsilon subunit); fludarabine and cyclophosphamide; with/without nivolumab and/or ipilimumab	Recurrent serous ovarian cancer; between one and five prior lines; tumor is positive for mesothelin
NCT05451849	A phase 1/2 trial of TC-510 in patients with advanced mesothelin-expressing cancer	1/2	TC-510 (engineered T cells expressing antibody for human mesothelin fused to the CD3-epsilon subunit, and a PD-1: CD28 switch receptor, which is expressed on the surface of the T cell, independently from the TCR); fludarabine and cyclophosphamide	Recurrent serous ovarian cancer; tumor positive for mesothelin; between one and five prior lines

(CAR) Chimeric antigen receptor, (TCR) T-cell receptor.
[a]"Ovarian cancer" refers to ovarian, fallopian tube, or primary peritoneal cancers.

Other studies have supported this idea by demonstrating the expression of LAG-3 cells in ovarian cancer and its models (Huang et al. 2015; Chen et al. 2020; Tu et al. 2020; Whitehair et al. 2020). TIM-3 is also a known marker of immune exhaustion and has been similarly found to be expressed in ovarian tumors (Fucikova et al. 2019; Tu et al. 2020; Niu et al. 2021). Thus, it is possible that concurrent targeting of multiple checkpoints may be beneficial (Lu et al. 2014; Huang et al. 2017), an idea supported by the increased efficacy seen in the doublet arm of the phase II trial of nivolumab and ipilimumab in ovarian cancer patients (Zamarin et al. 2020).

TIGIT is another immune checkpoint that contributes to the immunosuppressive network in HGSOC. It delivers inhibitory signals to T cells by binding to CD155 or CD112, and this can prevent T-cell-mediated tumor elimination (Wu et al. 2019) and sustain immune evasion (Freed-Pastor et al. 2021). TIGIT binds CD155 with the highest affinity, making it the primary ligand for TIGIT. In addition, TIGIT inhibits CD226 (DNAM-1) signaling, and enhances immunosuppression by Tregs. In HGSOC, CD155 and CD112 are highly expressed on tumor cells, APCs, and tumor vasculature (Smazynski et al. 2020). Expression of CD155 and TIGIT is substantially more frequent than expression of PD-

L1 and PD-1 in HGSOC, with elevated CD155 levels detected in immunologically "cold" tumors lacking infiltrating lymphocytes (Smazynski et al. 2020). These results suggest the CD155 and PD-L1 axis represent nonredundant immunosuppressive mechanisms in ovarian cancer. Moreover, the expression of CD155 has been associated with a stem cell–like gene expression signature in tumors and a TIL-deficient phenotype (Miranda et al. 2019).

Tregs, classically defined by expression of $CD4^+$, $CD25^+$, and FOXP3, are associated with an immunosuppressive landscape in ovarian carcinomas and have been associated with poorer survival outcomes and more aggressive tumors (Curiel et al. 2004; Barnett et al. 2010). Recent papers have discussed the importance of the relationship between T-cell populations, with tumors showing high CD8 or CD4 to Treg ratios being associated with the best outcomes (Sato et al. 2005; Knutson et al. 2015). One related study evaluated circulating Tregs and intratumoral Tregs in patients with ovarian cancer and noted that differences occurred in these two Treg populations even within the same patient (Toker et al. 2018). Miyara et al. (2009) reported that human $FoxP3^+$ CD4 T cells were composed of three functionally and phenotypically distinct subpopulations. $CD45RA^+$ FoxP3lo resting/naive Tregs and $CD45RA^-$ FoxP3hi activated/effector Tregs were suppressive, while a $CD45RA^-$ FoxP3lo population was made up of nonsuppressive, non-Tregs. A newer subset of T cells that are $CD25^+$ but $FOXP3^-$ have now also been identified in ovarian cancer patients. The presence of this immune cell population was associated with an exhausted phenotype and improvement in survival outcomes (deLeeuw et al. 2015). In combination, the above findings suggest an even more complex relationship between the tumor itself and the host immune system, with ongoing feedback occurring between the tumor and the host immune system resulting in a dynamic, bidirectional effect. Additionally, a more recent study found that the Tregs present in ovarian tumors had a more highly immunosuppressive phenotype compared to the Tregs found in a cohort of melanoma tumors (Toker et al. 2018). The Tregs in ovarian tumors had a higher surface expression of several surface receptors including PD-1, CD137 (also known as 4-1BB), and ICOS, consistent with a highly activated Treg-high phenotype. In contrast, the Tregs in the melanoma tumors were more consistent with a Treg-low phenotype and showed lower expression of multiple surface markers. Given the differences between responsiveness to immunotherapy between these two tumor types, it has been hypothesized that overcoming the increased immunosuppression related to the highly activated Tregs in ovarian tumors (i.e., blocking the other surface markers such as 4-1BB or ICOS) concurrently with immune checkpoint blockade could improve clinical responses (Toker et al. 2018; Saleh and Elkord 2020). Some preclinical and clinical studies evaluating inhibition of Tregs are underway and suggest this may be feasible in the future (Kurose et al. 2015; Torrey et al. 2017), although available data also suggest that this may be more difficult than initially thought (Zou 2006).

Shifts in tumor immunologic characteristics may also occur during treatment (Chang et al. 2013; Dijkgraaf et al. 2013; Galluzzi et al. 2015; Vankerckhoven et al. 2021; Sun et al. 2022) or in response to biologic changes that occur after metastases (Dötzer et al. 2019; Parvathareddy et al. 2021). Up-regulation of other factors such as TGF-β (Kao et al. 2003; Kobie et al. 2003; Ghiringhelli et al. 2005; Roane et al. 2019), IDO (Inaba et al. 2009; Moon et al. 2015; Amobi-McCloud et al. 2021), and COX2 and PGE_2 (Albu et al. 2017; Hennequart et al. 2017) could potentially diminish responses to immunotherapy. MDSCs appear to induce cancer cells with stem cell–like properties through the production of PGE_2 and increase expression of the immune checkpoint ligand PD-L1 (Komura et al. 2020). MHC I expression loss on tumor cells, leading to the inability of dendritic cells to efficiently present antigen, has also been described (Dhatchinamoorthy et al. 2021). Additionally, the expression of antigens that are initially recognized by the immune system can be lost, particularly those that are not essential for tumor cell survival. This immune sculpting may be more common in tumors with low mutational burdens to start, such as high-grade serous ovarian cancer, or those with fewer immunogenic antigens (Dhatchinamoorthy et al. 2021).

POTENTIAL STRATEGIES FOR IMPROVING IMMUNOTHERAPY SUCCESS

Given the up-regulation of many immunosuppressive factors in ovarian tumors either at baseline or in response to treatment with immunotherapy agents, new combinations of therapies have been proposed. The most robust subset of new combinatorial approaches target T-cell function and frequently include the use of an immune checkpoint inhibitor with another agent that sensitizes the immune system. IDO inhibitors are a rational consideration, given the association between the up-regulation of IDO and increasing immunosuppressive properties discussed above. Although clinical trials of IDO inhibition have not been successful in melanomas, a preclinical study of an IDO inhibitor with paclitaxel in ovarian cancer was promising (Inaba et al. 2009). The combination of an IDO inhibitor with PD-(L)1 blockade, such as pembrolizumab, showed some success in melanoma (Zakharia et al. 2021) and has been proposed as a rational combination in ovarian cancer. OX40 is also a relevant immune checkpoint for ovarian cancer. The combination of a TGF-β inhibitor and an OX40 agonist has been studied in preclinical models of breast cancer (Inaba et al. 2009), and may represent a potentially relevant combination for ovarian cancers. Similarly, as TGF-β has been hypothesized to contribute to resistance to immune checkpoint inhibition, other TGF-β inhibitors given in combination with immune checkpoint blockade have also been explored preclinically with some promising results (de Streel et al. 2020; Martin et al. 2020).

Given the immunosuppressive role of Tregs, some studies have specifically focused on targeting Tregs. Several trials evaluated the use of low-dose cyclophosphamide with the goal of modulating the tumor immune environment, as this had previously been shown to be associated with a reduction in Treg populations (Lutsiak et al. 2005). Unfortunately, other studies have not been able to confirm these findings (Chu et al. 2012; Vermeij et al. 2012; Ning et al. 2021). The involvement of CCR4 and CCR4-associated chemokines, TARC/CCL17 and MDC/CCL22, for $FoxP3^+$ Tregs migration has been documented (Sugiyama et al. 2013), and this has prompted clinical studies of antihuman CCR4 mAb in other solid tumors (Sugiyama et al. 2013). Targeting of certain immune checkpoints such as CTLA-4, GITR, and the T-cell costimulatory OX40 has also been associated with the suppression of Treg populations (Wing et al. 2008; Simpson et al. 2013; Zhang et al. 2018; Tanaka and Sakaguchi 2019; Amoozgar et al. 2021). However, most of this work has been performed in tumor types other than ovarian cancer, and further research in ovarian tumors is needed.

Given the baseline immune cell infiltrates present in many ovarian tumors, finding ways to capitalize on what may already be an immune-primed environment could be critical. After lysis of the cell membrane, there is known to be a rapid increase in TAAs available for presentation to T cells. In a primed immune environment, this may create strong antitumor activity. Using the knowledge that luteinizing hormone-releasing hormone (LHRH) receptor is up-regulated in ovarian cancer (Westphalen et al. 2000), the use of a lytic peptide-based agent attached to the LHRH ligand (EP-100) was, therefore, evaluated as a single agent and in combination with an anti-PD-1 agent in preclinical models. In this study, the use of EP-100 with PD-L1 blockade increased antitumor efficacy in preclinical ovarian cancer models (Kim et al. 2020). Additionally, analyses of immune cell profiles after treatment showed a more pronounced decrease in the number of Tregs and monocytic MDSCs, and an increased number of NK cells when mice were treated with the combination therapy (Kim et al. 2020), supporting the hypothesized rationale. A selection of the recently proposed immunotherapy approaches is summarized in Table 3.

Non-T-cell-based therapies have also been explored. Tumor-associated macrophages are an immunosuppressive population found in tumor cells, and research is similarly being done to evaluate strategies for overcoming this mechanism (Pathria et al. 2019; Schweer et al. 2022). One historical approach to targeting tumor-associated macrophages in ovarian cancer has been through the use of IFN-γ (Pujade-Lauraine et al. 1996; Windbichler et al. 2000), although this was ultimately not found to be a successful approach in

Table 3. Selection of proposed new immunotherapy approaches for ovarian cancer patients

Immune modulator	Second agent	References
Immunotherapy approaches		
IDO inhibitor	Paclitaxel	Tanyi et al. 2018
IDO inhibitor	Anti-PD-(L)1	Chu et al. 2012; Odunsi et al. 2014; Tanyi et al. 2018; Zimmer et al. 2019; Chow et al. 2020; Smazynski et al. 2020
OX-40		Zou 2006; deLeeuw et al. 2015; Kurose et al. 2015; Torrey et al. 2017; Saleh and Elkord 2020
OX-40	TGF-β	Tanyi et al. 2018
TGF-β	Anti-PD-(L)1	Knutson et al. 2015; Miranda et al. 2019
GITR		Zou 2006; deLeeuw et al. 2015; Kurose et al. 2015; Torrey et al. 2017; Saleh and Elkord 2020
Anti-PD-(L)1	EP-100	Vankerckhoven et al. 2021
Toll-like receptor agonists		Roane et al. 2019
CSF-1R inhibitors		Kao et al. 2003
CD47/SIRP-α		Kobie et al. 2003
Possible new cell therapy targets		
MUC16 (CA-125)		Dhatchinamoorthy et al. 2021
IDO1		Dhatchinamoorthy et al. 2021
FOLR1		Dhatchinamoorthy et al. 2021
EYA2		Dhatchinamoorthy et al. 2021

ovarian cancer patients in a phase III trial (Alberts et al. 2008). Newer strategies for targeting tumor-associated macrophages include Toll-like receptor agonists (promote macrophage activation, specifically with an M1 phenotype) (Kang et al. 2021), CSF-1R inhibition (blocks differentiation into the M2 phenotype) (Moughon et al. 2015), and CD47/SIRP-α (blocks avoidance of macrophage phagocytosis) (Sikic et al. 2019), but the longer-term clinical success of these strategies remains to be seen. Last, therapies targeting MDSCs have also been proposed (Li et al. 2021; Mabuchi et al. 2021). However, unlike other immune cell populations, there is not currently an effective inhibitor of human MDSCs available, likely because MDSCs represent a diverse subset of cell populations with differing roles. Studies evaluating low-dose chemotherapy have shown some benefits in reducing MDSC populations (one study showed a reduction in only gMDSC, the other study showed a reduction in both gMDSC and mMDSC) (Vincent et al. 2010; Eriksson et al. 2016), although the effect was not always consistent (Iida et al. 2017). In general, despite limited success thus far, there is great interest in identifying strategies that target these other immune cell populations.

As MHC loss of tumor cells has been described as a mechanism for avoiding immune cell recognition, overcoming this loss may be beneficial to improving the success of immunotherapy agents (Dhatchinamoorthy et al. 2021). Frequently, the loss of MHC expression may be due to epigenetic changes. These changes may be able to be overcome by interventions such as reversing epigenetic changes with the use of demethylating agents, histone deacetylase inhibitors, or blocking miRNAs, which may be serving to silence the transcription of these proteins (Dhatchinamoorthy et al. 2021). One preclinical study showed that treatment with epigenetic modulation increased the expression of MHC II pathway components on tumor cells (Turner et al. 2017). As such, a recent preclinical study evaluated the combinations of epigenetic modification and immune checkpoint blockade in preclinical models. However, the authors found no improvement in response, suggesting these pathways and interactions are complex and additional work is needed (Moufarrij et al. 2020).

It is also possible that better antigens may be able to be targeted for cell therapy trials. A 2017 study characterized the peptides that are most commonly associated with HLA molecules in epithelial ovarian cancer (i.e., immunopeptidome). This study demonstrated that the most common targets to date did not necessarily have the highest HLA expression rates (Schuster et al. 2017). Not surprisingly, MUC16 (CA-125) showed the largest differential relative to benign tubal and ovarian tissue, suggesting that this might be a prime future target. Other antigens were also identified, including IDO1, FOLR1, and EYA2. Some commonly seen antigens, such as WT-1, TP53, and mesothelin were identified but not exclusive to ovarian cancer (Schuster et al. 2017; Ning et al. 2021). This latter antigen is particularly interesting as it is a known ligand for MUC16. Folate receptor has also been identified as a potential target (Peoples et al. 1998). Additionally, pairing these cell therapy trials with immune checkpoint inhibitors may also improve efficacy (Matsuzaki et al. 2010; Ning et al. 2021).

CONCLUSION

Although immunotherapy for the treatment of ovarian cancer has been disappointing to date, it is a tumor type ripe for further development. As our understanding of the molecular heterogeneity of ovarian cancer increases, our ability to consider these molecular subtypes as distinct entities and ultimately correlate these findings with the immune microenvironment will also improve. By harnessing our rapidly expanding scientific understanding of the immune microenvironment of epithelial ovarian carcinomas and building on the successes and shortcomings of treatment strategies thus far, we are optimistic that the next decade will usher in new, durable approaches for patients with this devastating disease.

REFERENCES

Alberts DS, Marth C, Alvarez RD, Johnson G, Bidzinski M, Kardatzke DR, Bradford WZ, Loutit J, Kirn DH, Clouser MC, et al. 2008. Randomized phase 3 trial of interferon γ-1b plus standard carboplatin/paclitaxel versus carboplatin/paclitaxel alone for first-line treatment of advanced ovarian and primary peritoneal carcinomas: results from a prospectively designed analysis of progression-free survival. *Gynecol Oncol* **109:** 174–181. doi:10.1016/j.ygyno.2008.01.005

Albu DI, Wang Z, Huang KC, Wu J, Twine N, Leacu S, Ingersoll C, Parent L, Lee W, Liu D, et al. 2017. EP4 antagonism by E7046 diminishes Myeloid immunosuppression and synergizes with Treg-reducing IL-2-diphtheria toxin fusion protein in restoring anti-tumor immunity. *Oncoimmunology* **6:** e1338239. doi:10.1080/2162402X.2017.1338239

Amobi-McCloud A, Muthuswamy R, Battaglia S, Yu H, Liu T, Wang J, Putluri V, Singh PK, Qian F, Huang RY, et al. 2021. IDO1 expression in ovarian cancer induces PD-1 in T cells via aryl hydrocarbon receptor activation. *Front Immunol* **12:** 678999. doi:10.3389/fimmu.2021.678999

Amoozgar Z, Kloepper J, Ren J, Tay RE, Kazer SW, Kiner E, Krishnan S, Posada JM, Ghosh M, Mamessier E, et al. 2021. Targeting Treg cells with GITR activation alleviates resistance to immunotherapy in murine glioblastomas. *Nat Commun* **12:** 2582. doi:10.1038/s41467-021-22885-8

André N, Carré M, Pasquier E. 2014. Metronomics: towards personalized chemotherapy? *Nat Rev Clin Oncol* **11:** 413–431. doi:10.1038/nrclinonc.2014.89

Azizi E, Carr AJ, Plitas G, Cornish AE, Konopacki C, Prabhakaran S, Nainys J, Wu K, Kiseliovas V, Setty M, et al. 2018. Single-cell map of diverse immune phenotypes in the breast tumor microenvironment. *Cell* **174:** 1293–1308.e36. doi:10.1016/j.cell.2018.05.060

Barnett JC, Bean SM, Whitaker RS, Kondoh E, Baba T, Fujii S, Marks JR, Dressman HK, Murphy SK, Berchuck A. 2010. Ovarian cancer tumor infiltrating T-regulatory (T_{reg}) cells are associated with a metastatic phenotype. *Gynecol Oncol* **116:** 556–562. doi:10.1016/j.ygyno.2009.11.020

Bradley A, Zheng H, Ziebarth A, Sakati W, Branham-O'Connor M, Blumer JB, Liu Y, Kistner-Griffin E, Rodriguez-Aguayo C, Lopez-Berestein G, et al. 2014. EDD enhances cell survival and cisplatin resistance and is a therapeutic target for epithelial ovarian cancer. *Carcinogenesis* **35:** 1100–1109. doi:10.1093/carcin/bgt489

Bronger H, Singer J, Windmüller C, Reuning U, Zech D, Delbridge C, Dorn J, Kiechle M, Schmalfeldt B, Schmitt M, et al. 2016. CXCL9 and CXCL10 predict survival and are regulated by cyclooxygenase inhibition in advanced serous ovarian cancer. *Br J Cancer* **115:** 553–563. doi:10.1038/bjc.2016.172

Cai Z, Ang X, Xu Z, Li S, Zhang J, Pei C, Zhou F. 2021. A pan-cancer study of PD-1 and CTLA-4 as therapeutic targets. *Transl Cancer Res* **10:** 3993–4001. doi:10.21037/tcr-21-561

Cancer Genome Atlas Research Network. 2011. Integrated genomic analyses of ovarian carcinoma. *Nature* **474:** 609–615. doi:10.1038/nature10166

Chang CL, Hsu YT, Wu CC, Lai YZ, Wang C, Yang YC, Wu TC, Hung CF. 2013. Dose-dense chemotherapy improves mechanisms of antitumor immune response. *Cancer Res* **73:** 119–127. doi:10.1158/0008-5472.CAN-12-2225

Chen DS, Mellman I. 2013. Oncology meets immunology: the cancer-immunity cycle. *Immunity* **39:** 1–10. doi:10.1016/j.immuni.2013.07.012

Chen F, Sherwood T, De Costa A, Yee-Toy N, Lung P, Easton A, Sumrow B, Bonvini E, Moore PA. 2020. Immunohistochemistry analyses of LAG-3 expression across different tumor types and co-expression with PD-1. *J Clin Oncol* **38** (Suppl). doi:10.1200/JCO.2020.38.15_suppl.e15086

Chow S, Berek JS, Dorigo O. 2020. Development of therapeutic vaccines for ovarian cancer. *Vaccines (Basel)* **8:** 657. doi:10.3390/vaccines8040657

Chu CS, Boyer J, Schullery DS, Gimotty PA, Gamerman V, Bender J, Levine BL, Coukos G, Rubin SC, Morgan MA, et al. 2012. Phase I/II randomized trial of dendritic cell vaccination with or without cyclophosphamide for consolidation therapy of advanced ovarian cancer in first or second remission. *Cancer Immunol Immunother* **61:** 629–641. doi:10.1007/s00262-011-1081-8

Cui TX, Kryczek I, Zhao L, Zhao E, Kuick R, Roh MH, Vatan L, Szeliga W, Mao Y, Thomas DG, et al. 2013. Myeloid-derived suppressor cells enhance stemness of cancer cells by inducing microRNA101 and suppressing the corepressor CtBP2. *Immunity* **39:** 611–621. doi:10.1016/j.immuni.2013.08.025

Curiel TJ, Coukos G, Zou L, Alvarez X, Cheng P, Mottram P, Evdemon-Hogan M, Conejo-Garcia JR, Zhang L, Burow M, et al. 2004. Specific recruitment of regulatory T cells in ovarian carcinoma fosters immune privilege and predicts reduced survival. *Nat Med* **10:** 942–949. doi:10.1038/nm1093

deLeeuw RJ, Kroeger DR, Kost SE, Chang PP, Webb JR, Nelson BH. 2015. CD25 identifies a subset of $CD4^{+}FoxP3^{-}$ TIL that are exhausted yet prognostically favorable in human ovarian cancer. *Cancer Immunol Res* **3:** 245–253. doi:10.1158/2326-6066.CIR-14-0146

de Streel G, Bertrand C, Chalon N, Liénart S, Bricard O, Lecomte S, Devreux J, Gaignage M, De Boeck G, Mariën L, et al. 2020. Selective inhibition of TGF-β1 produced by GARP-expressing Tregs overcomes resistance to PD-1/PD-L1 blockade in cancer. *Nat Commun* **11:** 4545. doi:10.1038/s41467-020-17811-3

Dhatchinamoorthy K, Colbert JD, Rock KL. 2021. Cancer immune evasion through loss of MHC class I antigen presentation. *Front Immunol* **12:** 636568. doi:10.3389/fimmu.2021.636568

Diefenbach CS, Gnjatic S, Sabbatini P, Aghajanian C, Hensley ML, Spriggs DR, Iasonos A, Lee H, Dupont B, Pezzulli S, et al. 2008. Safety and immunogenicity study of NY-ESO-1b peptide and montanide ISA-51 vaccination of patients with epithelial ovarian cancer in high-risk first remission. *Clin Cancer Res* **14:** 2740–2748. doi:10.1158/1078-0432.CCR-07-4619

Dijkgraaf EM, Heusinkveld M, Tummers B, Vogelpoel LT, Goedemans R, Jha V, Nortier JW, Welters MJ, Kroep JR, van der Burg SH. 2013. Chemotherapy alters monocyte differentiation to favor generation of cancer-supporting M2 macrophages in the tumor microenvironment. *Cancer Res* **73:** 2480–2492. doi:10.1158/0008-5472.CAN-12-3542

Disis ML, Taylor MH, Kelly K, Beck JT, Gordon M, Moore KM, Patel MR, Chaves J, Park H, Mita AC, et al. 2019. Efficacy and safety of avelumab for patients with recurrent or refractory ovarian cancer: phase 1b results from the JAVELIN solid tumor trial. *JAMA Oncol* **5:** 393–401. doi:10.1001/jamaoncol.2018.6258

Dong HP, Elstrand MB, Holth A, Silins I, Berner A, Trope CG, Davidson B, Risberg B. 2006. NK- and B-cell infiltration correlates with worse outcome in metastatic ovarian carcinoma. *Am J Clin Pathol* **125:** 451–458. doi:10.1309/15B66DQMFYYM78CJ

Dötzer K, Schlüter F, Schoenberg MB, Bazhin AV, von Koch FE, Schnelzer A, Anthuber S, Grab D, Czogalla B, Burges A, et al. 2019. Immune heterogeneity between primary tumors and corresponding metastatic lesions and response to platinum therapy in primary ovarian cancer. *Cancers (Basel)* **11:** 1250. doi:10.3390/cancers11091250

Duncan TJ, Al-Attar A, Rolland P, Scott IV, Deen S, Liu DT, Spendlove I, Durrant LG. 2008. Vascular endothelial growth factor expression in ovarian cancer: a model for targeted use of novel therapies? *Clin Cancer Res* **14:** 3030–3035. doi:10.1158/1078-0432.CCR-07-1888

El-Arabey AA, Denizli M, Kanlikilicer P, Bayraktar R, Ivan C, Rashed M, Kabil N, Ozpolat B, Calin GA, Salama SA, et al. 2020. GATA3 as a master regulator for interactions of tumor-associated macrophages with high-grade serous ovarian carcinoma. *Cell Signal* **68:** 109539. doi:10.1016/j.cellsig.2020.109539

Eriksson E, Wenthe J, Irenaeus S, Loskog A, Ullenhag G. 2016. Gemcitabine reduces MDSCs, tregs and TGFβ-1 while restoring the teff/treg ratio in patients with pancreatic cancer. *J Transl Med* **14:** 282. doi:10.1186/s12967-016-1037-z

Freed-Pastor WA, Lambert LJ, Ely ZA, Pattada NB, Bhutkar A, Eng G, Mercer KL, Garcia AP, Lin L, Rideout WM 3rd, et al. 2021. The CD155/TIGIT axis promotes and maintains immune evasion in neoantigen-expressing pancreatic cancer. *Cancer Cell* **39:** 1342–1360.e14. doi:10.1016/j.ccell.2021.07.007

Fucikova J, Rakova J, Hensler M, Kasikova L, Belicova L, Hladikova K, Truxova I, Skapa P, Laco J, Pecen L, et al. 2019. TIM-3 dictates functional orientation of the immune infiltrate in ovarian cancer. *Clin Cancer Res* **25:** 4820–4831. doi:10.1158/1078-0432.CCR-18-4175

Galanis E, Hartmann LC, Cliby WA, Long HJ, Peethambaram PP, Barrette BA, Kaur JS, Haluska PJ Jr, Aderca I, Zollman PJ, et al. 2010. Phase I trial of intraperitoneal administration of an oncolytic measles virus strain engineered to express carcinoembryonic antigen for recurrent ovarian cancer. *Cancer Res* **70:** 875–882. doi:10.1158/0008-5472.CAN-09-2762

Galluzzi L, Buqué A, Kepp O, Zitvogel L, Kroemer G. 2015. Immunological effects of conventional chemotherapy and targeted anticancer agents. *Cancer Cell* **28:** 690–714. doi:10.1016/j.ccell.2015.10.012

Garaud S, Taher TE, Debant M, Burgos M, Melayah S, Berthou C, Parikh K, Pers JO, Luque-Paz D, Chiocchia G, et al. 2018. CD5 expression promotes IL-10 production through activation of the MAPK/Erk pathway and upregulation of TRPC1 channels in B lymphocytes. *Cell Mol Immunol* **15:** 158–170. doi:10.1038/cmi.2016.42

Ghiringhelli F, Ménard C, Terme M, Flament C, Taieb J, Chaput N, Puig PE, Novault S, Escudier B, Vivier E, et al. 2005. $CD4^{+}$ $CD25^{+}$ regulatory T cells inhibit natural killer cell functions in a transforming growth factor-β-dependent manner. *J Exp Med* **202:** 1075–1085. doi:10.1084/jem.20051511

Godin-Ethier J, Hanafi LA, Piccirillo CA, Lapointe R. 2011. Indoleamine 2,3-dioxygenase expression in human cancers: clinical and immunologic perspectives. *Clin Cancer Res* **17:** 6985–6991. doi:10.1158/1078-0432.CCR-11-1331

Gonzalez VD, Huang YW, Delgado-Gonzalez A, Chen SY, Donoso K, Sachs K, Gentles AJ, Allard GM, Kolahi KS, Howitt BE, et al. 2021. High-grade serous ovarian tumor cells modulate NK cell function to create an immune-tolerant microenvironment. *Cell Rep* **36:** 109632. doi:10.1016/j.celrep.2021.109632

Groth C, Hu X, Weber R, Fleming V, Altevogt P, Utikal J, Umansky V. 2019. Immunosuppression mediated by myeloid-derived suppressor cells (MDSCs) during tumour progression. *Br J Cancer* **120:** 16–25. doi:10.1038/s41416-018-0333-1

Guo Z, Wang X, Cheng D, Xia Z, Luan M, Zhang S. 2014. PD-1 blockade and OX40 triggering synergistically protects against tumor growth in a murine model of ovarian cancer. *PLoS ONE* **9:** e89350. doi:10.1371/journal.pone.0089350

Guo T, Li B, Gu C, Chen X, Han M, Liu X, Xu C. 2019. PGC-1α inhibits polyamine metabolism in Cyclin E1-driven ovarian cancer. *Cancer Med* **8:** 7754–7761. doi:10.1002/cam4.2637

Gupta P, Chen C, Chaluvally-Raghavan P, Pradeep S. 2019. B cells as an immune-regulatory signature in ovarian cancer. *Cancers (Basel)* **11:** 894. doi:10.3390/cancers11070894

Hamanishi J, Mandai M, Iwasaki M, Okazaki T, Tanaka Y, Yamaguchi K, Higuchi T, Yagi H, Takakura K, Minato N, et al. 2007. Programmed cell death 1 ligand 1 and tumor-infiltrating CD8$^+$ T lymphocytes are prognostic factors of human ovarian cancer. *Proc Natl Acad Sci* **104:** 3360–3365. doi:10.1073/pnas.0611533104

Hamanishi J, Takeshima N, Katsumata N, Ushijima K, Kimura T, Takeuchi S, Matsumoto K, Ito K, Mandai M, Nakai H, et al. 2021. Nivolumab versus gemcitabine or pegylated liposomal doxorubicin for patients with platinum-resistant ovarian cancer: open-label, randomized trial in Japan (NINJA). *J Clin Oncol* **39:** 3671–3681. doi:10.1200/JCO.21.00334

Hennequart M, Pilotte L, Cane S, Hoffmann D, Stroobant V, Plaen E, Van den Eynde BJ. 2017. Constitutive IDO1 expression in human tumors is driven by cyclooxygenase-2 and mediates intrinsic immune resistance. *Cancer Immunol Res* **5:** 695–709. doi:10.1158/2326-6066.CIR-16-0400

Henriksen JR, Nederby L, Donskov F, Waldstrøm M, Adimi P, Jakobsen A, Steffensen KD. 2020. Prognostic significance of baseline T cells, B cells and neutrophil-lymphocyte ratio (NLR) in recurrent ovarian cancer treated with chemotherapy. *J Ovarian Res* **13:** 59. doi:10.1186/s13048-020-00661-4

Hinchcliff E, Patel A, Fellman B, Westin S, Sood A, Soliman P, Shafer A, Meyer L, Fleming N, Bathala T, et al. 2021. Randomized phase II trial of durvalumab (anti-PDL1) and tremelimumab (anti-CTLA4) administered in combination versus sequentially for the treatment of recurrent platinum-resistant non-clear cell ovarian cancer (NCT03026062). *Gynecol Oncol* **162:** S39. doi:10.1016/S0090-8258(21)00718-6

Hoare J, Campbell N, Carapuça E. 2018. Oncolytic virus immunotherapies in ovarian cancer: moving beyond adenoviruses. *Porto Biomed J* **3:** e7. doi:10.1016/j.pbj.0000000000000007

Hong DS, Asch A, Calvo E, Zugazagoitia J, Charlson J, Butler MO, Moreno Garcia V, Cervantes A, Van Tine BA, Lawtrence DP, et al. 2022. 735MO updated safety and efficacy from SURPASS, the phase I trial of ADP-A2M4CD8, a next-generation autologous T-cell receptor T-cell therapy, in previously treated patients with unresectable or metastatic tumors. *Ann Oncol* **33:** S879–S880. doi:10.1016/j.annonc.2022.07.861

Hoogstad-van Evert JS, Maas RJ, van der Meer J, Cany J, van der Steen S, Jansen JH, Miller JS, Bekkers R, Hobo W, Massuger L, et al. 2018. Peritoneal NK cells are responsive to IL-15 and percentages are correlated with outcome in advanced ovarian cancer patients. *Oncotarget* **9:** 34810–34820. doi:10.18632/oncotarget.26199

Hornyák L, Dobos N, Koncz G, Karányi Z, Páll D, Szabó Z, Halmos G, Székvölgyi L. 2018. The role of indoleamine-2,3-dioxygenase in cancer development, diagnostics, and therapy. *Front Immunol* **9:** 151. doi:10.3389/fimmu.2018.00151

Huang RY, Eppolito C, Lele S, Shrikant P, Matsuzaki J, Odunsi K. 2015. LAG3 and PD1 co-inhibitory molecules collaborate to limit CD8$^+$ T cell signaling and dampen antitumor immunity in a murine ovarian cancer model. *Oncotarget* **6:** 27359–27377. doi:10.18632/oncotarget.4751

Huang RY, Francois A, McGray AR, Miliotto A, Odunsi K. 2017. Compensatory upregulation of PD-1, LAG-3, and CTLA-4 limits the efficacy of single-agent checkpoint blockade in metastatic ovarian cancer. *Oncoimmunology* **6:** e1249561. doi:10.1080/2162402X.2016.1249561

Iida Y, Harashima N, Motoshima T, Komohara Y, Eto M, Harada M. 2017. Contrasting effects of cyclophosphamide on anti-CTL-associated protein 4 blockade therapy in two mouse tumor models. *Cancer Sci* **108:** 1974–1984. doi:10.1111/cas.13337

Inaba T, Ino K, Kajiyama H, Yamamoto E, Shibata K, Nawa A, Nagasaka T, Akimoto H, Takikawa O, Kikkawa F. 2009. Role of the immunosuppressive enzyme indoleamine 2,3-dioxygenase in the progression of ovarian carcinoma. *Gynecol Oncol* **115:** 185–192. doi:10.1016/j.ygyno.2009.07.015

Kandalaft LE, Odunsi K, Coukos G. 2019. Immunotherapy in ovarian cancer: are we there yet? *J Clin Oncol* **37:** 2460–2471. doi:10.1200/JCO.19.00508

Kao JY, Gong Y, Chen CM, Zheng QD, Chen JJ. 2003. Tumor-derived TGF-β reduces the efficacy of dendritic cell/tumor fusion vaccine. *J Immunol* **170:** 3806–3811. doi:10.4049/jimmunol.170.7.3806

Kang Y, Flores L, Ngai HW, Cornejo YR, Haber T, McDonald M, Moreira DF, Gonzaga JM, Abidi W, Zhang Y, et al. 2021. Large, anionic liposomes enable targeted intraperitoneal delivery of a TLR 7/8 agonist to repolarize ovarian tumors' microenvironment. *Bioconjug Chem* **32:** 1581–1592. doi:10.1021/acs.bioconjchem.1c00139

Kim KH, Dmitriev IP, Saddekni S, Kashentseva EA, Harris RD, Aurigemma R, Bae S, Singh KP, Siegal GP, Curiel DT, et al. 2013. A phase I clinical trial of Ad5/3-Δ24, a novel serotype-chimeric, infectivity-enhanced, conditionally-replicative adenovirus (CRAd), in patients with recurrent ovarian cancer. *Gynecol Oncol* **130:** 518–524. doi:10.1016/j.ygyno.2013.06.003

Kim MS, Ma S, Chelariu-Raicu A, Leuschner C, Alila HW, Lee S, Coleman RL, Sood AK. 2020. Enhanced immunotherapy with LHRH-R targeted lytic peptide in ovarian cancer. *Mol Cancer Ther* **19:** 2396–2406. doi:10.1158/1535-7163.MCT-20-0030

Knutson KL, Maurer MJ, Preston CC, Moysich KB, Goergen K, Hawthorne KM, Cunningham JM, Odunsi K, Hartmann LC, Kalli KR, et al. 2015. Regulatory T cells, inherited variation, and clinical outcome in epithelial ovarian cancer. *Cancer Immunol Immunother* **64:** 1495–1504. doi:10.1007/s00262-015-1753-x

Kobie JJ, Wu RS, Kurt RA, Lou S, Adelman MK, Whitesell LJ, Ramanathapuram LV, Arteaga CL, Akporiaye ET. 2003. Transforming growth factor β inhibits the antigen-presenting functions and antitumor activity of dendritic cell vaccines. *Cancer Res* **63:** 1860–1864.

Kolomeyevskaya N, Eng KH, Khan AN, Grzankowski KS, Singel KL, Moysich K, Segal BH. 2015. Cytokine profiling of ascites at primary surgery identifies an interaction of tumor necrosis factor-α and interleukin-6 in predicting reduced progression-free survival in epithelial ovarian cancer. *Gynecol Oncol* **138:** 352–357. doi:10.1016/j.ygyno.2015.05.009

Komura N, Mabuchi S, Shimura K, Yokoi E, Kozasa K, Kuroda H, Takahashi R, Sasano T, Kawano M, Matsumoto Y, et al. 2020. The role of myeloid-derived suppressor cells in increasing cancer stem-like cells and promoting PD-L1 expression in epithelial ovarian cancer. *Cancer Immunol Immunother* **69:** 2477–2499. doi:10.1007/s00262-020-02628-2

Konstantinopoulos PA, Waggoner S, Vidal GA, Mita M, Moroney JW, Holloway R, Van Le L, Sachdev JC, Chapman-Davis E, Colon-Otero G, et al. 2019. Single-arm phases 1 and 2 trial of niraparib in combination with pembrolizumab in patients with recurrent platinum-resistant ovarian carcinoma. *JAMA Oncol* **5:** 1141–1149. doi:10.1001/jamaoncol.2019.1048

Kurose K, Ohue Y, Wada H, Iida S, Ishida T, Kojima T, Doi T, Suzuki S, Isobe M, Funakoshi T, et al. 2015. Phase Ia study of FoxP3$^+$ CD4 Treg depletion by infusion of a humanized anti-CCR4 antibody, KW-0761, in cancer patients. *Clin Cancer Res* **21:** 4327–4336. doi:10.1158/1078-0432.CCR-15-0357

Kverneland AH, Pedersen M, Westergaard MCW, Nielsen M, Borch TH, Olsen LR, Aasbjerg G, Santegoets SJ, van der Burg SH, Milne K, et al. 2020. Adoptive cell therapy in combination with checkpoint inhibitors in ovarian cancer. *Oncotarget* **11:** 2092–2105. doi:10.18632/oncotarget.27604

Larkin J, Chiarion-Sileni V, Gonzalez R, Grob JJ, Rutkowski P, Lao CD, Cowey CL, Schadendorf D, Wagstaff J, Dummer R, et al. 2019. Five-year survival with combined nivolumab and ipilimumab in advanced melanoma. *N Engl J Med* **381:** 1535–1546. doi:10.1056/NEJMoa1910836

Ledermann JA. 2019. Do increased tumor infiltrating lymphocytes co-existing with homologous recombination deficiency provide clues to enhance immunotherapy of ovarian cancer? *Gynecol Oncol* **153:** 213–214. doi:10.1016/j.ygyno.2019.04.014

Lee W, Ko SY, Mohamed MS, Kenny HA, Lengyel E, Naora H. 2019. Neutrophils facilitate ovarian cancer premetastatic niche formation in the omentum. *J Exp Med* **216:** 176–194. doi:10.1084/jem.20181170

Li K, Shi H, Zhang B, Ou X, Ma Q, Chen Y, Shu P, Li D, Wang Y. 2021. Myeloid-derived suppressor cells as immunosuppressive regulators and therapeutic targets in cancer. *Signal Transduct Target Ther* **6:** 362. doi:10.1038/s41392-021-00670-9

Liu JF, Herold C, Gray KP, Penson RT, Horowitz N, Konstantinopoulos PA, Castro CM, Hill SJ, Curtis J, Luo W, et al. 2019. Assessment of combined nivolumab and bevacizumab in relapsed ovarian cancer: a phase 2 clinical trial. *JAMA Oncol* **5:** 1731–1738. doi:10.1001/jamaoncol.2019.3343

Liu R, Hu R, Zeng Y, Zhang W, Zhou HH. 2020. Tumour immune cell infiltration and survival after platinum-based chemotherapy in high-grade serous ovarian cancer subtypes: a gene expression-based computational study. *EBioMedicine* **51:** 102602. doi:10.1016/j.ebiom.2019.102602

Lu L, Xu X, Zhang B, Zhang R, Ji H, Wang X. 2014. Combined PD-1 blockade and GITR triggering induce a potent antitumor immunity in murine cancer models and synergizes with chemotherapeutic drugs. *J Transl Med* **12:** 36. doi:10.1186/1479-5876-12-36

Lutsiak ME, Semnani RT, De Pascalis R, Kashmiri SV, Schlom J, Sabzevari H. 2005. Inhibition of CD4$^+$25$^+$ T regulatory cell function implicated in enhanced immune response by low-dose cyclophosphamide. *Blood* **105:** 2862–2868. doi:10.1182/blood-2004-06-2410

Mabuchi S, Sasano T, Komura N. 2021. Targeting myeloid-derived suppressor cells in ovarian cancer. *Cells* **10:** 329. doi:10.3390/cells10020329

Mackensen A, Haanen JBAG, Koenecke C, Alsdorf W, Wagner-Drouet E, Heudobler D, Borchmann P, Bokemeyer C, Klobuch S, Smit E, et al. 2022. LBA38 BNT211-01: a phase I trial to evaluate safety and efficacy of CLDN6 CAR T cells and CLDN6-encoding mRNA vaccine-mediated in vivo expansion in patients with CLDN6-positive advanced solid tumours. *Ann Oncol* **33:** S1404–S1405. doi:10.1016/j.annonc.2022.08.035

Macpherson AM, Barry SC, Ricciardelli C, Oehler MK. 2020. Epithelial ovarian cancer and the immune system: biology, interactions, challenges and potential advances for immunotherapy. *J Clin Med* **9:** 2967. doi:10.3390/jcm9092967

Makker V, Taylor MH, Aghajanian C, Oaknin A, Mier J, Cohn AL, Romeo M, Bratos R, Brose MS, DiSimone C, et al. 2020. Lenvatinib plus pembrolizumab in patients with advanced endometrial cancer. *J Clin Oncol* **38:** 2981–2992. doi:10.1200/JCO.19.02627

Markman M, Webster K, Zanotti K, Kulp B, Peterson G, Belinson J. 2003. Phase 2 trial of single-agent gemcitabine in platinum-paclitaxel refractory ovarian cancer. *Gynecol Oncol* **90:** 593–596. doi:10.1016/s0090-8258(03)00399-8

Martin CJ, Datta A, Littlefield C, Kalra A, Chapron C, Wawersik S, Dagbay KB, Brueckner CT, Nikiforov A, Danehy FT Jr, et al. 2020. Selective inhibition of TGFβ1 activation overcomes primary resistance to checkpoint blockade therapy by altering tumor immune landscape. *Sci Transl Med* **12:** eaay8456. doi:10.1126/scitranslmed.aay8456

Matsuzaki J, Gnjatic S, Mhawech-Fauceglia P, Beck A, Miller A, Tsuji T, Eppolito C, Qian F, Lele S, Shrikant P, et al. 2010. Tumor-infiltrating NY-ESO-1-specific CD8$^+$ T cells are negatively regulated by LAG-3 and PD-1 in human ovarian cancer. *Proc Natl Acad Sci* **107:** 7875–7880. doi:10.1073/pnas.1003345107

Matulonis UA, Shapira-Frommer R, Santin AD, Lisyanskaya AS, Pignata S, Vergote I, Raspagliesi F, Sonke GS, Birrer M, Provencher DM, et al. 2019. Antitumor activity and safety of pembrolizumab in patients with advanced recurrent ovarian cancer: results from the phase II KEYNOTE-100 study. *Ann Oncol* **30:** 1080–1087. doi:10.1093/annonc/mdz135

Milne K, Köbel M, Kalloger SE, Barnes RO, Gao D, Gilks CB, Watson PH, Nelson BH, et al. 2009. Systematic analysis of immune infiltrates in high-grade serous ovarian cancer reveals CD20, FoxP3 and TIA-1 as positive prognostic factors. *PLoS ONE* **4:** e6412. doi:10.1371/journal.pone.0006412

Miranda A, Hamilton PT, Zhang AW, Pattnaik S, Becht E, Mezheyeuski A, Bruun J, Micke P, de Reynies A, Nelson BH. 2019. Cancer stemness, intratumoral heterogeneity, and immune response across cancers. *Proc Natl Acad Sci* **116:** 9020–9029. doi:10.1073/pnas.1818210116

Miyara M, Yoshioka Y, Kitoh A, Shima T, Wing K, Niwa A, Parizot C, Taflin C, Heike T, Valeyre D, et al. 2009. Functional delineation and differentiation dynamics of human $CD4^+$ T cells expressing the FoxP3 transcription factor. *Immunity* **30:** 899–911. doi:10.1016/j.immuni.2009.03.019

Mizoguchi A, Mizoguchi E, Takedatsu H, Blumberg RS, Bhan AK. 2002. Chronic intestinal inflammatory condition generates IL-10-producing regulatory B cell subset characterized by CD1d upregulation. *Immunity* **16:** 219–230. doi:10.1016/s1074-7613(02)00274-1

Mohd Jaya FN, Garcia SG, Borras FE, Guerrero D, Chan GCF, Franquesa M. 2021. In vitro characterization of human $CD24^{hi}CD38^{hi}$ regulatory B cells shows CD9 is not a stable breg cell marker. *Int J Mol Sci* **22:** 4583. doi:10.3390/ijms22094583

Monk BJ, Colombo N, Oza AM, Fujiwara K, Birrer MJ, Randall L, Poddubskaya EV, Scambia G, Shparyk YV, Lim MC, et al. 2021. Chemotherapy with or without avelumab followed by avelumab maintenance versus chemotherapy alone in patients with previously untreated epithelial ovarian cancer (JAVELIN Ovarian 100): an open-label, randomised, phase 3 trial. *Lancet Oncol* **22:** 1275–1289. doi:10.1016/S1470-2045(21)00342-9

Moon YW, Hajjar J, Hwu P, Naing A. 2015. Targeting the indoleamine 2,3-dioxygenase pathway in cancer. *J Immunother Cancer* **3:** 51. doi:10.1186/s40425-015-0094-9

Moore KN, Bookman M, Sehouli J, Miller A, Anderson C, Scambia G, Myers T, Taskiran C, Robison K, Mäenpää J, et al. 2021. Atezolizumab, bevacizumab, and chemotherapy for newly diagnosed stage III or IV ovarian cancer: placebo-controlled randomized phase III trial (IMagyn050/GOG 3015/ENGOT-OV39). *J Clin Oncol* **39:** 1842–1855. doi:10.1200/JCO.21.00306

Moroney JW, Powderly J, Lieu CH, Bendell JC, Eckhardt SG, Chang CW, Molinero L, Spahn J, Williams P, Lin YG, et al. 2020. Safety and clinical activity of atezolizumab plus bevacizumab in patients with ovarian cancer: a phase Ib study. *Clin Cancer Res* **26:** 5631–5637. doi:10.1158/1078-0432.CCR-20-0477

Morse CB, Toukatly MN, Kilgore MR, Agnew KJ, Bernards SS, Norquist BM, Pennington KP, Garcia RL, Liao JB, Swisher EM. 2019. Tumor infiltrating lymphocytes and homologous recombination deficiency are independently associated with improved survival in ovarian carcinoma. *Gynecol Oncol* **153:** 217–222. doi:10.1016/j.ygyno.2019.02.011

Moufarrij S, Srivastava A, Gomez S, Hadley M, Palmer E, Austin PT, Chisholm S, Diab N, Roche K, Yu A, et al. 2020. Combining DNMT and HDAC6 inhibitors increases anti-tumor immune signaling and decreases tumor burden in ovarian cancer. *Sci Rep* **10:** 3470. doi:10.1038/s41598-020-60409-4

Moughon DL, He H, Schokrpur S, Jiang ZK, Yaqoob M, David J, Lin C, Iruela-Arispe ML, Dorigo O, Wu L. 2015. Macrophage blockade using CSF1R inhibitors reverses the vascular leakage underlying malignant ascites in late-stage epithelial ovarian cancer. *Cancer Res* **75:** 4742–4752. doi:10.1158/0008-5472.CAN-14-3373

Müller S, Kohanbash G, Liu SJ, Alvarado B, Carrera D, Bhaduri A, Watchmaker PB, Yagnik G, Di Lullo E, Malatesta M, et al. 2017. Single-cell profiling of human gliomas reveals macrophage ontogeny as a basis for regional differences in macrophage activation in the tumor microenvironment. *Genome Biol* **18:** 234. doi:10.1186/s13059-017-1362-4

Mustea A, Könsgen D, Braicu EI, Pirvulescu C, Sun P, Sofroni D, Lichtenegger W, Sehouli J. 2006. Expression of IL-10 in patients with ovarian carcinoma. *Anticancer Res* **26:** 1715–1718.

Nakayama N, Nakayama K, Shamima Y, Ishikawa M, Katagiri A, Iida K, Miyazaki K. 2010. Gene amplification *CCNE1* is related to poor survival and potential therapeutic target in ovarian cancer. *Cancer* **116:** 2621–2634. doi:10.1002/cncr.24987

Nersesian S, Schwartz SL, Grantham SR, MacLean LK, Lee SN, Pugh-Toole M, Boudreau JE. 2021. NK cell infiltration is associated with improved overall survival in solid cancers: a systematic review and meta-analysis. *Transl Oncol* **14:** 100930. doi:10.1016/j.tranon.2020.100930

Nielsen JS, Sahota RA, Milne K, Kost SE, Nesslinger NJ, Watson PH, Nelson BH. 2012. $CD20^+$ tumor-infiltrating lymphocytes have an atypical $CD27^-$ memory phenotype and together with $CD8^+$ T cells promote favorable prognosis in ovarian cancer. *Clin Cancer Res* **18:** 3281–3292. doi:10.1158/1078-0432.CCR-12-0234

Ning F, Cole CB, Annunziata CM. 2021. Driving immune responses in the ovarian tumor microenvironment. *Front Oncol* **10:** 604084. doi:10.3389/fonc.2020.604084

Nirschl CJ, Drake CG. 2013. Molecular pathways: co-expression of immune checkpoint molecules: signaling pathways and implications for cancer immunotherapy. *Clin Cancer Res* **19:** 4917–4924. doi:10.1158/1078-0432.CCR-12-1972

Niu N, Shen W, Zhong Y, Bast RC Jr, Jazaeri A, Sood AK, Liu J. 2021. Expression of B7-H4 and IDO1 is associated with drug resistance and poor prognosis in high-grade serous ovarian carcinomas. *Hum Pathol* **113:** 20–27. doi:10.1016/j.humpath.2021.04.003

Obermajer N, Muthuswamy R, Odunsi K, Edwards RP, Kalinski P. 2011. PGE_2-induced CXCL12 production and CXCR4 expression controls the accumulation of human MDSCs in ovarian cancer environment. *Cancer Res* **71:** 7463–7470. doi:10.1158/0008-5472.CAN-11-2449

O'Brien PM, Davies MJ, Scurry JP, Smith AN, Barton CA, Henderson MJ, Saunders DN, Gloss BS, Patterson KI, Clancy JL, et al. 2008. The E3 ubiquitin ligase EDD is an adverse prognostic factor for serous epithelial ovarian cancer and modulates cisplatin resistance in vitro. *Br J Cancer* **98:** 1085–1093. doi:10.1038/sj.bjc.6604281

Odunsi K. 2017. Immunotherapy in ovarian cancer. *Ann Oncol* **28**(Suppl 8)**:** viii1–viii7. doi:10.1093/annonc/mdx444

Odunsi K, Qian F, Matsuzaki J, Mhawech-Fauceglia P, Andrews C, Hoffman EW, Pan L, Ritter G, Villella J, Thomas B, et al. 2007. Vaccination with an NY-ESO-1 peptide of HLA class I/II specificities induces integrated humoral and T cell responses in ovarian cancer. *Proc Natl Acad Sci* **104:** 12837–12842. doi:10.1073/pnas.0703342104

Odunsi K, Matsuzaki J, James SR, Mhawech-Fauceglia P, Tsuji T, Miller A, Zhang W, Akers SN, Griffiths EA, Miliotto A, et al. 2014. Epigenetic potentiation of NY-ESO-1 vaccine therapy in human ovarian cancer. *Cancer Immunol Res* **2:** 37–49. doi:10.1158/2326-6066.CIR-13-0126

Okamoto A, Nikaido T, Ochiai K, Takakura S, Saito M, Aoki Y, Ishii N, Yanaihara N, Yamada K, Takikawa O, et al. 2005. Indoleamine 2,3-dioxygenase serves as a marker of poor prognosis in gene expression profiles of serous ovarian cancer cells. *Clin Cancer Res* **11:** 6030–6039. doi:10.1158/1078-0432.CCR-04-2671

Olkhanud PB, Damdinsuren B, Bodogai M, Gress RE, Sen R, Wejksza K, Malchinkhuu E, Wersto RP, Biragyn A. 2011. Tumor-evoked regulatory B cells promote breast cancer metastasis by converting resting CD4$^+$ T cells to T-regulatory cells. *Cancer Res* **71:** 3505–3515. doi:10.1158/0008-5472.CAN-10-4316

Ostrand-Rosenberg S, Beury DW, Parker KH, Horn LA. 2020. Survival of the fittest: how myeloid-derived suppressor cells survive in the inhospitable tumor microenvironment. *Cancer Immunol Immunother* **69:** 215–221. doi:10.1007/s00262-019-02388-8

Ouzounova M, Lee E, Piranlioglu R, El Andaloussi A, Kolhe R, Demirci MF, Marasco D, Asm I, Chadli A, Hassan KA, et al. 2017. Monocytic and granulocytic myeloid derived suppressor cells differentially regulate spatiotemporal tumour plasticity during metastatic cascade. *Nat Commun* **8:** 14979. doi:10.1038/ncomms14979

Ovarian Tumor Tissue Analysis (OTTA) Consortium, Goode EL, Block MS, Kalli KR, Vierkant RA, Chen W, Fogarty ZC, Gentry-Maharaj A, Tołoczko A, Hein A, et al. 2017. Dose-response association of CD8$^+$ tumor-infiltrating lymphocytes and survival time in high-grade serous ovarian cancer. *JAMA Oncol* **3:** e173290. doi:10.1001/jamaoncol.2017.3290

Parvathareddy SK, Siraj AK, Al-Badawi IA, Tulbah A, Al-Dayel F, Al-Kuraya KS. 2021. Differential expression of PD-L1 between primary and metastatic epithelial ovarian cancer and its clinico-pathological correlation. *Sci Rep* **11:** 3750. doi:10.1038/s41598-021-83276-z

Pathria P, Louis TL, Varner JA. 2019. Targeting tumor-associated macrophages in cancer. *Trends Immunol* **40:** 310–327. doi:10.1016/j.it.2019.02.003

Peoples GE, Anderson BW, Fisk B, Kudelka AP, Wharton JT, Ioannides CG. 1998. Ovarian cancer-associated lymphocyte recognition of folate binding protein peptides. *Ann Surg Oncol* **5:** 743–750. doi:10.1007/BF02303486

Peres LC, Cushing-Haugen KL, Köbel M, Harris HR, Berchuck A, Rossing MA, Schildkraut JM, Doherty JA. 2019. Invasive epithelial ovarian cancer survival by histotype and disease stage. *J Natl Cancer Inst* **111:** 60–68. doi:10.1093/jnci/djy071

Price TH, Dale DC. 1977. Neutrophil preservation: the effect of short-term storage on in vivo kinetics. *J Clin Invest* **59:** 475–480. doi:10.1172/JCI108662

Pujade-Lauraine E, Guastalla JP, Colombo N, Devillier P, François E, Fumoleau P, Monnier A, Nooy M, Mignot L, Bugat R, et al. 1996. Intraperitoneal recombinant interferon γ in ovarian cancer patients with residual disease at second-look laparotomy. *J Clin Oncol* **14:** 343–350. doi:10.1200/JCO.1996.14.2.343

Pujade-Lauraine E, Hilpert F, Weber B, Reuss A, Poveda A, Kristensen G, Sorio R, Vergote I, Witteveen P, Bamias A, et al. 2014. Bevacizumab combined with chemotherapy for platinum-resistant recurrent ovarian cancer: the AURELIA open-label randomized phase III trial. *J Clin Oncol* **32:** 1302–1308. doi:10.1200/JCO.2013.51.4489

Pujade-Lauraine E, Fujiwara K, Ledermann JA, Oza AM, Kristeleit R, Ray-Coquard IL, Richardson GE, Sessa C, Yonemori K, Banerjee S, et al. 2021. Avelumab alone or in combination with chemotherapy versus chemotherapy alone in platinum-resistant or platinum-refractory ovarian cancer (JAVELIN Ovarian 200): an open-label, three-arm, randomised, phase 3 study. *Lancet Oncol* **22:** 1034–1046. doi:10.1016/S1470-2045(21)00216-3

Qian F, Villella J, Wallace PK, Mhawech-Fauceglia P, Tario JD Jr, Andrews C, Matsuzaki J, Valmori D, Ayyoub M, Frederick PJ, et al. 2009. Efficacy of levo-1-methyl tryptophan and dextro-1-methyl tryptophan in reversing indoleamine-2,3-dioxygenase-mediated arrest of T-cell proliferation in human epithelial ovarian cancer. *Cancer Res* **69:** 5498–5504. doi:10.1158/0008-5472.CAN-08-2106

Qiu X, Cheng JC, Chang HM, Leung PC. 2014. COX2 and PGE2 mediate EGF-induced E-cadherin-independent human ovarian cancer cell invasion. *Endocr Relat Cancer* **21:** 533–543. doi:10.1530/ERC-13-0450

Rabinovich A, Medina L, Piura B, Huleihel M. 2010. Expression of IL-10 in human normal and cancerous ovarian tissues and cells. *Eur Cytokine Netw* **21:** 122–128. doi:10.1684/ecn.2010.0188

Rask K, Zhu Y, Wang W, Hedin L, Sundfeldt K. 2006. Ovarian epithelial cancer: a role for PGE2-synthesis and signalling in malignant transformation and progression. *Mol Cancer* **5:** 62. doi:10.1186/1476-4598-5-62

Reck M, Rodríguez-Abreu D, Robinson AG, Hui R, Csőszi T, Fülöp A, Gottfried M, Peled N, Tafreshi A, Cuffe S, et al. 2016. Pembrolizumab versus chemotherapy for PD-L1-positive non-small-cell lung cancer. *N Engl J Med* **375:** 1823–1833. doi:10.1056/NEJMoa1606774

Restivo G, Tastanova A, Balázs Z, Panebianco F, Diepenbruck M, Ercan C, Preca BT, Hafner J, Weber WP, Kurzeder C, et al. 2022. Live slow-frozen human tumor tissues viable for 2D, 3D, ex vivo cultures and single-cell RNAseq. *Commun Biol* **5:** 1144. doi:10.1038/s42003-022-04025-0

Roane BM, Arend RC, Birrer MJ. 2019. Review: targeting the transforming growth factor-β pathway in ovarian cancer. *Cancers (Basel)* **11:** 668. doi:10.3390/cancers11050668

Rodriguez GM, Galpin KJC, McCloskey CW, Vanderhyden BC. 2018. The tumor microenvironment of epithelial ovarian cancer and its influence on response to immunotherapy. *Cancers (Basel)* **10:** 242. doi:10.3390/cancers10080242

Ryan MC, Kostner H, Gordon KA, Duniho S, Sutherland MK, Yu C, Kim KM, Nesterova A, Anderson M, McEarchern JA, et al. 2010. Targeting pancreatic and ovarian carcinomas using the auristatin-based anti-CD70 antibody-drug conjugate SGN-75. *Br J Cancer* **103:** 676–684. doi:10.1038/sj.bjc.6605816

Sabbatini P, Tsuji T, Ferran L, Ritter E, Sedrak C, Tuballes K, Jungbluth AA, Ritter G, Aghajanian C, Bell-McGuinn K, et al. 2012. Phase I trial of overlapping long peptides from a tumor self-antigen and poly-ICLC shows rapid induction of integrated immune response in ovarian cancer patients.

Clin Cancer Res 18: 6497–6508. doi:10.1158/1078-0432.CCR-12-2189

Saleh R, Elkord E. 2020. Foxp3$^+$ T regulatory cells in cancer: prognostic biomarkers and therapeutic targets. *Cancer Lett* **490:** 174–185. doi:10.1016/j.canlet.2020.07.022

Sarivalasis A, Morotti M, Mulvey A, Imbimbo M, Coukos G. 2021. Cell therapies in ovarian cancer. *Ther Adv Med Oncol* **13:** 175883592110083. doi:10.1177/17588359211008399

Sato E, Olson SH, Ahn J, Bundy B, Nishikawa H, Qian F, Jungbluth AA, Frosina D, Gnjatic S, Ambrosone C, et al. 2005. Intraepithelial CD8$^+$ tumor-infiltrating lymphocytes and a high CD8$^+$/regulatory T cell ratio are associated with favorable prognosis in ovarian cancer. *Proc Natl Acad Sci* **102:** 18538–18543. doi:10.1073/pnas.0509182102

Schuster H, Peper JK, Bösmüller HC, Röhle K, Backert L, Bilich T, Ney B, Löffler MW, Kowalewski DJ, Trautwein N, et al. 2017. The immunopeptidomic landscape of ovarian carcinomas. *Proc Natl Acad Sci* 114: E9942–E9951. doi:10.1073/pnas.1707658114

Schweer D, McAtee A, Neupane K, Richards C, Ueland F, Kolesar J. 2022. Tumor-associated macrophages and ovarian cancer: implications for therapy. *Cancers (Basel)* **14:** 2220. doi:10.3390/cancers14092220

Shaul ME, Levy L, Sun J, Mishalian I, Singhal S, Kapoor V, Horng W, Fridlender G, Albelda SM, Fridlender ZG. 2016. Tumor-associated neutrophils display a distinct N1 profile following TGFβ modulation: a transcriptomics analysis of pro- vs. antitumor TANs. *Oncoimmunology* **5:** e1232221. doi:10.1080/2162402X.2016.1232221

Siegel RL, Miller KD, Fuchs HE, Jemal A. 2022. Cancer statistics. *CA Cancer J Clin* **72:** 7–33. doi:10.3322/caac.21708

Sikic BI, Lakhani N, Patnaik A, Shah SA, Chandana SR, Rasco D, Colevas AD, O'Rourke T, Narayanan S, Papadopoulos K, et al. 2019. First-in-human, first-in-class phase I trial of the anti-CD47 antibody Hu5F9-G4 in patients with advanced cancers. *J Clin Oncol* **37:** 946–953. doi:10.1200/JCO.18.02018

Simpson TR, Li F, Montalvo-Ortiz W, Sepulveda MA, Bergerhoff K, Arce F, Roddie C, Henry JY, Yagita H, Wolchok JD, et al. 2013. Fc-dependent depletion of tumor-infiltrating regulatory T cells co-defines the efficacy of anti-CTLA-4 therapy against melanoma. *J Exp Med* **210:** 1695–1710. doi:10.1084/jem.20130579

Singel KL, Emmons TR, Khan ANH, Mayor PC, Shen S, Wong JT, Morrell K, Eng KH, Mark J, Bankert RB, et al. 2019a. Mature neutrophils suppress T cell immunity in ovarian cancer microenvironment. *JCI Insight* **4:** e122311. doi:10.1172/jci.insight.122311

Singel KL, Grzankowski KS, Khan ANMNH, Grimm MJ, D'Auria AC, Morrell K, Eng KH, Hylander B, Mayor PC, Emmons TR, et al. 2019b. Mitochondrial DNA in the tumour microenvironment activates neutrophils and is associated with worse outcomes in patients with advanced epithelial ovarian cancer. *Br J Cancer* **120:** 207–217. doi:10.1038/s41416-018-0339-8

Smazynski J, Hamilton PT, Thornton S, Milne K, Wouters MCA, Webb JR, Nelson BH. 2020. The immune suppressive factors CD155 and PD-L1 show contrasting expression patterns and immune correlates in ovarian and other cancers. *Gynecol Oncol* **158:** 167–177. doi:10.1016/j.ygyno.2020.04.689

Song M, Yeku OO, Rafiq S, Purdon T, Dong X, Zhu L, Zhang T, Wang H, Yu Z, Mai J, et al. 2020. Tumor derived UBR5 promotes ovarian cancer growth and metastasis through inducing immunosuppressive macrophages. *Nat Commun* **11:** 6298. doi:10.1038/s41467-020-20140-0

Strickland KC, Howitt BE, Shukla SA, Rodig S, Ritterhouse LL, Liu JF, Garber JE, Chowdhury D, Wu CJ, D'Andrea AD, et al. 2016. Association and prognostic significance of BRCA1/2-mutation status with neoantigen load, number of tumor-infiltrating lymphocytes and expression of PD-1/PD-L1 in high grade serous ovarian cancer. *Oncotarget* **7:** 13587–13598. doi:10.18632/oncotarget.7277

Sugiyama D, Nishikawa H, Maeda Y, Nishioka M, Tanemura A, Katayama I, Ezoe S, Kanakura Y, Sato E, Fukumori Y, et al. 2013. Anti-CCR4 mAb selectively depletes effector-type FoxP3$^+$CD4$^+$ regulatory T cells, evoking antitumor immune responses in humans. *Proc Natl Acad Sci* **110:** 17945–17950. doi:10.1073/pnas.1316796110

Sun J, Yan C, Xu D, Zhang Z, Li K, Li X, Zhou M, Hao D. 2022. Immuno-genomic characterisation of high-grade serous ovarian cancer reveals immune evasion mechanisms and identifies an immunological subtype with a favourable prognosis and improved therapeutic efficacy. *Br J Cancer* **126:** 1570–1580. doi:10.1038/s41416-021-01692-4

Tanaka A, Sakaguchi S. 2019. Targeting Treg cells in cancer immunotherapy. *Eur J Immunol* **49:** 1140–1146. doi:10.1002/eji.201847659

Tanyi JL, Bobisse S, Ophir E, Tuyaerts S, Roberti A, Genolet R, Baumgartner P, Stevenson BJ, Iseli C, Dangaj D, et al. 2018. Personalized cancer vaccine effectively mobilizes antitumor T cell immunity in ovarian cancer. *Sci Transl Med* **10:** eaao5931. doi:10.1126/scitranslmed.aao5931

Toker A, Nguyen LT, Stone SC, Yang SYC, Katz SR, Shaw PA, Clarke BA, Ghazarian D, Al-Habeeb A, Easson A, et al. 2018. Regulatory T cells in ovarian cancer are characterized by a highly activated phenotype distinct from that in melanoma. *Clin Cancer Res* **24:** 5685–5696. doi:10.1158/1078-0432.CCR-18-0554

Torrey H, Butterworth J, Mera T, Okubo Y, Wang L, Baum D, Defusco A, Plager S, Warden S, Huang D, et al. 2017. Targeting TNFR2 with antagonistic antibodies inhibits proliferation of ovarian cancer cells and tumor-associated T_{regs}. *Sci Signal* **10:** eaaf8608. doi:10.1126/scisignal.aaf8608

Truxova I, Kasikova L, Hensler M, Skapa P, Laco J, Pecen L, Belicova L, Praznovec I, Halaska MJ, Brtnicky T, et al. 2018. Mature dendritic cells correlate with favorable immune infiltrate and improved prognosis in ovarian carcinoma patients. *J Immunother Cancer* **6:** 139. doi:10.1186/s40425-018-0446-3

Tu L, Guan R, Yang H, Zhou Y, Hong W, Ma L, Zhao G, Yu M. 2020. Assessment of the expression of the immune checkpoint molecules PD-1, CTLA4, TIM-3 and LAG-3 across different cancers in relation to treatment response, tumor-infiltrating immune cells and survival. *Int J Cancer* **147:** 423–439. doi:10.1002/ijc.32785

Turner TB, Meza-Perez S, Londoño A, Katre A, Peabody JE, Smith HJ, Forero A, Norian LA, Straughn JM Jr, Buchsbaum DJ, et al. 2017. Epigenetic modifiers upregulate MHC II and impede ovarian cancer tumor growth. *Oncotarget* **8:** 44159–44170. doi:10.18632/oncotarget.17395

Vankerckhoven A, Baert T, Riva M, De Bruyn C, Thirion G, Vandenbrande K, Ceusters J, Vergote I, Coosemans A. 2021. Type of chemotherapy has substantial effects on the immune system in ovarian cancer. *Transl Oncol* **14:** 101076. doi:10.1016/j.tranon.2021.101076

van Wagensveld L, van Baal JOAM, Timmermans M, Gaillard D, Borghuis L, Coffelt SB, Rosenberg EH, Lok CAR, Nijman HW, et al. 2022. Homologous recombination deficiency and cyclin E1 amplification are correlated with immune cell infiltration and survival in high-grade serous ovarian cancer. *Cancers (Basel)* **14:** 5965. doi:10.3390/cancers14235965

Vasey PA, Shulman LN, Campos S, Davis J, Gore M, Johnston S, Kirn DH, O'Neill V, Siddiqui N, Seiden MV, et al. 2002. Phase I trial of intraperitoneal injection of the *E1B*-55-kd-gene-deleted adenovirus ONYX-015 (dl1520) given on days 1 through 5 every 3 weeks in patients with recurrent/refractory epithelial ovarian cancer. *J Clin Oncol* **20:** 1562–1569. doi:10.1200/JCO.2002.20.6.1562

Vermeij R, Leffers N, Hoogeboom BN, Hamming IL, Wolf R, Reyners AK, Molmans BH, Hollema H, Bart J, Drijfhout JW, et al. 2012. Potentiation of a p53-SLP vaccine by cyclophosphamide in ovarian cancer: a single-arm phase II study. *Int J Cancer* **131:** E670–E680. doi:10.1002/ijc.27388

Vincent J, Mignot G, Chalmin F, Ladoire S, Bruchard M, Chevriaux A, Martin F, Apetoh L, Rébé C, Ghiringhelli F. 2010. 5-Fluorouracil selectively kills tumor-associated myeloid-derived suppressor cells resulting in enhanced T cell-dependent antitumor immunity. *Cancer Res* **70:** 3052–3061. doi:10.1158/0008-5472.CAN-09-3690

Webb JR, Milne K, Watson P, Deleeuw RJ, Nelson BH. 2014. Tumor-infiltrating lymphocytes expressing the tissue resident memory marker CD103 are associated with increased survival in high-grade serous ovarian cancer. *Clin Cancer Res* **20:** 434–444. doi:10.1158/1078-0432.CCR-13-1877

Webb JR, Milne K, Nelson BH. 2015. PD-1 and CD103 are widely coexpressed on prognostically favorable intraepithelial CD8 T cells in human ovarian cancer. *Cancer Immunol Res* **3:** 926–935. doi:10.1158/2326-6066.CIR-14-0239

Webb JR, Milne K, Kroeger DR, Nelson BH. 2016. PD-L1 expression is associated with tumor-infiltrating T cells and favorable prognosis in high-grade serous ovarian cancer. *Gynecol Oncol* **141:** 293–302. doi:10.1016/j.ygyno.2016.03.008

Wei X, Jin Y, Tian Y, Zhang H, Wu J, Lu W, Lu X. 2016. Regulatory B cells contribute to the impaired antitumor immunity in ovarian cancer patients. *Tumour Biol* **37:** 6581–6588. doi:10.1007/s13277-015-4538-0

Westphalen S, Kotulla G, Kaiser F, Krauss W, Werning G, Elsasser HP, Nagy A, Schulz KD, Grundker C, Schally AV, et al. 2000. Receptor mediated antiproliferative effects of the cytotoxic LHRH agonist AN-152 in human ovarian and endometrial cancer cell lines. *Int J Oncol* **17:** 1063–1069. doi:10.3892/ijo.17.5.1063

Whitehair R, Peres LC, Mills AM. 2020. Expression of the immune checkpoints LAG-3 and PD-L1 in high-grade serous ovarian carcinoma: relationship to tumor-associated lymphocytes and germline BRCA status. *Int J Gynecol Pathol* **39:** 558–566. doi:10.1097/PGP.0000000000000657

Windbichler GH, Hausmaninger H, Stummvoll W, Graf AH, Kainz C, Lahodny J, Denison U, Müller-Holzner E, Marth C. 2000. Interferon-γ in the first-line therapy of ovarian cancer: a randomized phase III trial. *Br J Cancer* **82:** 1138–1144. doi:10.1054/bjoc.1999.1053

Wing K, Onishi Y, Prieto-Martin P, Yamaguchi T, Miyara M, Fehervari Z, Nomura T, Sakaguchi S. 2008. CTLA-4 control over Foxp3$^+$ regulatory T cell function. *Science* **322:** 271–275. doi:10.1126/science.1160062

Wu L, Deng Z, Peng Y, Han L, Liu J, Wang L, Li B, Zhao J, Jiao S, Wei H. 2017. Ascites-derived IL-6 and IL-10 synergistically expand CD14$^+$HLA-DR(-/low) myeloid-derived suppressor cells in ovarian cancer patients. *Oncotarget* **8:** 76843–76856. doi:10.18632/oncotarget.20164

Wu J, Sun H, Yang L, Deng Y, Yan Y, Wang S, Yang G, Ma H. 2018. Improved survival in ovarian cancer, with widening survival gaps of races and socioeconomic status: a period analysis, 1983-2012. *J Cancer* **9:** 3548–3556. doi:10.7150/jca.26300

Wu L, Mao L, Liu JF, Chen L, Yu GT, Yang LL, Wu H, Bu LL, Kulkarni AB, Zhang WF, et al. 2019. Blockade of TIGIT/CD155 signaling reverses T-cell exhaustion and enhances antitumor capability in head and neck squamous cell carcinoma. *Cancer Immunol Res* **7:** 1700–1713. doi:10.1158/2326-6066.CIR-18-0725

Yang C, Lee H, Jove V, Deng J, Zhang W, Liu X, Forman S, Dellinger TH, Wakabayashi M, Yu H, et al. 2013. Prognostic significance of B-cells and pSTAT3 in patients with ovarian cancer. *PLoS ONE* **8:** e54029. doi:10.1371/journal.pone.0054029

Yang M, Zhang G, Wang Y, He M, Xu Q, Lu J, Liu H, Xu C. 2020. Tumour-associated neutrophils orchestrate intratumoural IL-8-driven immune evasion through Jagged2 activation in ovarian cancer. *Br J Cancer* **123:** 1404–1416. doi:10.1038/s41416-020-1026-0

Yuan X, Zhang J, Li D, Mao Y, Mo F, Du W, Ma X. 2017. Prognostic significance of tumor-associated macrophages in ovarian cancer: a meta-analysis. *Gynecol Oncol* **147:** 181–187. doi:10.1016/j.ygyno.2017.07.007

Zakharia Y, McWilliams RR, Rixe O, Drabick J, Shaheen MF, Grossmann KF, Kolhe R, Pacholczyk R, Sadek R, Tennant LL, et al. 2021. Phase II trial of the IDO pathway inhibitor indoximod plus pembrolizumab for the treatment of patients with advanced melanoma. *J Immunother Cancer* **9:** e002057. doi:10.1136/jitc-2020-002057

Zamarin D, Burger RA, Sill MW, Powell DJ Jr, Lankes HA, Feldman MD, Zivanovic O, Gunderson C, Ko E, Mathews C, et al. 2020. Randomized phase II trial of nivolumab versus nivolumab and ipilimumab for recurrent or persistent ovarian cancer: an NRG oncology study. *J Clin Oncol* **38:** 1814–1823. doi:10.1200/JCO.19.02059

Zhang L, Conejo-Garcia JR, Katsaros D, Gimotty PA, Massobrio M, Regnani G, Makrigiannakis A, Gray H, Schlienger K, Liebman MN, et al. 2003. Intratumoral T cells, recurrence, and survival in epithelial ovarian cancer. *N Engl J Med* **348:** 203–213. doi:10.1056/NEJMoa020177

Zhang X, Xiao X, Lan P, Li J, Dou Y, Chen W, Ishii N, Chen S, Xia B, Chen K, et al. 2018. OX40 costimulation inhibits Foxp3 expression and treg induction via BATF3-dependent and independent mechanisms. *Cell Rep* **24:** 607–618. doi:10.1016/j.celrep.2018.06.052

Zimmer AS, Nichols E, Cimino-Mathews A, Peer C, Cao L, Lee MJ, Kohn EC, Annunziata CM, Lipkowitz S, Trepel JB, et al. 2019. A phase I study of the PD-L1 inhibitor, durvalumab, in combination with a PARP inhibitor, olaparib, and a VEGFR1–3 inhibitor, cediranib, in recurrent women's cancers with biomarker analyses. *J Immunother Cancer* **7:** 197. doi:10.1186/s40425-019-0680-3

Zou W. 2006. Regulatory T cells, tumour immunity and immunotherapy. *Nat Rev Immunol* **6:** 295–307. doi:10.1038/nri1806

Zsiros E, Lynam S, Attwood KM, Wang C, Chilakapati S, Gomez EC, Liu S, Akers S, Lele S, Frederick PJ, et al. 2021. Efficacy and safety of pembrolizumab in combination with bevacizumab and oral metronomic cyclophosphamide in the treatment of recurrent ovarian cancer: a phase 2 nonrandomized clinical trial. *JAMA Oncol* **7:** 78–85. doi:10.1001/jamaoncol.2020.5945

Index

H

I

K

L

Index